AF652926

HERBAL MEDICINE FOR HUMAN DISEASES

VOLUME - III

HERBAL MEDICINE FOR HUMAN DISEASES

VOLUME - III

EDITORS

IRFAN ALI KHAN AND ATIYA KHANUM

NAWAB SHAH ALAM KHAN CENTRE FOR POST GRADUATE
STUDIES AND RESEARCH (AFFILIATED TO OSMANIA UNIVERSITY)
ANWARUL ULOOM COLLEGE CAMPUS, MALLEPALLY, HYDERABAD-1 (A.P.), INDIA

UKAAZ PUBLICATIONS

16-11-511/D/408, Shalivahana Nagar, Moosarambagh,
Hyderabad-36, Andhra Pradesh. India (Ph:24547392 and 65704477)
E-mail : ukaaz@yahoo.com and Website : www.ukaazpublications.com

© UKAAZ PUBLICATIONS

First Edition : 2007
Price : Rs. 950=00

All rights reserved. No part of this publication may be reproduced, stored in any retrieval system or transmitted in any form or by any means, without the prior written permission of the publisher

DISTRIBUTOR

THE BOOK SYNDICATE, BANK STREET, KOTI, HYDERABAD-500 095. (INDIA)
Fax : 91+ 40 - 23445611 Ph: 23445622, 44, 77 E-mail : booksynd@hd2.dot.net.in

ISBN 81-88279-42-0

Published by : **UKAAZ PUBLICATIONS**
16-11-511/D/408, Shalivahana Nagar, Moosarambagh, Hyderabad-36, Andhra Pradesh. (Ph:24547392)

Typeset by : **UKAAZ GRAPHICS**
16-11-511/D/408, Shalivahana Nagar, Moosarambagh, Hyderabad-36, Andhra Pradesh. (Ph:24547392)

Printed by : **ROWSHNI GRAPHICS**
Nallakunta, Hyderabad. (Ph: 65162576)

Binding by : **Y.V.REDDY BINDING WORKS**
Moosarambagh, Hyderabad-36 (Ph: 65162429)

Title cover design : **Dr.Irfan Ali Khan and Dr.Atiya Khanum : Editors**
Dr.Adnan Ahmad Khan

PREFACE

Global estimates indicate that over 3/4th of the five billion world population cannot afford the products of the western pharmaceutical industry and have to rely upon the use of traditional medicines, which are mainly derived from plants. As a part of strategy to reduce financial burden on developing countries which spend 40-50% of their total health budget on drugs, W.H.O. currently encourages, recommends and promotes the inclusion of herbal drugs in national health care programmes because such drugs are easily available at a price within the reach of a common man and as such are time tested and thus considered to be much safer than the modern synthetic drugs.

Plants have curative measures for all the ailments but man has to discover it out. Herbs act in almost magical and astonishing ways. Since early Neanderthal man, plants and herbs have been used for healing purposes and maintaining good health. Even as medical science has progressed, methods and ideas based on herbal healing have sustained and grown in different countries, across different cultures, often being used in exactly the same way. Traditional herbal remedies have led scientists to the development of numerous modern drugs, establishing beyond doubt the efficacy of 'herbal medicine'.

Herbs are used in many different ways. However, the ultimate objective of their use is that they should interact directly with our body chemistry. Their active constituents must be absorbed into the body for deriving the required benefits. Once they are absorbed in the blood stream, they circulate to influence our whole system. Herbs are considered food for the body. They are valuable sources of natural medicine, vitamins, minerals and phytochemicals that have a remarkable history of curative effects, when used under the supervision of an experienced and knowledgeable practitioner are generally safe and do not produce side effects.

This book is the outcome of efforts of a large number of experts who have not only recorded their ideas in the form of review articles but have also shared their thoughts which would be valuable to the users of this very useful text. The wide coverage, expertise of the contributors and potential for practical use of the contents of this book, we expect, will be of immense utility. This book will cater to the immediate needs of students, researchers, faculty members and pharmaceutical industries in India and abroad.

Though meticulous care has been taken in editing and printing of the material, some mistakes might have crept in. We, therefore, close with the request to all who may use this book to be free to pass on to us their comments or suggestions, to enables us to improve our future prints.

Hyderabad
2007

IRFAN ALI KHAN
ATIYA KHANUM

ACKNOWLEDGEMENTS

We are deeply grateful to our benefactors, Nawab Shah Alam Khan, Chairman and Nawab Mahboob Alam Khan, Hon.Secretary, Anwarul Uloom Educational Association, for their unwavering and enthusiastic encouragement in bringing out this project to its present zenith.

We are immensely thankful to Late Professor Jafar Nizam, former Vice Chancellor of the Kakatiya University, Warangal and Late Professor M. Hashim, former Head, Department of Botany, Osmania University, Hyderabad who inspired us to edit books on new frontiers which will cater to the immediate needs of the students, the researchers, the faculty members and the pharmaceutical industries in India and abroad.

We are extremely grateful to Dr. E.A.Siddiq, Professor G.M.Reddy, Professor A.R.Zafar, Professor S.Y.Anwar and Dr. S.I. Rizvi for their continuous encouragement and also unwavering support.

Throughout its preparation, many well wishers and colleagues have freely given their help, advice, knowledge and insight. In this respect, our thanks are especially due to Dr. Rizwana Mubeen, Dr. Farhath Khanum and Dr. Sadia Fatima - all of whose continuous encouragement has largely contributed to bring out this publication. It is a particularly pleasant duty to appreciate and acknowledge the painstaking effort of A. Rajkumar for type setting and M/s Rowshni Graphics for nice printing with great perseverance. We are also thankful to M/s Y.V.Reddy Binding Works for the nice binding and attractive getup.

CONTENTS

HERBAL CURE FOR HUMAN DISEASES

IRFAN ALI KHAN AND ATIYA KHANUM
P.G. DEPARTMENT OF BOTANY, NAWAB SHAH ALAM KHAN CENTRE FOR POST GRADUATE STUDIES AND RESEARCH, ANWARUL ULOOM COLLEGE CAMPUS, NEW MALLEPALLY, HYDERABAD-500 001

Chapter Outline

IN: HERBAL MEDICINE FOR HUMAN DISEASES: VOLUME-III, PAGES: 1-177
(EDITORS : IRFAN ALI KHAN AND ATIYA KHANUM), UKAAZ PUBLICATIONS - HYDERABAD (A.P)-INDIA

1. INTRODUCTION

World population is nearing 5 billion and with this rate of growth it is likely to touch 7.5 billion by the year 2020. Global estimates indicate that over 3/4th of the five billion world population cannot afford the products of the western pharmaceutical industry and have to rely upon the use of traditional medicines, which are mainly derived from plants. As a part of strategy to reduce financial burden on developing countries which spend 40-50% of their total health budget on drugs, W.H.O. currently encourages, recommends and promotes the inclusion of herbal drugs in national health care programmes because such drugs are easily available at a price within the reach of a common man and as such are time tested and thus considered to be much safer than the modern synthetic drugs.

From time immemorial man has been interested in trying to control diseases by utilizing many plant species as natural remedies. In accordance with the World Health Organization, more than 20,000 plant species are used medicinally and 80% of the world's total population relies chiefly on herbal traditional medicine to their Primary Health Care. Even in the developed countries, plants are the source of ingredients in one - fourth of the prescriptions prescribed by pharmacists. It is neither possible nor desirable to replace the herbal medicine with modern medicine, as the phytomedicines are relatively inexpensive, therapeutically effective and probably with minimal side effects. The medicinal properties of herbs have been effectively used not only to heal and rejuvenate the sick, but also to protect the healthy against disease and infection.

Primitive man lived in a constant fear of diseases and had to depend on tribal priests, and witch doctors, who used various plants, minerals, and animal organs in association with strange rituals and incantation, to drive out the evil spirits, which they believed were the cause of disease.

Plants are one of the most important sources of medicine. The application of plants as medicine, dates back to prehistoric period. The early civilization reveals that a considerable number of drugs used in modern medicine have figured in ancient manuscripts such as *The Rigveda, The Bible, The Quran, The Iliad, The Odyssey* and the *History of Herodotus*. Over 6000 years ago, the ancient Chinese were the first to use the natural vegetation as medicine.

In India, the Ayurvedic system of medicine has been in use for over three thousand years. *Charaka* and *Susruta,* two of the earliest Indian authors had sufficient knowledge of the properties of the Indian medicinal plants. The two treatises, the *Charaka Samhita* and the *Susruta Samhita* are esteemed even to this day as the treasures of literature on indigenous medicines.

The Greeks and the Romans, have given voluminous information of the present day drugs which is evident from the works of *Hippocrates* (460-360 B.C.), *Aristotle* (384-322 B.C.) and *Theophrastus* (327-287 B.C.). They wrote extensively about medicinal herbs, giving their names, putative healing properties, and also complex descriptions for the interpretation of medicines. *Hippocrates*, the 'Father of Medicine' was the first to give a scientific explanation of diseases. His influence remains even today in the Hippocratic oath taken by young doctors upon their graduation from medical schools. *Dioscoride's* treatise on medicinal plants, *De Materia Medica* remained the supreme authority for over sixteen centuries. In the centuries that followed 'Doctrine of Signatures' was advocated, that all plants useful for man possessed certain sign's given by God which indicated their usefulness in treating the disease of similarly shaped organs in the human body. For instance, plants with heart-shaped leaves were used for cardio disorders; the walnut with numerous invaginations and convolutions for brain diseases and pomegranate seeds for dental diseases. With the advancement of knowledge, such superstitions gradually were lost, and useful remedies were discovered.

With the development of synthetic drugs, plant products lost their significance. In the last few decades, however, there has been probably more interest in drugs obtained from vegetative sources than at any time in history, because of the success with the antibiotics and other plant drugs, such as *Rauwolfia* (for treatment of mental diseases), *Podophyllum* (a cathartic, as well as for the treatment of atomic radiation burn), *Veratrum* (hypertensive agent), *Peyote* (psychoactive drug) sundry and others. Sapogenins (closely related to steroids), obtained from many members of Dioscoreaceas and Agavaceae, can be converted into cortisone, into male hormone (testosferone) and female hormones (estrogens and progesterone). Sapogenins have many potential uses in the treatment of rheumatoid arthritis and the female hormones are used in contraceptive pills.

Nature has provided a rich store house of herbal remedies to cure all mankind's ailments. Ancient people have utilized thousands of different plants and plant products for human ailments. Some of them are widely cultivated and others are in a wild state.

Studies of medicinal plants based on ancient literature and its investigation in the modern light is known as Ethnology. However, the branch of medicine dealing with history, collection, selection, identification and preservation of crude drugs and raw materials is Pharmacognosy, while the branch dealing with the study of action of drugs is Pharmacology. The information on drugs and drug plants whose efficacy in medicine has been established is available in various authentic books known as Pharmacopoeia, and the drugs included therein are described as 'official'. The most important of these Pharmacopoeia is, India Pharmaceutical Codex, and the work is constantly being revised and kept up-to-date.

India has a vast and inexhaustible resource of drugs of plant origin. The systematic investigation of these drugs used in indigenous medicine on modern scientific line, gained considerable momentum since independence. It was *Dr. Shanti Swarup Bhatnagar,* the first Director General of Council of Scientific and Industrial Research (CSIR) without whose continuous efforts and foresight, the indigenous system of medicine would not have flourished manifold in recent decades. A number of important medicinal and aromatic plants prescribed by the

Vaids and *Hakims* have been carefully investigated from every point of view. Their chemical composition has been determined, by the pharmacological action of active principles, worked out by animal experimentation, and it is only by such a thorough enquiry that the real merits of these drugs have been proved.

Medicinal plants have their values in the substance or substances present in various plant tissues. These produce specific physiological action in the human body. The more important of these substances, glucosides, essential and fatty oils, resins, gums, mucilage, tannins *etc.*, are *viz.,* roots, seeds, leaves, bark, wood *etc.*

2. CONCEPTS OF HEALTH AND DISEASE

In the middle of the 20th century a profound revolution was brought in "allopathic medicine", which has been defined as "treatment of disease by the use of a drug which produces a reaction that itself neutralises the disease" by the introduction of antibacterial and antibiotic agents. In recent past, a new concept - concept of disease eradication - began to take shape. This concept found ready application in the eradication of smallpox, and certain other diseases are on the anvil.

The 30th World Health Assembly resolved that "the main social target of governments and WHO in the coming decades should be the attainment to health by all citizens of the world. Medicine is also a science for the prevention of disease, and the promotion of health. The scope of medicine has expanded during the last few decades to include not only health problems of individuals, but those of communities as well. This is how medicine has evolved down the centuries. Medicine will continue to evolve so long as man's quest for better health continues.

2.1 HEALTH

"Health" is one of those terms which most people find it difficult to define although they are confident of its meaning. Therefore, many definitions of health have been offered from time to time. The widely accepted definition of health is that given by the World Health Organisation (1948) in the preamble to its constitution, which is as follows: "Health is a state of complete physical mental and social well being and not merely an absence of disease or infirmity". Health is multidimentional. The definition envisages three specific dimentions - the physical, the mental, and the social. Besides this, many more may be cited, *viz.,* spiritual dimension, emotional dimension, vocational dimension, and political dimensions.

Health and disease lie along a continuum, and there is no single cut-off point. Health is multifactorial and is multidimensional, and each dimension is influenced by numerous factors, some are known and many unknown.

2.2 DISEASE

There have been many attempts to define disease. *Webster* defines disease as "a condition in which body health is impaired, a departure from a state of health, an altteration of the human body interrupting the performance of vital functions". The Oxford English Dictionary defines disease as "a condition of the body or some part or organ of the body in which its functions are disrupted or deranged". The WHO has defined health, but not disease. This is because it has many shades ("Spectrum of disease")ranging from inapparent (subclinical) cases to severe manifest illness. Some diseases commence acutely (*e.g.,* food poisoning), and some insidiously (*e.g.,* mental illness, rheumatoid arthritis). In some diseases, a "carrier" state occurs in which the individual remains outwardly healthy, and is able to infect others (*e.g.,* typhoid fever). In some instances, the same organism may cause more than one clinical manifestation (*e.g.,* streptococcus). In some cases, the same disease may be caused by more than one organism (*e.g.* diarrhoea). Some diseases have a short course, and some a prolonged course. It is easy to determine illness when the signs and symptoms are manifest, but in many diseases the border-line between normal and abnormal is indistinct as in the case of diabetes, hypertension, and mental illness.

The concept that disease is due to multiple factors is not a new one. It is now known that diseases such as coronary heart disease, and cancer are due to multiple factors. For example, excess of fat intake, smoking, lack of physical exercise, and obesity are all involved in the pathogenesis of coronary heart disease. Most of the factors are linked to life styles and human behaviour.

3. SCREENING FOR DISEASE

It is the search for unrecognised disease or defect by means of rapidly applied tests. The basic purpose of screening, is to sort out from a large group of apparently healthy persons, those likely to have the disease under study, and to bring those who are "apparently abnormal" under medical supervision or treatment. However the criteria for screening are based on two considerations:

- the disease to be screened, and
- the test to be applied.

The screening test must satisfy the criteria of acceptability, repeatability and validity, besides, others such as yield, simplicity, safety, rapidity, ease of administration and cost. However, validity expresses the ability of a test to separate or distinguish those who have the disease from those who do not. One must consider the validity components - sensitivity and specificity when assesssing the accuracy of a diagnostic test. In addition to sensitivity and specificity, the performance of a screening test is measured by its "predictive value" which reflects the diagnostic power of the test. The predictive value of a positive result falls, as disease prevalence declines. Taking diabetes as an example, if the cut-off point for blood glucose is lowered to detect diabetes (say less than 120 mg per cent) the sensitivity of the test is increased at the cost of specificity. If the cut-off point is raised (say to 180 mg percent), the sensitivity is decreased. In other words there is no blood sugar level which will ensue the separation of all those with the disease from those without the disease.

4. CLASSIFICATION OF DISEASES

The broad line of the classification is as :

4.1 COMMUNICABLE DISEASES

RESPIRATORY INFECTIONS

Smallpox, Chickenpox, Measles, Rubella, Mumps, Influenza, Diphtheria, Whooping cough, Meningococcal meningitis, Acute respiratory infections, SARS and Tuberculosis.

INTESTINAL INFECTIONS

Poliomyelitis, Viral hepatitis, Cholera, Acute diarrheal diseases, Typhoid fever, Food poisoning, Amoebiasis, Ascariasis, Hookworm infection and Dracunculiasis.

ARTHROPOD - BORNE INFECTIONS

Dengue syndrome, Malaria, Lymphatic and filariasis.

ZOONOSES

- Viral: Rabies, Yellow fever, Japanese encephalitis and KFD.
- Bacterial: Brucellosis, Leptospirosis, Plague and Human salmonellosis
- Rickettsial diseases: Rickettsial zoonoses, Scrub typhus, Murine typhus, Tick typhus and Q fever.
- Parasitic zoonoses: Tarniasis, Hydatid disease and Leishmaniasis.

SURFACE INFECTIONS

Trachoma, Tetanus, Leprosy, STD, Yaws and AIDS.

Emerging and re-emerging infections diseases

Hospital acquired infections

4.2 NON-COMMUNICABLE DISEASES

Cardiovascular diseases, Coronary heart disease, Hypertensions, Stroke, Rheumatic heart disease, Cancer, Diabetes, Obesity, Blindness and Accidents and injuries.

5. BRIEF DESCRIPTION OF COMMON DISEASES

5.1 AIDS

AIDS, the acquired immuno-deficiency syndrome (sometimes called "slim disease") is a fatal illness caused by a retrovirus known as the human immuno-deficiency virus (HIV) which breaks down the body's immune system, leaving the victim vulnerable to a host of life-threatening opportunistic infections, neurological disorders, or unusual malignancies (1). Among the special features of HIV infection are that once infected, it is probable that a person will be infected for life. Strictly speaking, the term AIDS can be called our modern pandemic, affecting both industrialised and developing countries.

5.2 ASTHMA

Respiratory disorder Asthma is a very common health problem in India and is increasing alarmingly with the rise in air pollution especially in the cities. It is caused by tightening of the small bronchial tubes and production of thick sticky mucus that makes breathing difficult with a characteristic wheeze. Difficulty in breathing, heaviness in the chest and restlessness are its main symptoms. It is so called as a deadly disorder, because you can only control asthma and not cure. Modern medicines only give symptomatic relief. Traditional herbal medicine, however, has some specific herbal products which can cure many of those respiratory disorders from their very root. There has been an increasing interest in the recent years in medical ethnobotany data mainly because of the renewed interest in natural drugs specially those derived from plants, started in the last two decades mainly because of the widespread belief that *green medicines* are healthier and safer than the synthetic ones.

5.3 ANTIOXIDANT

Antioxidants are substances that may protect cells from damage caused by unstable molecules known as free radicals. Exposure to various environmental factors lead to formation of free radicals, which are actually electrically charged oxygen molecules. These electrically charged oxygen molecules take up electrons from other molecules causing an array of disorders. Antioxidants interact with these free radicals and stabilize them and thereby prevent them from damaging the cells. Some antioxidants stimulate the immune system, and increase the activity of detoxifying enzymes in the liver.

5.4 ASTRINGENT

Astringents are any of a group of medicines that shrink mucous membranes, and stop or slow secretion of blood, mucous, or other fluids from human body. Astringents decrease fluids by narrowing small blood vessels, drawing water away from organ, or coagulating the superficial layers of organ into a crust. They usually contain tannins that precipitate the proteins when they come into contact with it. Thus, in a remedy, they will tend to tone up the mucous membranes and reduce secretions and discharge, and have an anti-catarrhal effect. Astringents are also anti-haemorrhagic and will form an eschar (scab) over a wound thus preventing the entry of bacteria. Sometimes they will act on tissues with which there is no direct contact.

5.5 APHRODISIAC

Since the beginning of time, people have searched high and low for substances they could use to stimulate and heighten sexual desire in themselves and others. Various foods have gained notoriety for being sexual stimulants, however, there is very little scientific evidence in their support. An aphrodisiac is defined as any food or drug that arouses sexual instinct, enhances sexual vitality, and helps to overcome sexual dysfunction naturally. Herbs have become increasingly fashionable for use as aphrodisiac and unlike substances like the Spanish Fly and Chan Su, it does not hurt to try and find out if they actually possess the said property. Most of the herbs are not only said to increase libido but they are quite healthy to eat. In fact some say that the true reason people believe these foods are aphrodisiacs is because good eating promotes better physical condition and, in turn, better sexual performance.

5.6 ABORTIFACIENT

Abortifacient are substances that causes or induces abortion. The mode of action alters the endometrium, so the uterus is not receptive to implantation of the fertilized egg. The developing embryo travels through the fallopian tube, reaches the uterus where it would normally be nourished and protected until birth. The uterus gets chemically altered so that there is no nourishment for the developing embryo, and hence the embryo is aborted. They may have other benefits such as regulation of menstrual cycle.

5.7 ANTIPERIODIC

These are agents, which prevent or check the return of diseases which recur periodically. Very little is known of their mode of action, however, it is possible that they have a toxic action upon the microbes in the blood, which are supposed to cause the disease. The typical antiperiodic, quinine, has, however, a decided effect upon the heart and brain, as well as other parts of the nervous system.

5.8 ANTI-INFLAMMATORY

Inflammation is a process that is accompanied by local liberation of chemical mediators like histamines, 5 – hydroxytryptamine, bradykinin and eicosanoids. They are formed in almost every tissue in the body. Inhibition of their biosynthesis is the main stay of anti-inflammatory therapy. Antiinflammatory drugs are used in a variety of conditions including arthritis, muscle and ligament pains, pains after operations, headaches, migraines, and some other types of pains. Antiinflammatory agents do not alter the course of painful conditions, however, they ease symptoms of pain and stiffness.

5.9 ANTISPASMODIC

Antispasmodic drugs also known as anticholinergics, relieve cramps, reduce uncontrollable movements, prevent bladder spasm, relax the lung airways and dry the nose and chest. They are used to treat stomach cramps, Parkinson's disease, colds, chronic obstructive pulmonary disease, and urinary incontinence and muscle spasms from cerebral palsy. Antispasmodics prevent the entry of choline in the nerve terminal by hemicholinium and triethylcholine. It also prevents the entry of acetylcholine into the synaptic vesicles by vesamicol. It prevents the release of acetylcholine by ecocytosis and blocks the cholinergic receptors.

5.10 ANTIPYRETIC (FEBRIFUGE)

Body temperature is regulated by a centre in the hypothalamus. Disturbances in this region lead to a rise in the body temperature and manifestation of pyrexia (fever). In fever there is an increase, in formation of various cytokines, which in turn increase the synthesis of PGE_2 in circumventricular organs in and near the preoptic hypothalamic area. This ultimately results in elevation of body temperature by promotion of heat generation and suppression of heat loss. Antipyretic agents inhibit the synthesis of PGE_2 thereby preventing rise in body temperature. Normal body temperature is not affected by antipyretic agents.

5.11 ANTIMICROBIAL

Antimicrobials destroy disease causing microorganism with minimal damage to host tissues. They act against bacteria, viruses, fungi and other invading organisms to inactivate or destroy them. This may be a direct effect on the microbe or it may be indirect, by way of stimulating or modifying the immune response. Broad spectrum antimicrobials act on a large number of microbes, whereas narrow spectrum antimicrobials are selective in action, acting on specific organisms.

5.12 ANTIMALARIAL

Malaria is one of the most significant and the fifth largest killer infectious diseases of the world. It is a protozoal disease caused by *Plasmodium vivax, Plasmodium malariae, Plasmodium ovale* and *Plasmodium falciparum.* The effectiveness of drug in malaria depends upon the efficacy of the particular drug in a particular parasite species and the stage in the life cycle of the parasite. Antimalarial drugs, if used appropriately, can cure malarial infection completely and suppress symptoms in individuals exposed to infection in endemic areas. Certain antimalarial inhibit the growth of the parasite in the pre- erythrocytic stages which prevents malarial fever and further transmission to mosquitoes. Second group of drug eliminates all the remaining parasites in the body after the primary infection is effectively treated. Third group of antimalarial drug kill the asexual erythrocytic stage of the malarial parasites and thus terminate the clinical attacks of the disease. Fourth group of antimalarial destroys the sexual stages of the parasite in blood, thereby, prevent the transmission of the parasite to the mosquito. The fifth group prevents further development of the malarial oocysts and sporozoites in the infected mosquito.

5.13 ANTIBACTERIAL

Antibacterial drugs either kill the bacteria directly or prevent them from multiplying, so that the body's immune system can destroy the invading bacteria. Antibacterial drugs act by interfering with some specific characteristics of bacteria. Bacterial cells possess rigid cell wall which maintains its shape. Certain antibacterial injure the wall or inhibits its formation leading to lysis of the bacterial cell thereby causing the death of the organism. One group of antibacterial inhibit cell membrane function by altering the permeability that results in leakage of intracellular macromolecules and ions leading to cell damage and cell death. A number of antibacterial inhibit protein synthesis through an action on ribosomes in the bacterial cells. Some antibacterial bind strongly to DNA dependant RNA polymerase of bacteria inhibiting RNA synthesis thus inhibiting bacterial growth.

5.14 ANTIFUNGAL

Fungal infections can have effects ranging from an irritating patch of itchy skin to a life threatening condition. In general fungal infections can be divided into topical (superficial) infection affecting the skin, nails, hair or mucous membranes, and systematic infections affecting deeper tissues and organs. Widespread use of immunosuppressive chemotherapy, broad spectrum antibiotics, corticosteroids, implants and the emergence of AIDS, compromise the host defense mechanism allowing infection by saprophytic fungi. Mild infections are usually susceptible to topical therapy, however severe or resistant infections may require systemic treatment. Certain antifungal bind with high affinity to ergosterol present in fungal membranes resulting in certain alterations in the fungal membrane with formation of microspores. Through these pores vital macromolecules and ions are lost leading to irreversible damage. Another group of antifungal inhibits DNA synthesis of the fungus exerting antifungal effect.

5.15 ANTIVIRAL

Viruses are the smallest microorganism infecting human beings. Virus invades the cell and is dependant on the cell's metabolic for its requirements, and hence, it is difficult to control or inhibit them. There are two types of viruses- DNA viruses that cause smallpox, chicken pox, herpes, glandular fever, and RNA viruses that cause influenza, measles, mumps etc. Antiviral drugs interfere with the life cycle of a virus by preventing its penetration into a host cell or by blocking the synthesis of new virus. Some antiviral stimulate the immune system so that the body can fight the viral infection itself.

5.16 ANTISEPTIC

Since time immemorial chemical substances were used to control the infection in wounds and spread of contagious diseases. Antiseptic agents kill or inhibit the growth of microorganisms on the external surfaces of the body. They are toxic both to the microorganism and the host and hence are used topically. There is a great variation in the ability of antiseptics to destroy microorganisms and in their effect on living tissue. Antiseptics are potent germicidal usually with broad spectrum activity. There is also a great difference in the time required for different antiseptics to work.

5.17 ANTHELMENTIC

Parasitic infections impose a substantial health problem and economic burden in under-developed countries. Anthelmentic are used in eradicating a number of helminthic parasites in the intestinal tracts of humans and other animals. There are two categories of anthelmentics:

- Vermicide which destroys the parasite without causing their expulsion from the bowels, and hence, a laxative or a cathartic has to be used to expel the dead parasite.

- Vermifuge which expels the parasite from the bowel. Anthelmentics inhibits cytoplasmic microtubule synthesis in nematodes and impair their glucose uptake and secretion of acetylcholinesterase. As a result the parasites are immobilized and die slowly.

5.18 ANTIJAUNDICE

Jaundice or Hepatitis A is an acute infectious disease caused by Hepatitis A virus (HAV). Jaundice means the yellow appearance of the skin and whites of the eyes that occurs when the blood contains an excess of the pigment called bilirubin. Bilirubin is a natural product arising from the normal breakdown of red blood cells in the body and is excreted in the bile, through the actions of the liver. Although jaundice is most often the result of a disorder affecting the liver it can be caused by a variety of other conditions affecting, for example, the blood or spleen.

The red blood cells in our circulation carry oxygen to all parts of the body and have a life span of about 120 days. At the end of their life they are broken down and removed from the circulation by special cells called phagocytes, which are found within the bone marrow, spleen and liver. Following breakdown of the red cells some of their component parts such as amino acids and iron can be re-used by the body. Other components such as bilirubin need to be removed. Bilirubin released from old red cells, passes through the bloodstream to the liver, where the liver cells process it. These cells carry out many complex chemical functions and also produce the liquid bile, which is the 'vehicle' by which the cells discharge their output to the bile duct system. Bile (and therefore bilirubin) then passes out through the small and large intestines and is excreted in the stool (faeces).Therefore, any failure of the bilirubin removal pathway will lead to a build-up of bilirubin in the blood. When this happens the individual's skin turns yellow, causing jaundice. The balance between manufacture and breakdown of red cells is normally precisely balanced and equal, but there are several conditions in which the rate of breakdown increases. If the amount of bilirubin thus released exceeds the liver's capacity to remove it, then jaundice will develop.

The commonest cause is a viral infection of the liver cells known as Hepatitis. Many different types of infection including glandular fever (mononucleosis) can also be responsible for this. Alcohol abuse and subsequent scarring of the liver (cirrhosis) can cause significant cell damage leading to jaundice.

The disease is heralded by non specific symptoms such as fever, chills, headache, fatigue, generalized weakness, followed by anorexia, nausea, vomiting and dark urine.

5.19 ANTICANCER

Cancer is commonly defined as an uncontrolled growth of cells, with loss of differentiation and commonly, with metastasis, spread of the cancer to other tissues and organs. Cancer is a malignant growth. Cancer treatment involves surgery, radiation and drugs, singly or in combination. Majority of anticancer drugs act by interfering with cancerous cell growth, however these drugs commonly affect not only the cancerous cells, but other cells that reproduce quickly like the cancer cells. Therapeutic effect of anticancer herbs is executed by inhibiting the cancer activating enzymes, stimulating DNA repair mechanism, promoting production of protective enzymes, inducing antioxidant action and by enhancing activity of the immune cells. Certain biological response modifiers derived from herbs are known to inhibit growth of cancer by modulating the activity of specific hormones and enzymes. Some herbs reduce toxic side effects of chemotherapy and radiotherapy.

5.20 ANTITUMOR

Tumors are benign growth that remain encapsulated and grow within a well defined area. Tumors may be fatal if untreated as they may exert pressure on essential organs. Antitumor agents work in the same way as anticancer agents.

5.21 ANTIULCER

Ulcer is caused by peptic ulceration that involves the stomach, duodenum, and lower oseophagus. Ulcers are caused by *Helicobacter pylori* infections and are treated with a combination treatment that incorporates antibiotic therapy with gastric acid suppression. Antiulcer drugs are a class of drugs used to treat ulcers in the stomach and the upper part of the small intestine. The objectives of antiulcers are relief of pain, promotion of ulcer healing and prevention of recurrence and complication. The agents used for treatment of ulcers are: (i) acid neutralizing agents that are basic in nature and neutralized acid in the lumen.

(ii) proton pump inhibitor that blocks the secretion of gastric acid by the gastric parietal cells inhibiting the secretion of gastric acid. (iii) ulcer insulators does not inhibit gastric acid, but rather react with the existing stomach acid to form a thick coating that covers the surface of an ulcer protecting the open area from further damage.

5.22 ANTIDIABETIC

Diabetes mellitus is a metabolic disorder characterized by hyperglycemia resulting from defects in insulin secretion, insulin action or both. The lock and key binding of insulin to the insulin receptors fails to initiate the intercellular signaling cascade that results both in glycosis and in synthesis of the carbohydrate reserve molecule glycogen from glucose. To compensate this down regulating of signaling pathway the body secretes greater amount of insulin. As a result of this over burdening the insulin secreting cells of the pancreas eventually become exhausted and cease to function. Anti-diabetics function in different ways. They may be substances that stimulate secretion of insulin, may be insulin sensitizers, biguanides, inhibitors of carbohydrate absorption, and inhibitors of fat absorption.

5.23 ANTIHYPERTENSION

Hypertension is defined as elevation of arterial blood pressure. Hypertension is a major factor for coronary artery disease and the most important risk factor for stroke. Hypertension is a multifactorial disease and is categorized as primary and secondary. Primary hypertension can be hereditary or can be caused by increased fluid volume, renal Na^+ transport deficiency, increased vascular tone and thickness, sympathetic nervous system, hyperactivity, chronic stress, obesity, excess or deficiency of minerals, alcohol etc. Secondary hypertension may be caused by renal, endocrine and neurological abnormalities, drug induced and cardiovascular structural defects. Untreated hypertension generally has no symptoms hence it is a silent killer.

5.24 ACNE

Acne is a skin problem that consists of mild to severe outbreaks of pimples and cysts - mainly on the face, but also on the back, arms and chest. Acne can cause a number of different types of spots. They may be blackheads that are caused by a blockage of the pores, which get their dark color through excess skin pigment or whiteheads that occur near the surface of the skin when excess sebum gets trapped inside the follicle. In more severe "inflammatory acne", cysts develop beneath the skin's surface. These acne cysts can rupture, spreading the infection into nearby skin tissue. This can result in scarring. Anti-acne can be an antibiotic which will kill the germs or it may be an agent that will dry out the skin and encourage it to shed the surface layer of dead skin. Medication may have the property to reduce the amount of oil being produced or to reduce the amount of androgen in the body.

5.25 CONTRACEPTIVE

The primary mechanism of action of contraceptives is the inhibition of ovulation. The release of an egg, which commonly occurs in the middle of the menstrual cycle, is prevented by them. Two hormones produced by the pituitary, a gland located at the base of the brain, coordinate the development and release of an egg from the ovary. One is follicle stimulating hormone, abbreviated FSH, and the other is luteinizing hormone, or LH. A surge in both of these hormones ordinarily occurs in the middle of a woman's menstrual cycle. The surge in LH is the trigger for ovulation. Oral contraceptives inhibit the production of both FSH and LH and consequently prevent ovulation. The contraceptive action of one group of contraceptives occurs primarily at the level of the pituitary and the hypothalamus. They interrupt the usual hormonal messages sent from the brain to the ovary that lead to ovulation.

5.26 COSMETICS AND TOILETRY

Herbs and spices have been used for enhancement and maintenance of human beauty since time immemorial. Sandalwood, turmeric, henna, and natural oils have found use in a wide variety of beauty treatments. Elaborate herbal beauty treatments are carried out to heighten sensual appeal and maintain general hygiene. A large number of cosmetics and toiletry formulation have been developed based on herbs.

5.27 CARDIOPROTECTIVE

Almost anything that causes the heart to increase its workload for a prolonged period or produces anatomic damage that makes it more difficult for the heart to function leads to cardiac disorder. Cardiac disorders manifest itself in various forms. Primary heart muscle diseases, and coronary artery disease, causes diminishing of the force of contraction of the ventricles. Mechanical failure in filling the ventricles during diastole occur due to narrowing of the mitral valve opening and accumulation of fluid in the pericardium. Narrowing and obstruction of aortic valve and incomplete closure of aortic valve causes overload of the ventricles during systole. These cause dilation of the ventricles, increase in the mass of cardiac muscle, increase in the activity of sympathetic nervous system and activation of renin- angiotensin system.

Cardiac glycosides causes increase in the force and velocity of cardiac contractions and decrease in the heart rate which results in increased cardiac output and increased renal perfusion, therefore increased fluid, resulting in elimination. Vasodilators decreases preload through venodilation and decreases after load through arteriolar dilation. Angiotensin converting enzyme inhibitors leads to (i) decreased peripheral resistance which in turn decreases afterload, (ii) decreased salt and water retention leading to decreased preload, (iii) increased kinin activity which leads to increased vasodilation and, (iv) decreased sympathetic activity by decreased angiotensin mediated norpinephrine release.

5.28 CARMINATIVE

These herbs have a settling effect on the gut wall and ease pains. They contain volatile oils which stimulate the expulsion from the gastrointestinal tract. Carminatives also increase the tone of the musculature and stimulate peristalsis.

5.29 COUGHS

Chest coughs are loose and produce white, yellow, or green phlegm. Colored phlegm may indicate an infection or bronchitis. Irritating, dry, or 'unproductive' coughs can be debilitating. They are often associated with nervous tension and anxiety, rather than infections, and may respond to soothing cough suppressants.

5.30 CONJUNCTIVITIS

Conjunctivitis, commonly known as "pink eye", is an inflammation of the mucous membrane covering the eyeball. It is usually caused by infection, although it can also be associated with dusty air, or a drying of the eye's normal secretions in old age. It may be caused by infections of bacteria, viruses or other microorganisms. It also may result from allergies or chemical burns. Most types of conjunctivitis caused by infection are contagious. Symptoms of conjunctivitis include burning, itching, watering and redness of the eye, and the sensation that an object is lodged on the eyeball. In addition, pus may form and the eyelids may stick together. Allergic conjunctivitis is frequently associated with hay fever.

5.31 DEPURATIVE

A depurative is effective in blood purification and detoxification. They assist the body in ridding itself of viral and bacterial toxins that the body has stored over the years. The blood performs many vital functions which sometimes become over-taxed during acute and chronic cellular disease. Likewise, many ailments and diseases are the direct result of impurities and toxins within the blood. The blood is, therefore, a target for effective medicinal intervention. Depurative changes the properties of the blood from an "unhealthy state" to a "healthy" one. It filters out the toxins and wastes, kills microbial organisms present in the blood, adjusts and balances vital salts, furnishes nutrients, strengthens and enhances important plasma substances.

5.32 DIURETIC

Diuresis means increase in urine volume with loss of solute and water. Agents that increase the rate of the urine formation are called diuretics. The primary function of these drugs is maintenance of normal volume and composition of the body fluid hence they act on the kidney. Most of the diuretics act mainly by blocking tubular reabsorption of sodium at a particular site along the nephrons. Diuretics are mainly used in strangury that may be caused by edema due to cardiac failure, renal diseases and cirrhosis of liver as in the treatment of hypertension. They are usually combined with a demulcent to sooth any irritation due to acids or gravel. Diuretic can also be used in the treatment of backache, prostatitis, sciatic, kidney stones, bladder ache, gonorrhea, and water retention.

5.33 DIGESTIVE

It is the agents that stimulates or strengthens the activity of the stomach. They effect solution (digestion) of food in the alimentary canal. They can be used as tonic to improve the appetite and digestive processes.

5.34 DYSENTERY / DIARRHOEA

Diarrhoea, characterized by loose and frequent stools is generally a symptom of imbalance rather than a primary disease. Food poisoning or bacterial infections are often responsible for sudden attacks, and the aim of treatment is to help the body to rid itself of toxins, rather than simply suppressing the symptoms.

5.35 EMMENAGOUGE

Emmenagouge stimulates the uterine muscular fibers and promotes menstrual flow. If used in higher doses they can act as abortifacients. Some of the emmenagouge acts as tonic in gynaecological disorders.

5.36 EXPECTORANT

Cough is one of the most common symptoms of respiratory diseases. It is a protective reflex and helps in clearing the airway of unwanted matter from upper respiratory tract. Cough reflex is elicited on stimulation of receptors in the mucosa of airway. The cough receptors are stimulated by inflammation, secretion, foreign bodies, chemical substances, and intrabronchial tumours. Expectorants augment the output of the respiratory tract and facilitate the excretion of mucous from the lungs and the throat.

5.37 ECZEMA

Eczema is a group of skin conditions that cause skin to become irritated. There are many forms of eczema, but atopic eczema is the most common form, however, may be caused by a difference in the way a person's immune system reacts to things. Skin allergies may be involved in some forms of eczema. Eczema usually breaks out where the elbow bends; on the backs of the knees, ankles, and wrists; and on the face, neck, and upper chest - although any part of the body can be affected. At first your skin may feel hot and itchy. Then, if you scratch, your skin may become red, inflamed, or blistered.

5.38 EPILEPSY

Epilepsy is a neurological condition, which affects the nervous system. Epilepsy is also known as *seizure disorder*. It is usually diagnosed after a person has had at least two seizures that were not caused by some known medical condition like alcohol withdrawal or extremely low blood sugar. The seizures in epilepsy may be related to a brain injury or a family tendency, but most of the time the cause is unknown. The word "epilepsy" does not indicate anything about the cause of person's seizures, what type they are, or how severe they are. Epilepsy is a disorder in which nerve cells of the brain, from time to time, release abnormal electrical impulses.

5.39 GENERAL TONIC

The term "general tonic" refers to a substance or medication that increases the tone of a tissue or an organ. They increase the vigor and tone of the system by improving the appetite, favoring digestion and assimilation, and adding strength to the circulatory system. Sometimes tonics are also taken to be herbs that have a nourishing and supportive effect.

5.40 GALACTAGOUGE

Galactagouge promotes the flow of milk in nursing mothers. Although their exact mode of action is unclear and probably diverse, some are known to act by inhibiting dopamine release, allowing for the unopposed secretion of prolactin.

5.41 HEPATOPROTECTIVE

Liver breaks down and neutralizes an array of toxins that enters our body. Natural substances like hormones are also broken down by the liver. Hepatitis and cirrhosis are two diseases that can badly damage the liver. Hepatitis is an inflammation of liver caused by certain viruses. Cirrhosis changes the structure of the liver and hence, it fails to function properly leading to retention of toxins in the blood. Therapeutic agents used in liver disorders promote the production of bile in the liver and promotes the release of bile from the gall bladder into the duodenum. Agents that stimulate the production and flow of bile often considered alternatives, and because bile promotes peristalsis, the net effect of it is usually a laxative effect. Hepatics are often liver trophorestoratives, acting to strengthen the liver, aid in pelvic decongestion, and generally improve digestion and elimination.

5.42 HYPERTENSION

Hypertension or high blood pressure can be defined as the force that the blood exerts on the veins and arteries while it circulates around the body. Although the causes are not always known, high blood pressure can often run in families, indicating a strong genetic component. Risk factors include smoking, alcohol abuse, obesity, a high salt intake, lack of exercise and stress. Hypertension is dangerous because it causes the heart to work extra hard. If it is left untreated, it can result in heart disease or even stroke. Carefully chosen herbal remedies and dietary supplements can help to lower the blood pressure, as well as to improve the overall functioning of the heart, arteries and the entire cardiovascular system.

5.43 HAEMORRHOIDS

Haemorrhoids are small, blood filled swellings caused by dilated varicose veins. Constipation and prolonged straining when using the toilet are thought to contribute to the formation of haemorrhoids by increasing the pressure in the veins. Haemorrhoids (often known as piles) are enlarged and engorged blood vessels in or around the back passage (anus). These may be associated with pain, bleeding, itching and a feeling as if a bump or lump is hanging down.

Haemorrhoids also known as piles are rather like varicose veins in the canal of the anus. Here, just under the mucous membrane inner lining, is a considerable network of veins extending upwards for an inch or so from the level of the skin to just above the anal canal, where it joins the rectum. When the veins of this network become swollen with blood, haemorrhoids occur.

5.44 IMMUNOMODULATOR

The immune system, resulting from millions of years of evolution, provides protection against microbial infections and the body's own damaged or cancerous cells. It is composed of the innate and the adaptive immune responses. The innate immune response involves processes that occur almost immediately after exposure to a foreign microorganism, and is now known to exhibit a degree of specificity. The adaptive immune response is triggered within a few hours to a few days, and provides exquisite specificity and a long-lasting protection through specialist memory cells.

An immunomodulator is any substance that helps to regulate the immune system. This "regulation" is a normalisation process, so that an immunomodulator helps to optimise immune response. Immunomodulators do not tend to boost immunity, but to normalize it. Part of their benefit appears to be their ability to naturally increase the body's production of messenger molecules, such as cytokines, which mediate and regulate the immune system making the immune system more efficient.

5.45 INSOMNIA

Insomnia is a sleep disorder characterized by an inability to sleep and/or to remain asleep for a reasonable period during the night. Sufferers typically complain of being unable to close their eyes for more than a few minutes at a time, or of 'tossing and turning' throughout the night. If insomnia continues for more than a few nights running, it can become chronic and cause a sleep deficit that is extremely detrimental to the sufferer's wellbeing. It interrupts the natural sleep cycle which can be hard to restore. Insomnia is a common side-effect of some medications, and it can also be caused by stress, emotional upheaval, physical or mental illness, dietary allergy and poor sleep hygiene. Insomnia can cause problems during the day, such as sleepiness, fatigue, difficulty in concentrating, and irritability. Insomnia tends to increase with age and affects about 40% of women and 30% of men.

5.46 LAXATIVE

Laxatives promote bowel action by stimulating evacuation of the bowels. Laxatives can cause retention of fluid in the colonic content by inhibiting electrolyte and water absorption from the colon by direct or indirect mechanism. Laxative may enhance the motility of the colon. They also cause looseness or relaxation of intestinal muscles. A laxative can cause cramping, hence, should be used with care. Usually, they can be used in short term, along with long term diet and lifestyle correction.

5.47 LEPROSY

Leprosy is characterized by multiple lesions accompanied by sensory loss in the affected areas. Usually, sensory loss begins in the extremities (toes, fingertips). In many advanced cases, gangrene sets in, causing parts of the body to "die" (necrosis) and become deformed. Leprosy in all ages has been considered as one of the more despicable diseases, and victims have been despised throughout the history, and kept in separate places (leper colonies, sanitariums). Even today, most people with leprosy are shunned by their neighbours and are held at arm's length. In the medieval period, leper colonies sprung up where victims of this disease resided, and thus left to themselves, the untreatable disease would go to die slowly from the illness.

5.48 MEMORY ENHANCERS

Certain types of mental decline result from exposure to toxins and from allergies, stress or low nutrient levels in the tissues, which appear to contribute to brain inflammation, scarring and cognitive function impairment. Memory is only one aspect of cognitive functioning. Cognitive functioning refers to the collection of brain functions that constitute our intellectual ability. Included in this are higher order sensory and motor processing, attention and concentration, language function, and executive functions. Executive functions refer to the ability to plan a task, execute the task according to your plan, and also the ability to change execution of the task after having acquired relevant new information.

Some memory enhancers reduce the age-related decline of neurotransmitters and receptors. Through these actions they may improve cognitive function and reduce central nervous system degeneration. Certain other memory enhancers appear to interact strongly, promoting cognitive performance, slowing vascular dementia and improving late-life brain function. Some memory enhancers have been shown to enhance the actions of acetylcholine through cholinergic activity.

5.49 MALARIA

Malaria is a protozoal disease transmitted by the Anopheles mosquito, caused by minute parasitic protozoa of the genus Plasmodium, which infect human and insect hosts alternatively. It is a very old time disease and prehistoric man is thought to have suffered from malaria. It probably originated in Africa and accompanied human migration to the Mediterranean shores, India and South East Asia. In the past it used to be common in the marshy areas around Rome and the name is derived from the Italian, (mal-aria) or "bad air"; it was also known as "Roman fever". Fishermen and traders, long before British colonization, probably introduced the disease into North Australia and in the past malaria was not uncommon in the northern parts of that country.

5.50 NAUSEA AND VOMITING

Nausea and vomiting are common symptoms of digestive upsets, fevers, and migraines. Many people suffer from nausea when travelling, and women suffer from nausea in their early pregnancy. Nausea is a disagreeable sensation in the area of the stomach. It may result from many other causes, both mental and physical. Mental causes of nausea include unpleasant sights, disgusting odors, and severe anxiety. Physical causes include severe pain, obstruction or irritation of the digestive tract, excessive physical exercise, and unnatural stimulation of the vestibular system, the organs of balance of the inner ear. It is often followed by vomiting.

5.51 PURGATIVE

A substance used to cleanse or purge especially causing the immediate evacuation of the bowel. Purgatives cause massive, explosive bowel movements. This function is frequently accompanied by severe cramps and abdominal pain, and can be harmful to the patient. Purgatives are to be used with extreme caution. These are usually combined with carminatives to reduce griping. They produce evacuation of the contents of the intestinal canal by increasing secretion along the tract, by exciting peristaltic action.

5.52 PSORIASIS

Psoriasis is a chronic skin condition. In simple terms, it is only an acceleration of the usual replacement processes of the skin. Normally a skin cell matures in 21 to 28 days during its passage to the surface where a constant invisible shedding of dead cells, as scales, takes place. Psoriatic cells, however, are believed to turn over in two to three days and in such profusion that even live cells reach the surface and accumulate with the dead cells in visible layers. It appears as raised red patches of skin covered with silvery scales. It can occur on any part of the body although elbows, knees, and the scalp are usual sites. There is often an accompanying irritation. Some parts of the body do not have this typical scale. These are areas where two skin surfaces come together as in the natural skin creases and folds e.g., the groin and genital area and underneath woman's breasts. Psoriasis, in these areas can look bright red and shiny rather than scaly. There are a variety of topical treatments available *i.e.,* creams and ointments that are applied to the skin. When used properly they can be most effective and have minimal side effects. Whatever treatment you use it is also vitally important to use a moisturiser to make the skin more comfortable.

5.53 PARKINSON'S DISEASE

Parkinson's disease is a degenerative neurological illness that gets worse over time. The names "Parkinson's Disease", "Shaking Palsy" and "Paralysis agitans" all refer to the same illness. It is a clinical syndrome characterized by slowness of movement, rigidity, tremor of the limbs at rest and disorders of posture. The persons suffering from this disease may also be affected with many nonmotor problems including depression, anxiety, sweating, and mental disturbance. The disease may afflict people from all classes of society and all races. It occurs throughout the world. Its rate of incidence has been found to increase with ageing. Men and women are equally affected by the illness.

5.54 RHEUMATISM

Also known as lumbago or fibrositis, muscular rheumatism is common from late middle age onward. Rheumatism is a type of disorder of joints which affects about 2-3 % of world population. In this condition, the connective tissues and tendons associated with leg or arm muscles become inflamed. Warming rubs can often help to relieve the discomfort, and internal remedies are also useful when the condition is persistent. Modern medicine, especially synthetic medicines give only symptomatic relief. The plant world comprises a rich store house of biochemicals that could be tapped for use as antirheumatic agents.

5.55 STOMACHIC

These are those herbs that stimulate and strengthen the functions of the stomach. They promote and improve digestion and appetite and are usually bitter in flavor. They also check fermentation and dispel accumulation of flatus.

5.56 URTICARIA

Urticaria and hives are names for a rash of red itchy lumps and blisters on the skin. They can be caused by contact with irritant allergens, such as those found in plants like stinging nettles, hops, runner beans, or borage. Chemicals such as salicylates, found in aspirin and in many foods, can have a similar effect, causing rashes that most often occur around the mouth. Urticaria results from antigen entering specific skin areas and causing localized anaphylactic reactions. Histamine released locally causes vasodilatation that induces an immediate red flare and increased local permeability of the capillaries that leads to local circumscribed areas of swelling of the skin in another few minutes. The swellings are commonly called hives. Administration of antihistamine drugs to a person before exposure will prevent the hives.

5.57 VIRAL HEPATITIS

The liver is clearly one of the largest and most important organs in our body, and it is not surprising, therefore, that inflammation of the organ can lead to numerous unpleasant symptoms and loss of vitality. Hepatitis means liver inflammation which usually produces swelling, tenderness and sometimes permanent damage. A viral infection of the liver makes the liver swell up and stops working well. In the long term it can cause liver cirrhosis and death. Firstly, there are a number of herbal remedies which protect liver cells from damage by poisons and viruses, and there are ample published reports of animal studies and clinical trials, which have demonstrated an ability of a herb to lower, levels of liver enzymes in affected individuals. The second means by which herbal remedies can be of help is in supporting the immune system's efforts to fight off the virus. Herbal treatments are not designed for acute stages of hepatitis. In this case, bed rest and low fat diet, along with gentle herbal diaphoretics are the limit of treatment recommended.

6. HERBALWEALTH FOR HUMAN HEALTH

The WHO estimates that 80% of people living in developing countries rely almost exclusively on traditional medicine for their primary health care needs. Medicinal plants form the back bone of traditional medicine, and hence, more than 3300 million people utilize medicinal plants on a regular basis. Demand for medicinal plants is increasing due to growing recognisation of natural products being non toxic, and having no side effects. Furthermore an increasing reliance on the use of medicinal plants in the industrialized societies has been traced to the extraction and development of several drugs, and chemotherapeutics from the plants as well as from traditionally used rural remedies. Moreover in these societies herbal remedies have become more popular in the treatment of minor ailments on account of the increasing cost of personal health maintenance.

Medicinal plants represent not only a valuable part of India's biodiversity, but also a source of great knowledge. The WHO has listed 21,000 plants that are used as medicine around the world. India has a rich medicinal plant flora of some 2500 species and out of these 150 species are used commercially on a fairly large scale.

India is well known as an Emporium of medicinal plants. Knowledge of medicinal use of plants in India is amassed over millennia by tribals. For thousands of years Indian plants have been attracting attention of foreign countries. People from countries like China, Cambodia, Indonesia and Baghdad, used to come to ancient universities of India like Takshila (700BC) and Nalanda (500BC) to learn health science of India. Dioscorides mentions many plants including datura smoke for treating asthma, nux vomica for paralysis and indigestion, and croton as purgatives.

It is evident that the Indian people have a tremendous passion for medicinal plants and use them for a wide range of health related applications from common cold to memory improvement and treatment of poisonous snake bites to a cure for muscular dystrophy and the enhancement of body's general immunity. There are estimated to be around 25,000 effective plant based formulations available in the indigenous medical text used in folk medicine and known to rural communities all over India. Medicinal plants provide raw material for use in all indigenous systems of medicine in India.

7. HISTORY OF HERBAL MEDICINE

Herbal medicine is the oldest form of healthcare known to mankind. Herbs had been used by all cultures throughout history. It was an integral part of the development of modern civilization. Primitive man observed and appreciated the great diversity of plants available to him. The plants provided food, clothing, shelter and medicine. Much of the medicinal use of plants seems to have been developed through observations of wild animals, and by trial and error. As time went on, the tribe added the medicinal power of herbs in their area to its knowledgebase. They methodically collected information on herbs and developed well-defined herbal pharmacopoeias. Indeed, well into the 20th century much of the pharmacopoeia of scientific medicine was derived from the herbal lore of native people. Many drugs commonly used today are of herbal origin. The World Health Organization (WHO) estimates that 4 billion people, 80 percent of the world population, presently use herbal medicine for some aspect of primary health care.

8. DIFFERENT SYSTEMS OF MEDICINE

The traditional medicine all over the world is nowadays revalued by an extensive activity of research on different plant species and their therapeutic principles. Experimental evidence suggests that free radicals (FR) and reactive oxygen species (ROS) can be involved in a high number of diseases. As plants produce a lot of antioxidants to control the oxidative stress caused by sunbeams and oxygen, they can represent a source of new compounds with antioxidant activity. The Indian system of medicine today uses across the various systems *i.e.,* folk and codified around 8,000 species of plants. The maximum numbers of medicinal plants are utilized by the folk traditions, followed by Ayurveda, Siddha, Unani, Homeopathy, Tibetan and Modern medicine, respectively.

8.1 AYURVEDA

Translated from Sanskrit, *Ayurveda* means 'the science of life'. It is the oldest medicinal system in the world and is being revived in its complete form under the name of Maharishi Ayurved. This system provides an approach to prevention and treatment of different diseases by a large number of medical procedures and pharmaceuticals. The central philosophy is that the mind and body are one and the same, and that physical health can not be achieved without emotional, mental and spiritual health. *Ayurveda* is an ancient Indian healing system that has been developing over the past 5,000 years. Illness is believed to be caused by an imbalance of the body's 3 vital forces or 'doshas'. Treatment options are varied and can include yoga, acupuncture, herbal medicine and dietary changes.

8.2 HOMEOPATHY

Translated from the Greek *homois* and *pathos*, the word homeopathy means 'the cure is like the disease'. The cornerstone of homeopathic philosophy is the Law of Similar. This law or principle is based on a long held belief that substances that produce symptoms in a healthy individual can be used to treat similar symptoms in a sick person. Homeopathic medicine deliberately mimics or provokes the symptoms of a patient's disease to strengthen the body's ability to heal itself. Homeopathic medicines are made from a variety of sources, such as plants, animals and minerals. Homeopathy aims to treat the whole person – taking into account personality, lifestyle and hereditary factors as well as the history of the disease.

8.3 SIDDHA

Siddha simply means perfection. *Siddha* proved to be the ultimate healing system for the southern part of the Indian subcontinent. The word '*Siddha*' comes from the word '*Siddhi*' that means 'an object to be attained' or 'achievement'. Siddha works towards the elimination of diseases and their symptoms, and to help rejuvenate and revitalize persons. The specialized area of Siddha was rejuvenation and longevity. Unlike Ayurveda, which mainly depends upon herbal medicine, Siddha used extensive research in chemical processes such as alchemy.

8.4 UNANI

'*Unani*' means medicines which are a symbol of life. The name is derived from the word 'Ionian' which originated in Greece. Unani medicine, like any other form of medical science strives to find the best possible ways by which a person can lead a healthy life with the least or zero sickness. It prescribes drugs, diet, drinks and other regiments including codes of conduct which are conducive to the maintenance and promotion of positive health, as well as the prevention and cure of disease. It emphasizes on retaining natural compounds which belong to the human body, and hence prescribes only natural remedies.

8.5 ALLOPATHY

Allopathy, also known as the modern system of medicine is developed in the west. It is a system which treats a disease with drugs having opposite effects to the existing symptoms. Each successive discovery and development in Allopathy is the result of extensive research. Each new remedy has helped alleviate pain and suffering and increased the life span of people.

9. CONCLUDING REMARKS

Plants have been used from time immemorial as a source of food, aphrodisiac, anti stress agent, in wound care, in beauty care, and as a curative agent against several diseases.

More and more people are curing their illnesses with the herbal treatments and natural preventatives that have been effectively used for thousands of years. It is also essential to have herbal medicines, which are tested for quality and authenticity. One way of ensuring this is to grow medicinal plants and to meet the ever-increasing demand for these plants. It is essential to use the biotechnological method of mass propagating plants via *in vitro* techniques. This will have a two-fold advantage in ensuring quality production of plant material and regular supply as per the market demand.

Recent developments in chromatographic and spectroscopic techniques together with development in pharmacological testing, have led to a resurgence of interest in plants as sources of new drugs and an explosion of agents isolated from plants. Many of these plant origin agents may prove toxic in humans. However, a promising approach to the development of new pharmaceutical products is to use these agents as templates for the design of new synthetic chemical entities with improved properties.

Since the herbal drugs have been in use in various systems of medicine including folklore in India and other countries for many centuries, pharmacological and clinical evaluation of these drugs has to be taken up systematically. Efforts should be made for the evaluation of therapeutic efficacy of reported drugs. Search for new biologically potent entities from the indigenous system of medicine and folklore has a substantial potential to offer.

Finally, a word of caution. While most herbs have little or no harmful side effects, some herbs may cause slightly undesirable reactions in some persons. Therefore, try only one herb at a time, beginning in small doses and wait and watch for side effects. If there are none, increase the use or dosage cautiously. Also, not all herbal applications are effective in every case in every person. And in no case these should be used as substitutes for professional medical attention in emergencies or serious chronic diseases.

10. PLANTS AND THEIR CURATIVE PROPERTIES

1. *Abelmoschus esculentus* (L.) Moench

Family : Malvaceae

Common names : S: Bhenda H: Bhindi E: Lady's finger

Description : An annual erect herb. Leaves simple, alternate, toothed. Flowers large, yellow. Staminal tube antheriferous. Fruit long, ribbed, capsular. Seeds many.

USEFUL PARTS AND THEIR CURATIVE PROPERTIES

Fruit : Sweet, emollient, cooling, aphrodisiac, stomachic, haematinic, demulscent, diuretic, constipating, tonic, gonorrhoea, urethror-rhoea, abdominal disorders, anaemia, pruritus, strangury, diarrhoea, general debility

2. *Abelmoschus moschatus* Medikus

Family : Malvaceae

Common names : S: Latakasturika H: Maskdana E: Ambrette

Description : An erect annual herb. Leaves simple, palmately lobed. Hairy on both surfaces, flowers large yellow with purple centre, fruits hairy, capsular, seeds sub-reniform, black, scented.

USEFUL PARTS AND THEIR CURATIVE PROPERTIES

Seed : Powder mixed with coffee enhances taste, flavouring agent for chewing tea and tobacco, uterine problems, throat pain, asthma, cough, respiratory troubles.

Root : Gonorrhoea, pain and swellings of testicles

Flowers : Flavouring agent in zarda and pan masala

Whole plant : Unconsciousness, epilepsy

Uses : Oil - soaps, chocolates, cakes, cool drinks, main constituent in aromatic preparations, perfumes, cosmetics, incense sticks, skin diseases, massaging, drugs, flavouring

3. *Abrus precatorius* L.

Family : Papilionaceae

Common names : S: Gunja H: Gunj E: Crab's eye

Description : Straggler; leaves paripinnate, leaflets 10-13 pairs, opposite, oblong, glabrous, entire; racemes terminal or axillary, flowers clustered, pink. Pod oblong, wrinkled; seeds blood red, with a black lateral blotch around the hilum.

USEFUL PARTS AND THEIR CURATIVE PROPERTIES

Root : Antifertility activity, anti-estrogenic, gonorrhoea, stomach pain, dysentery, removing maggots in wounds, impotency, leucorrhoea, night blindness, syphilis, conception, abortion, hyper diuresis

Aerial part : CVS active

Seed : Cytotoxic, antifertility activity, contraception, abortion, leucorrhoea, leucoderma, hair tonic, snake bite, menstrual disorders, skin diseases

Leaf juice : White leucorrhoea, cough and other throat troubles, diabetes, leprosy, blood purifier, emetic, ulcers, hair tonic.

Roots : Sore mouth

Fresh leaves : Sore mouth

4. *Abutilon indicum* (L.) Sweet

Family : Malvaceae

Common names : S: Atibala H: Tepari E: Country mallow

Description : Shrub to 1 m, with spreading branches. Leaves orbicular, ovate, 7-9 nerved, minutely stellately hairy above, glaucous below, cordate, crenate-dentate, apex acute-acuminate. Flowers yellow, solitary; calyx much shorter than petals, spreading in fruit. Mericarps stellate - pubescent.

USEFUL PARTS AND THEIR CURATIVE PROPERTIES

Plant : Hypothermic, CVS active, gonorrhoea, showed significant analgesic activity

Leaves : Burning micturition, boils, abscesses, scabies, carbuncles, itches, gonorrhoea, syphilis, blood dysentery, leucorrhoea, piles, psoriasis, loose motions, fever, diabetes, snake bite, scorpion sting Root decoction – epilepsy, menstrual disorders, galactagogue.

Seeds : Laxative, piles, syphilis.

5. *Acacia catechu* (L. f.) Willd.

Family : Mimosaceae

Common names : S: Khadirah H: Khair E: Cutch tree

Description : A moderate sized deciduous tree. Leaves bipinnately compound. Flowers pale yellow, sessile in axillary spikes. Fruits flat brown, pods shiny, seeds 3-10 per pod.

USEFUL PARTS AND THEIR CURATIVE PROPERTIES

Bark : Melancholia, conjunctivitis, haemoptysis. Heartwood – astringent, antiseptic, acrid, cooling, tonic, depurative, anthelmintic, antidysentric, anti-inflammatory, catarrh, cough, anorexia, leprosy, pruritus, leucoderma, skin diseases, foul ulcers, wounds, anaemia, diabetes, splenomegaly, pharyngodynia

Kath : Thermogenic, digestive, appetizer, aphrodisiac, depurative, tonic, flatulence, laryngopathy, ulcers, wounds, urorrhoea, odontopathy, erysipelas

6. *Acacia chundra* (Roxb. ex Rottl.) Willd.

Family : Mimosaceae

Common names : S: Khadira H: Khair E: Red cutch

Description : Medium sized tree. Leaves spiral, leaflets 35-50 pairs, elliptic, oblique, entire, apex subacute. Stipular thorns short, hooked. Spikes axillary, 1-3 in a cluster, shorter than leaves. Petals white. Pod flat, thin, apically horned. Seeds ovoid.

USEFUL PARTS AND THEIR CURATIVE PROPERTIES

Bark : Spasmolytic, antifertility activity, ephemeral fever, dysentery, asthma, antipyretic

Leaf : Boils, blisters

Gum : Wounds

7. *Acacia leucophloea* (Roxb.) Willd.

Family : Mimosaceae

Common names : S: Arimeda H: Safed-babul E: White Babool

Description : Medium sized tree. Bark grey-white, spines short. Leaflets 10-30 pairs, linear, crowded. Flower heads small, pale yellow, in densely tomentose panicles. Pods pale brown, lomentum.

USEFUL PARTS AND THEIR CURATIVE PROPERTIES

Aerial part : Hypotensive, CVS depressant

Stem bark : Toothache, cold, cough, diabetes

Leaf : Boils

8. *Acacia nilotica* (L.) Willd. ex Del.

Family : Mimosaceae

Common names : S: Babbuka H: Babul E: Black Babool

Description : Tree upto 10 m, young branches pubescent. Stipular spines straight. Leaflets 18-26 pairs. Flowers sessile. Pod stalked, pubescent, moniliform, 10-12 seeded.

USEFUL PARTS AND THEIR CURATIVE PROPERTIES

Stem bark : Hypoglycaemic, antiprotozoal, spasmolytic, CVS active and analgesic, eczema, toothache, sore throat, diabetes, gonorrhoea, leucorrhoea, viper bite

Leaves	:	Epiphora, diarrhoea, venereal diseases, dysentery, dog bite
Gum-resin	:	Syphilis, diarrhoea, dysentery, diabetes, astringent, styptic
Flowers	:	Ear discharge
Seed	:	Impotency, urinogenital diseases

9. *Acacia pennata* (L.) Willd.

Family	:	Mimosaceae
Common names	:	S: Valli khadira H: Agla-bel
Description	:	Prickly, climbing shrub to tree. Gland on the petiole. Leaflets 50-60 pairs. Corolla white. Pod strap-shaped, flat, stalked.

USEFUL PARTS AND THEIR CURATIVE PROPERTIES

Stem sap	:	Asthma
Root	:	Menstrual disorders

10. *Acacia polyantha* Willd.

Family	:	Mimosaceae
Common names	:	S: Kadarah H: Svetakhair E: White cutch tree
Description	:	A medium sized tree with bark exfoliating as papery flakes. Leaves bipinnate, linear-oblong, pubescent. Flowers sessile, white, spikes. Fruits flat pods. Seeds many.

USEFUL PARTS AND THEIR CURATIVE PROPERTIES

Heartwood	:	Astringent, acrid, thermogenic, depurative, anthelmintic, revulsive, leprosy, leucoderma, pruritus, skin diseases, diabetes, helminthiasis, ulcers, epilepsy, insanity, rheumatism and obesity

11. *Acacia sinuata* (Lour.) Merr.

Family	:	Mimosaceae
Common names	:	S: Saptala H: Satala E: Soapnut Acacia
Description	:	A stout prickly climbing shrub. Leaves bipinnate, large gland on petiole, flowers small on globose heads. Fruits pods, flat, coriaceous. Seeds 6-10 per pod.

USEFUL PARTS AND THEIR CURATIVE PROPERTIES

Saponins from bark	:	Spermicidal, haemolytic, spasmolytic
Aerial part	:	Diuretic, spasmolytic and CVS active
Leaves	:	Malarial fever, jaundice, cough, bone fracture
Pods	:	Dandruff, eczema, helminthiasis, leucoderma, skin diseases, fractures

12. *Acacia torta* Craib

Family	:	Mimosaceae
Common names	:	S: Nikumhika E: Oily Wattle
Description	:	A large prickly climbing shrub, sometimes very pubescent, glands near the base of the petiole, conical, leaflets 25-40 pairs, oblong-falcate, pubescent beneath.

USEFUL PARTS AND THEIR CURATIVE PROPERTIES

Aerial part : Hypothermic and CVS active
Root bark : Fever, ulcerous wounds
Stem : Whooping cough

13. *Acalypha indica* L.

Family : Euphorbiaceae
Common names : S: Haritamanjari H: Khokali E: Indian Acalypha
Description : Erect herb to 75 cm; branchlets striate, thinly pubescent. Leaves broadly ovate, rounded to shortly attenuate, crenate-serrate, apex acute; staminate flowers from above the middle; pistillate ones 10-15 at the lower half.

USEFUL PARTS AND THEIR CURATIVE PROPERTIES

Plant : Antibacterial and antidiabetic, cough, constipation, scorpion sting, skin diseases, snake bite, toothache, bronchitis
Leaves : Emetic, skin diseases, intestinal worms, constipation, aphthous ulcers, diabetes, dysmenorrhoea, eczema, headache, scorpion sting, snake bite, toothache, swelling of eyes, jaundice, wounds, asthma, pneumonia, bronchitis
Root : Antiemetic

14. *Acanthospermum hispidum* DC.

Family : Asteraceae
Description : Herb to undershrub. Leaves opposite, obovate, spathulate, scabrous, cuneate, serrate, apex acute. Heads sessile, solitary in the forks of dichotomous branches, greenish yellow. Achenes 5-10, triangular, spinescent with 2 large, horn-like, erect, apical spines. Pappus absent.

USEFUL PARTS AND THEIR CURATIVE PROPERTIES

Oil from leaves : Antibacterial and antifungal
Leaf paste : Cuts, wounds
Fresh root juice : Jaundice

15. *Achyranthes aspera* L.

Family : Amaranthaceae
Common names : S: Apamarga H: Latjira E: Prickly chaff flower plant
Description : Erect stiff herb upto 1 m; branches spreading. Leaves opposite, velvety-tomentose; flowers pink or greenish-white, in long spikes, fruit deflexed.

USEFUL PARTS AND THEIR CURATIVE PROPERTIES

Leaf : Antibiotic, chicken pox, measles, blood dysentery, malaria, conjunctivitis, cuts and wounds, corns, deafness, piles, diarrhoea, rheumatism, ulcers, removal of spines, earache, foot cracks, headache, liver enlargement, dermal diseases, tooth infection, migraine.

Seeds : Bleeding piles, urinary troubles, gastric trouble, night blindness
Root powder : Cough, tumours, leucorrhoea, tuberculosis, gonorrhoea, fever, diarrhoea, antifertility, hastens delivery, wounds, swelling of eyes.
Whole plant : Snake bite, asthma with cough, hypo-glycaemic, body swellings, piles, leprosy, dysentery, skin diseases, cuts, wounds, scorpion sting, dog bite
Leaf paste : Insects bite (wasps, bees), snake bite, scorpion sting
Root paste : Stops bleeding after termination of foetus, haemorrhoids, teeth infection, easy delivery, dog bite, post partum treatment, leprosy, leucoderma, stomachache, toothache, snake bite, scorpion sting, cholera
Stem bark : Pain during delivery

16. *Aconitum napellus* L.

Family : Ranunculaceae
Common names : H: Vachnag E: Indian Aconite
Description : A biennial herb with tuberous roots. Leaves scattered, reniform. Flowers blue, in loose racemes, floral leaves much reduced. Sepals blue, hairy. Fruits oblong, follicles. Seeds obovoid.

USEFUL PARTS AND THEIR CURATIVE PROPERTIES

Plant : Antiarthritis, debility, diaphoretic, diuretic, expectorant, febrifuge, narcotic, nervine tonic, stomachic, asthma, diabetes, dyspepsia, ear and nose discharges, leprosy, paralysis, rheumatism, spermatorrhoea, typhoid

17. *Acorus calamus* L.

Family : Araceae
Common names : S: Vacha H: Bach E: Sweet flag
Description : Aromatic marsh herbs. Leaves distichous, spadix sessile, dense flowered. Flowers hermaphrodite. Perianth 6, stamens 6. ovary 2-3 celled.

USEFUL PARTS AND THEIR CURATIVE PROPERTIES

Rhizome : Insecticidal, spasmolytic, hypothermic, CNS active, analgesic, common cold, hoarseness of voice, constipation, snake bite
Essential oil : Anticonvulsant
Root extract : Exhibited antimicrobial activity, malaria, snake bites, headache, giddiness.The dried rhizome of the plant contains the drug 'calamus' which is used as emetic in diarrhoea, dysentery, as a household remedy for flatulence and colic, painful menstruation, paralytic fevers, conjunctivitis, asthma, backache, constipation, piles, cough, increase in appetite, stomachache, improves speaking ability in children, epilepsy.
Root bark : Snake bite
Stem bark : Toothache

18. *Actinopteris radiata* (Swartz) Link.

Family : Actinopteridaceae
Common names : E: Peacock's tail
Description : Fronds fan like, sori placed on each side of narrow segment of the frond, linear, elongated, opening towards midrib.

USEFUL PARTS AND THEIR CURATIVE PROPERTIES

Whole plant : Diarrhoea, dysentery, fever, cancer, stomachache, blood pressure, tuberculosis
Leaves : Tuberculosis

19. *Adenanthera pavonina* L.

Family : Mimosaceae
Common names : S: Kucandanah H: Baragunci E: Coralwood tree
Description : A medium sized, deciduous tree. Leaves bipinnate, opposite, obtuse, dark green. Flowers pale yellow, in peduncled racemes. Fruits falcately curved pointed pods. Seeds shining, lenticular globose.

USEFUL PARTS AND THEIR CURATIVE PROPERTIES

Bark and leaves : Astringent, vulnenary, aphrodisiac, colonorrhoea, haematuria, ulcers, gout, pharyngopathy
Seeds : Astringent, cooling, aphrodisiac, suppurative, antiemetic, febrifuge, burning sensation, vomiting, fever, giddiness.
Heartwood : Astringent, aphrodisiac, haemostatic, dysentery, haemorrhages

20. *Adiantum incisum* Forsk.

Family : Adiantaceae
Common names : S: Nilkanthashikha

USEFUL PARTS AND THEIR CURATIVE PROPERTIES

Et.OH (50 %) extract of plant : Hypoglycaemic and spasmogenic.
Plant : Antibiotic, cough, pneumonia, diabetes
Root : Bone fracture

21. *Adiantum philippense* L.

Family : Adiantaceae
Description : Rhizome short, erect or suberect with narrow black scales, unipinnately compound leaves, sori linear, coriaceous, entire.

USEFUL PARTS AND THEIR CURATIVE PROPERTIES

Whole plant : Typhoid, asthma, bronchitis
Rhizome paste : Scorpion sting, centipede bite, herpes

22. *Adina cordifolia* (Willd. ex Roxb.) Hook. f. ex Brandis

Family : Rubiaceae
Common names : S: Girikadambali H: Haldu

Description : A large and beautiful deciduous tree with large leaves. Flowers yellow in small heads and capsular fruits with small narrow seeds.

USEFUL PARTS AND THEIR CURATIVE PROPERTIES

Plant : Antibacterial

Bark : Febrifuge, scar formation of skin, malarial fever, sores, stomach disorder

23. *Aegle marmelos* (L.) Correa

Family : Rutaceae

Common names : S: Bilva H: Bel E: The Bael tree

Description : Small or medium sized, evergreen tree. Flowers greenish-white, sweet scented in short lateral panicles. Petals gland dotted.

USEFUL PARTS AND THEIR CURATIVE PROPERTIES

Root : CVS active, dysentery, high blood pressure, diarrhoea, snake bite, jaundice

Root bark : Hypoglycaemic, diarrhoea

Root and fruit : Hypoglycaemic

Fruit : Antiviral, useful in chronic dysentery and diarrhoea, dandruff, snake bite, haemorrhoids, blood dysentery, gastritis, colic pains, alterative, cooling, laxative, nutritive, stomach pain, heart palpitation

Seed : Antifungal, antihelmintic, antibacterial

Tender shoots : Asthma, intermittent fever, cholera, chest pain

Leaf : Diabetes, eczema, scabies, general debility in children, ulcers in throat, cold, peptic ulcer, jaundice, leprosy, leucoderma, ophthalmia, wounds, migraine, cataract, deafness

Epicarp : Excess of heat, leprosy, hiccups, joint pains, piles, of fruit air purifier, good for heart and brain

24. *Aerva lanata* (L.) Juss.

Family : Amaranthaceae

Common names : S: Astamabayda H: Chaya

Description : Much branched herb with the base woody and the branches erect or creeping. Leaves spiral, woolly-tomentose. Flowers bisexual, greenish-white, minute, borne in axillary panicles.

USEFUL PARTS AND THEIR CURATIVE PROPERTIES

Root : Diuretic, anti-inflammatory, antihelmintic, antibacterial, analgesic, burning micturition, headache, white leucorrhoea, diarrhoea

Leaf : Pimples, skin diseases, urinary troubles, earache, kidney stones, stones in urinary bladder

Whole plant : Nephrocalcinosis, ureteral stones, leucorrhoea, cutaneous infections, malarial fever, diabetes

Flowers : Gonorrhoea

Fruit : Pyorrhoea

25. *Agaricus campestris* L. ex Fries

Family : Agaricaceae
Common names : S: Chatrakah H: Kumbi E: Mushroom
Description : Fungus appears as buttons on the surface of the ground when young. When mature, it has underground rhizomorphs, a stipe, umbrella shaped pileus. It has many gills.

USEFUL PARTS AND THEIR CURATIVE PROPERTIES

Fungus : Cooling, laxative, aphrodisiac, tonic, nasitis, ophthalmopathy, paralysis, constipation, hepatodynia, seminal weakness, general debility, hydrocele

26. *Agave cantula* Roxb.

Family : Agavaceae
Description : Stem stout, short, woody , hidden by thick leaf bases, leaves linear, margin spinulose, scape stout, flowers greenish white, capsules oblong-cylindric.

USEFUL PARTS AND THEIR CURATIVE PROPERTIES

Leaf juice : Gonorrhoea, syphilis, bruises, diuretic, laxative, diaphoretic

27. *Ageratum conyzoides* L.

Family : Asteraceae
Common names : S: Visamustih H: Visadodi E: Goat weed
Description : Annual, erect, foetid herb. Leaves ovate to triangular, rounded or truncate, serrate, apex acute or acuminate. Heads in terminal corymbs. Florets pale blue. Achenes black, 5-angled.

USEFUL PARTS AND THEIR CURATIVE PROPERTIES

Whole Plant : Insecticidal, massaging body swelling, tumours, cuts and wounds
Leaves oil : Antifungal, antibacterial
Leaf paste : Wounds, typhoid and high temperature fevers, snake bite, emetic, leprous sores, skin diseases, flatulent colic, controls bed wetting, cuts
Leaves / fruits : Prevents bleeding
Root : Dysmenorrhoea, anthelmintic

28. *Ailanthus excelsa* Roxb.

Family : Simarubaceae
Common names : S: Mahanimba H: Arua E: Tree of heaven
Description : Large tree, bark grey. Leaves imparipinnate, leaflets 17-25, densely tomentose, acute or acuminate, base unequal. Flowers greenish yellow, panicles.samara membranous, elliptic, 1-seeded.

USEFUL PARTS AND THEIR CURATIVE PROPERTIES

Root bark : Anticancer, abortion, diarrhoea, antipyretic, astringent, expectorant, tonic
Stem bark : CVS active, spasmolytic, dysentery, chicken-pox, contraceptive, post partum treatment, constipation, jaundice, liver disorders, stomach pain
Leaf juice : Pains after delivery, constipation, malaria, asthma, bronchitis, dyspepsia, toothache

29. *Alangium salvifolium* (L.f.) Wang.

Family : Alangiaceae
Common names : S: Ankota H: Ankola E: Sage-leaved alangium
Description : Deciduous small tree with spinescent branches and grey bark. Leaves simple, spiral, membranous, acuminate, entire-wavy, acute or rounded. Flowers in axillary clusters, small, white, fragrant, woolly. Berry globular, crowned with persistent calyx- limb, purplish-red to black.

USEFUL PARTS AND THEIR CURATIVE PROPERTIES

Leaf : Antiprotozoal, hypoglycaemic and spasmolytic, fissures, swellings, cuts, dog bite, inflammations, arthritis, piles, bone fractures
Stem bark : Snake bite, bone fractures, fevers, cuts, wounds, sciatica
Root bark : Mad dog bite, rib muscle pain, fever, snake bite, leprosy, cat bite, anthelmintic, astringent, antipyretic, laxative, piles, body swellings, menstrual disorders, epilepsy
Fruit : Conjunctivitis, laxative, refrigerant, tonic

30. *Albizzia amara* (Roxb.) Boivin

Family : Mimosaceae
Common names : S: Krishna sirish
Description : Small, deciduous tree. Petiolar gland near the middle or above it. Leaflets 15-25 pairs, sessile. Heads 1-few fascicled. Flowers sub-sessile, yellowish white. Pod greyish-brown, pubescent.

USEFUL PARTS AND THEIR CURATIVE PROPERTIES

Leaf paste : Body swellings
Stem bark : Bone fracture

31. *Albizzia lebbeck* (L.) Willd.

Family : Mimosaceae
Common names : S: Sirisaha H: Siris E: Siris tree
Description : Large deciduous tree upto 12 m, petiolar gland near base. Leaflets 3-4 pairs, obliquely oblong, retuse, shining. Flowers heads large, white, fragrant, forming short corymbose racemes. Pod flat, straw-coloured.

USEFUL PARTS AND THEIR CURATIVE PROPERTIES

Root : CVS active, spasmolytic, dental powder
Stem bark /pod : Hypoglycaemic, fertility, sprains, gonorrhoea, piles, diarrhoea, jaundice
Pod and root : Anticancer, spermicidal
Pod : Antiprotozoal, antifertility, piles, infected teeth
Stem : Antiallergic, antianaphylactic, asthma with cough
Flowers : Boils, eruptions, carbuncles, swellings
Leaf : Night blindness

32. *Albizzia odoratissima* (L.f.) Benth.

Family : Mimosaceae
Common names : S: Bhusirisah H: Kala siris E: Black siris
Description : Tree. Petiolar gland near base. Leaflets 12-18 pairs, obliquely oblong, obtuse at apex. Panicles large. Flowers sessile. Corolla white. Pod brown flat.

USEFUL PARTS AND THEIR CURATIVE PROPERTIES

Extract of seeds : Semen coagulant and diuretic
Leaves : Dry cough, eye diseases, night blindness
Stem bark : Skin diseases, cold, fever, diabetes, leprosy, ulcers, bronchitis, body pains

33. *Allium cepa* L.

Family : Alliaceae
Common names : S: Palanduh H: Pyaj E: Onion
Description : Biennial or perennial herb with aromatic, fleshy underground bulb. Leaves linear, hollow, cylindric and fleshy. Flowers many, white in globular umbels.

USEFUL PARTS AND THEIR CURATIVE PROPERTIES

Bulbs : Acrid, sweet, aromatic, thermogenic, antiperiodic, antibacterial, aphrodisiac, emollient, emmenagogue, expectorant, carminative, stomachic, diuretic, anodyne, tonic, haemorrhoids, dysentery, flatulence, dyspepsia, colic, jaundice, splenopathy, hepatopathy, pneumopathy, asthma, bronchitis, ophthalmia, vomiting, otalgia, pharyngodynia, malarial fever, lumbago, epilepsy, tumours, wounds, paralysis, arthralgia, leucoderma, skin diseases

34. *Allium sativum* L.

Family : Alliaceae
Common names : S: Lasuna H: Lasun E: Garlic
Description : Bulbs short, with bulblets enclosed in a pink or white envelope. Leaves flat. Flowers often displaced by bulbils, pink on a long, terete scape. Anthers and style exerted.

USEFUL PARTS AND THEIR CURATIVE PROPERTIES

Bulb : Anti-inflammatory, antibacterial, antimicrobial, antifungal, gastric trouble, asthma, hypertension, facial paralysis, epilepsy, impotency, cuts, wounds, anti-patrum treatment, headache, joint pains, night blindness Juice, essential oil - hypocholes-terolemic, hypotensive, antitumour, antidiabetic.

35. *Allophylus serratus* (Roxb.) Kurz.

Family : Sapindaceae
Common names : S: Triputah H: Tippani

Description : A small tree or a large shrub. Leaves trifoliate, alternate, ovate, dentate. Flowers small, white, in fascicles on spicate axillary racemes. Stamens 8. Fruit globose.

USEFUL PARTS AND THEIR CURATIVE PROPERTIES

Whole plant : Astringent, anti-inflammatory, vulnerary, digestive, carminative, constipating, bone fractures, dislocations, inflammations, ulcers, wounds, dyspepsia, anorexia, diarrhoea

Fruits : Sweet, cooling, nourishing tonic

36. *Aloe barbadensis* Mill.

Family : Liliaceae

Common names : S: Kumari H: Ghikanvar E: Indian Aloe

Description : Erect herb. Leaves radical in rosettes, succulent, truncate, spiny, apex gradually tapering, spine tipped. Scapes 1-3. flowers orange. Capsule ellipsoid.

USEFUL PARTS AND THEIR CURATIVE PROPERTIES

Stem : Insect repellant

Barbaloin : Antitubercular

Root : Venereal diseases, wounds

Plant juice : Stomachache, anthelmintic, piles, rectal fissures, dandruff, itching of scalp

Pulp : Minimizes excess of heat, piles, shrinkage of skin

Leaves : Irregular menstruation, cold, cough, chest pain, diabetes, impotency, black patches, burns, joint pains, piles, gonorrhoea, syphilis, aphrodisiac, boils, blisters, wounds, oxytocic, purgative, antibacterial, antifertility, viral jaundice

37. *Alpinia galanga* (L.) Willd.

Family : Zingiberaceae

Common names : S: Kulanjan H: Kulinjan E: Major Galangal

Description : Herbaceous plant. Rhizomes aromatic. Leaves long, narrow, green. Flowers long, greenish white. In compound dense bunches, lip of corolla white. Fruit orange red.

USEFUL PARTS AND THEIR CURATIVE PROPERTIES

Rhizome : Rheumatism, respiratory complaints, bronchial catarrh, stomach complaints, tonic, disinfectant

Uses : Deodorants

38. *Alstonia scholaris* (L.) R. Br. ex DC.

Family : Apocynaceae

Common names : S: Saptaparnah H: Satiun E: Dita bark tree

Description : A large evergreen tree with greenish white flowers and long very narrow, pendulous follicles 1-2 ft long. Seeds papillose.

USEFUL PARTS AND THEIR CURATIVE PROPERTIES

Stem bark	: Hypotensive and anticancer, pain during delivery, fever with chills, galactagogue, lactation, tonic, febrifuge, lactagogue, skin diseases, gonorrhoea, malaria
Root bark	: Stomach ulcers
Whole plant	: Earache, ulcers
Latex	: Stomach troubles, sexually transmitted diseases, fungal infections, earaches, malaria, fever, asthma, leprosy, filariasis
Leaf	: Stomach ulcers, gastric disorders, cholera, dysentery, lactation

39. *Alternanthera sessilis* (L.) R. Br. ex DC.

Family	: Amaranthaceae
Common names	: S: Matsyaksi H: Gudrisag E: Khaki weed
Description	: Annual or perennial herb; rooting at the nodes, with many spreading branches. Leaves opposite, linear-lanceolate, oblong or ovate, pilose at lower mid rib. Inflorescence axillary to terminal globose spikes; flowers bisexual. Seed orbicular, black.

USEFUL PARTS AND THEIR CURATIVE PROPERTIES

Plant	: Hypothermic, antiulcer, galactagogue, bone fracture and swellings, blood diseases, unconsciousness, haemostatic for cuts and injuries
Tender shoots	: Snake bite, stomach disorder, dysentery
Root	: Emetic, tuberculosis
Leaves	: Corneal diseases, blood purifier, cooling

40. *Alysicarpus monilifer* (L.) DC.

Family	: Papilionaceae
Description	: Much prostrate herb. Leaves oblong-elliptic. Stipules scarious. Flowers in axillary racemes. Pod moniliform, turgid.

USEFUL PARTS AND THEIR CURATIVE PROPERTIES

Whole plant	: Jaundice, boils, blisters, diuretic

41. *Amaranthus spinosus* L.

Family	: Amaranthaceae
Common names	: S: Marish H: Katalichauli E: Prickly Amaranth
Description	: Erect herb upto 1 m; stem stout, spines axillary, paired, clustered, subtending the inflorescence. Leaves elliptic obovate to rhomboid, acute, apex acutely emarginate. Inflorescence axillary or aggregated into terminal panicles. Seed orbicular, black.

USEFUL PARTS AND THEIR CURATIVE PROPERTIES

Root paste	: Scabies, indigestion, haemorrhage, chronic diarrhoea, gonorrhoea
Whole plant	: Snake bite
Leaf paste	: Wounds, burns, dental caries, pyorrhoea, fever, laxative

42. *Amaranthus viridis* L.

Family : Amaranthaceae

Common names : S: Tanduliya E: Chinese spinach

Description : Erect herb to 1 m, leaves deltoid ovate to rhomboid, truncate to attenuate; acutely emarginated, glabrous above, glaucous beneath. Inflorescence axillary and terminal panicles, pendulous. Seed orbicular.

USEFUL PARTS AND THEIR CURATIVE PROPERTIES

Whole plant : Plant shows vit B_{12} like activity; juvenomimetic activity, diarrhoea, dental caries, dizziness

Root paste : Appetizer, kidney stones, abortion

Leaf : Constipation

43. *Ammania baccifera* L.

Family : Lythraceae

Common names : S: Kurandika H: Dadamari E: Blistering ammania

Description : Erect annual herb, leaves opposite, linear, flowers green, corolla absent, capsule globose, seeds minute, numerous.

USEFUL PARTS AND THEIR CURATIVE PROPERTIES

Plant decoction : Haematuria, urinary infections, boils on the breasts

Leaf : Cancerous ulcers

44. *Amomum subulatum* Roxb.

Family : Zingiberaceae

Common names : S: Sthulaila H: Badi Ilayaci E: Greater cardamom

Description : A herb with leafy stem. Leaves oblong-lanceolate, bright green. Flowers white in globose shortly, peduncled spikes, filaments very short. Fruits brown, globose capsules. Seeds, many held together by sugary pulp.

USEFUL PARTS AND THEIR CURATIVE PROPERTIES

Seeds : Thermogenic, aromatic, deodorant, carminative, digestive, stomachic, constipating, depurative, vulnerary, anodyne, cardiac, liver tonic, expectorant, febrifuge, sudorific, hypnotic, anorexia, dyspepsia, colic, flatulence, hyperacidity, vomiting, diarrhoea, gonorrhoea

45. *Amorphophallus paeoniifolius* (Dennst) Nicolson

Family : Araceae

Common names : S: Surana H: Gandira E: Elephant foot yam Stout cormous herb.

Description : Corm depressed globose. Leaves pinnate, petiole dark green with paler blotches. Spathes broadly campanulate. Flowers pale yellow. Berries obovoid, red, 2-3 seeded.

USEFUL PARTS AND THEIR CURATIVE PROPERTIES

Corm paste : Scorpion sting, stomach pain, rheumatism, haemorrhoids

46. *Ampelocissus latifolia* (Roxb.) Planch.

Family : Vitaceae

Common names : S: Sitalata H: Pani bel

Description : Large climber; stem soft, very porous, tendrils forked. Leaves simple, suborbicular, Berry black, 2-seeded. Seeds elliptic, rugose.

USEFUL PARTS AND THEIR CURATIVE PROPERTIES

Leaf paste : Boils, wounds, swellings due to snake bite

47. *Anacyclus pyrethrum* DC.

Family : Asteraceae

Common names : S: Agragrahi H: Akarkara E: Pellitory

Description : Perennial, procumbent with numerous stems. Leaves radical, stalked, brown. Flowers white, receptacle convex.

USEFUL PARTS AND THEIR CURATIVE PROPERTIES

Roots : Astringent, sialogogue, tonic, anti-inflammatory, depurative, irritant, dental caries, odontalgia, pharyngitis, tonsilitis, paralysis, cephalalgia, epilepsy, cholera, rheumatism, typhus fever

48. *Anamirta cocculus* (L.) Wt. & Arn.

Family : Menispermaceae

Common names : S: Garalaphala H: Kakamari E: Levant berries

Description : Large, woody, climbing, shrub. Leaves simple, alternate, ovate. Flowers greenish in long panicles. Fruit drupe, kidney shaped.

USEFUL PARTS AND THEIR CURATIVE PROPERTIES

Fruits : Astringent, thermogenic, antifungal, antihelmintic, depurative, bronchitis, ulcers, chronic skin diseases

Leaves : Contraction of uterus after delivery

49. *Ananas comosus* (L.) Merrill

Family : Bromeliaceae

Common names : S: Anamnasam H: Ananas E: Pineapple

Description : Herbaceous perennial. Leaves spirally arranged, linear, lanceolate. Head terminal, ovoid, numerous. Fruits composite, succulent.

USEFUL PARTS AND THEIR CURATIVE PROPERTIES

Unripe fruits : Cooling, appetizer, digestive, antihelmintic, cathartic, cardiotonic, uterine tonic, emmenagogue, febrifuge, anorexia, dyspepsia, amenorrhoea, dysmenorrhoea, fever

Ripe fruits : Cooling, emollient, diuretic, carminative, digestive, styptic, colic, hyperacidity, cardiac debility, haemoptysis, jaundice, scabies, pruritus, fever, general debility

Leaves : Anthelmintic, abortifacient, helminthiasis, amenorrhoea, whooping cough

50. *Andrographis paniculata* (Burm. f.) Wall. ex Nees

Family : Acanthaceae
Common names : S: Kirata H: Mahatita E: Kalmegh
Description : Erect branched annual herb to 70 cm. Leaves linear-obovate, acute at both ends. Panicle branches zig-zag. Flowers white with pink tinge. Capsule oblong, compressed, minutely hairy, acute.

USEFUL PARTS AND THEIR CURATIVE PROPERTIES

Plant : Antityphoid, antifungal, hepatoprotective, antidiabetic and cholenergic,malaria, jaundice, fractures, snake bite, cough, cold, asthma, fever, tuberculosis, anthelmintic, febrifuge, tonic, alterative, debility, dysentery, dyspepsia, ulcers, leprosy, skin diseases, anti-inflammatory, antibiotic
Shoot : Antibacterial, vermicide, malaria, asthma, snake bite, cough, cold
Leaf : Hypotensive, fever, malaria, diarrhoea, sexual weakness in males, stomach pain, bile and gastric troubles, sneezing, eczema, scabies, body pain, cold, cough, cuts, wounds
Fruit : Heart diseases
Root and leaves : Diarrhoea, intestinal worms, stomach pain, paralysis, ulcers, whooping cough, piles, influenza, snake bite

51. *Anethum graveolens* L.

Family : Apiaceae
Common names : S: Satapuspa H: Soya E: Garden dill
Description : A glabrous, aromatic, annual herb. Leaves compound. Flowers flat, compound umbels. Fruits winged, vittae large, conspicuous.

USEFUL PARTS AND THEIR CURATIVE PROPERTIES

Fruit : Bitter, thermogenic, digestive, carminative, stomachic, anthelmintic, anodyne, anti-inflammatory, diuretic, emmenagogue, galactagogue, expectorant, cardiotonic, febrifuge, dysentery, colic, flatulence, dyspepsia, strangury, amenorrhoea, dysmenor-rhoea, hiccups, cough, asthma, bronchitis, fever, spermatorrhoea, ulcers, skin diseases, syphilis, piles, cardiac debility
Uses : Culinary purposes, drugs, flavouring, perfumery

52. *Angelica archangelica* L.

Family : Apiaceae
Common names : E: Angelica

USEFUL PARTS AND THEIR CURATIVE PROPERTIES

Uses : Perfumery, confectionary, flavouring, cosmetics

53. *Anisochilus carnosus* (L.f.) Wall. ex Benth.

Family : Lamiaceae
Common names : S: Induparni H: Panjiri-ka-patta

Description : Annual aromatic erect herb to 50 cm; stems quadrangular. Leaves ovate, pubescent below, cordate, serrate, apex acute. Flowers purple or pale-violet, in terminal long spikes. Fruits strobilus like, enlarging with maturity.

USEFUL PARTS AND THEIR CURATIVE PROPERTIES

Tender shoots : Cold, cough
Leaf paste : Wounds, fissures, cracks

54. *Anisomeles indica* (L.) Kuntze

Family : Lamiaceae
Common names : S: Kala bhangra
Description : Perennial, pubescent, aromatic, bushy undershrub to 1.5 m. stems and branches acutely quadrangular. Leaves ovate to obovate, truncate, deeply crenate-serrate, apex acute to shortly acuminate. Flowers in dense whorls in axils of distal leaves; corolla pink. Nutlets ovoid, shining black.

USEFUL PARTS AND THEIR CURATIVE PROPERTIES

Leaf : Eczema, ephemeral fever, intermittent fevers, catarrhal affections, disorders in stomach and bowels, cold
Root powder : poisonous bites

55. *Annona squamosa* L.

Family : Annonaceae
Common names : S: Seethaphalam H: Sitaphal E: Custard apple
Description : Small tree upto 4 m; bark brown. Leaves elliptic or oblong-lanceolate. Flowers on short pedicels. Fruit globose, green; pulp sweet. Seeds many, angular, black and shiny.

USEFUL PARTS AND THEIR CURATIVE PROPERTIES

Aerial part : Insecticidal, anticancer
Plant : Antifertility
Alkaloid : P-hydroxybenzyl – 6,7 dihydroxyl – 1, 2, 3, 4 – tetrahydroisoquinoline from
Leaves : Cardiotonic, toothache
Root alkaloid : Antihypertensive, antispasmidic, antihista-mine, bronchodilator.
Alkaloid corydine : Anticancer
Stem bark : Asthma, snake bite
Leaf paste : Jaundice, wounds, pyorrhoea, dental carries, diarrhoea, kills lice.
Root paste : Abortion, diarrhoea, syphilis, epilepsy, drastic purgative, dysentery Seed paste – dandruff, kills lice.
Fruit : Constipation.

56. *Anogeissus latifolia* (Roxb. ex DC.)Wall. ex Guill. & Perr.

Family : Combretaceae
Common names : S: Dhavah H: Bankli E: Button tree

Description	: Large deciduous tree upto 25 m, bark white, smooth with rounded patches. leaves spiral, oblong or obovate, nerves 7-12 paired, rusty below, rotund to cuneate, entire, apex obtuse. Flowers pale yellow, axillary, aggregated in cymose heads.

USEFUL PARTS AND THEIR CURATIVE PROPERTIES

Stem bark	: Hypothermic, CNS active, antagonism of amphetamine hyperactivity, cough, asthma, headache, diarrhoea, lumbago and bowel pain, scorpion sting.
Gum	: Urinary disorders, leucorrhoea
Seed paste	: Snake bite
Leaf	: Scorpion sting, snake bite

57. *Anthemis nobilis* L.

Family	: Asteraceae
Common names	: E: Chamomile
Description	: Annual, erect, herbaceous aromatic plant. Leaves doubly pinnate, linear.Flower heads terminal, solitary, yellow. Ovary inferior, bicarpellary. Fruit achene.

USEFUL PARTS AND THEIR CURATIVE PROPERTIES

Uses	: Beverages, confectionery, cosmetics, drugs, flavouring and perfumery.

58. *Antidesma ghaesembilla* Gaertn.

Family	: Euphorbiaceae
Common names	: S: Janupulisaru H: Umtova
Description	: A small deciduous tree. Leaves alternate. Flowers dioecious, spikes.Stamens 2-5, inserted within the disc. Ovary 1-celled. Fruit drupe.

USEFUL PARTS AND THEIR CURATIVE PROPERTIES

Aerial part	: Hypotensive, diuretic.

59. *Aphanamixis polystachya* (Wall.) Parker

Family	: Meliaceae
Common names	: S: Rohitakah H: Harin-hara E: Rohituka tree
Description	: A medium to large sized tree. Leaves large, imparipinnate, elliptic-oblong. Male flowers numerous in axillary panicles. Female or bisexual flowers larger in spikes. Fruits globular, smooth, yellow when ripe. Seeds with scarlet aril.

USEFUL PARTS AND THEIR CURATIVE PROPERTIES

Bark	: Astringent, vulnerary, antihelmintic, depurative, urinary astringent,ophthalmic, refrigerant, splenomegaly, liver disorders, dyspepsia, leprosy, diabetes, skin diseases, rheumatoid arthritis, leucorrhoea
Seeds	: Refrigerant, laxative, anodyne, anthelmintic, ulcers, myalgia, otopathy

60. *Apium graveolens* L.

Family : Apiaceae
Common names : E: Celery
Description : Herbaceous annual or biennial erect herb. Leaves reduced, pinnate, large, deeply divided. Inflorescence compound umbel. Fruit schizocarp with 2 mericarps.

USEFUL PARTS AND THEIR CURATIVE PROPERTIES

Uses : Culinary, drugs, flavouring, food, perfumery

61. *Aquilaria agallocha* Roxb.

Family : Thymeleaceae
Common names : S: Aguruh H: Agar E: Aloe wood
Description : Large evergreen tree. Leaves linear lanceolate. Flowers small greenish on peduncled umbels, filaments red at the apex. Ovary tomentose. Fruits slightly compressed, yellowish, tomentose capsules.

USEFUL PARTS AND THEIR CURATIVE PROPERTIES

Wood : Fragrant, acrid, thermogenic, carminative, deodorant, sudorific, anorexia, cardiac debility, skin diseases, leprosy, albuminuria, general debility, vomiting
Oil : Astringent, alexeteric, antileprotic, asthma, cough, skin diseases, foul ulcers

62. *Argemone mexicana* L.

Family : Papaveraceae
Common names : S: Svarnaksiri H: Brahmadundi E: Mexican Poppy
Description : Erect prickly annual herb; latex yellow. Leaves bristly, with slightly incised undulated white veins. Flowers bright yellow. Fruit oblong, prickly; seeds blackish to brown.

USEFUL PARTS AND THEIR CURATIVE PROPERTIES

Plant : Effect on respiration, antiviral, psoriasis, wounds, toothache. Protopine fraction of plant extract stimulant heart, respiration, skeletal muscles and blood pressure, whereas the total alkaloid fraction stimulated all the smooth muscles and antagonized the actions of acetylcholine, histamine and 5 –hydroxytryptamine
Latex : Conjunctivitis, scabies, intestinal worms, eye diseases, rat bite, syphilis, piles, night blindness
Root : Leucoderma, menstrual disorders, spermatorrhoea, gonorrhoea, piles, fever. Leaf juice – leprous skin, boils, leucorrhoea, vermifuge, syphilis, ulcers, skin diseases
Stem : Syphilis, rheumatism
Seed : Pyorrhoea, leprotic spots, nauseant, purgative, dropsy, jaundice, cutaneous troubles, malaria

63. *Argyreia nervosa* (Burm. f.) Boj.

Family : Convolvulaceae
Common names : S: Samudrapalaka H: Samandar ka-pat E: The Elephant creeper
Description : Large woody climbing shrub with woolly white, tomentose stems. Leaves simple, large, ovate, acute, cordate, glabrous above, white tomentose beneath; flowers rose purple, in axillary clustered cymes; corolla tubular, infundibuliform.

USEFUL PARTS AND THEIR CURATIVE PROPERTIES

Seed : CVS active, syphilis, piles, anaemia
Roots : Migraine, healing wounds, muscular pain, skin diseases, aphrodisiac, rheumatism
Leaf : Rheumatism, carbuncles, boils, blisters, diabetes, abscess, gonorrhoea, eczema

64. *Aristolochia bracteolata* Lam.

Family : Aristolochiaceae
Common names : S: Kitamari H: Kiramar E: Bracteated birthwort
Description : Slender decumbent glabrous, perennial herb with long stems and striate branches. Leaves entire or undulate, usually widely and shallowly cordate, broadly ovate to reniform. Flowers solitary. Perianth tube cylindrical with trumpet shaped mouth and lip dark purple; linear, glandular, hairy within.

USEFUL PARTS AND THEIR CURATIVE PROPERTIES

Leaves : Eczema, deworming, cuts and wounds , night blindness, psoriasis, menstrual troubles, stomach ulcers, dental caries, appetizer
Root : Expelling roundworms, aphthous ulcers, snake bite, abortifacient, scorpion sting
Stem juice : Leucorrhoea
Whole plant : Indigestion, flatulence, abnormal menstruation, excessive bleeding, snake bite, helminthiasis, diabetes.

65. *Aristolochia indica* L.

Family : Aristolochiaceae
Common names : S: Nakuli H:Ishramul E: The Indian birthwort
Description : Twining shrub to 2 m. Leaves very variable, oblong to obovate, 3 nerved from base, lateral nerves 3-4, converging towards apex, truncate to subcordate or panduriform, apex obtuse to acuminate. Racemes axillary or terminal, 8-15 flowered, dark purple.

USEFUL PARTS AND THEIR CURATIVE PROPERTIES

Plant : Diuretic, anticancer, insecticidal, antiimplan-tation, interceptive and antifertility, eczema, snake bite. Dried stems and roots contain the

		drug 'Aristolochin' which promotes digestion and regulates menstruation in small doses; large doses causes dangerous irritation in the digestive system and in kidneys; leads to even abortion in pregnant women
Root bark	:	Snake bite, chest pain, stomach pain, scorpion and other insect stings
Leaves	:	Leucorrhoea and skin diseases, fever, leucoderma, toothache, boils, blisters, cholera, diarrhoea
Root	:	Wounds, diarrhoea, fever, snake bite, rheumatism, abortion

66. *Artemisia dracunculus* L.

Family	:	Asteraceae
Common names	:	E: Tarragon

USEFUL PARTS AND THEIR CURATIVE PROPERTIES

Uses	:	Cooling agent, cosmetics, flavouring beverages, perfumery

67. *Artemisia nilagirica* (Clarke) Pamp.

Family	:	Asteraceae
Common names	:	S: Davanam H: Dona E: Indian Wormwood
Description	:	A tall aromatic shrub, often gregarious. Leaves often long. Heads small, heterogamous. Disc florets fertile. Achenes very small.

USEFUL PARTS AND THEIR CURATIVE PROPERTIES

Whole plant	:	Herb steeped in hot vinegar is bound round a sprain or bruise and juice or the herb is applied to the head to prevent convulsions, itches, leprosy, skin diseases, perfume and cosmetics.
Leaves	:	Nervous disorders, whooping cough, haemorrhage, urinary troubles
Uses	:	Oil-aromatic, pleasant, cooling agent, cosmetics, flavouring beverages, confectionery and tobacco, perfumery.

68. *Artocarpus heterophyllus* Lam.

Family	:	Moraceae
Common names	:	S: Panasah H: Kanthal E: Jack fruit tree
Description	:	Evergreen tree to 15 m, leaves entire, coriaceous, base rounded, apex obtuse. Flowers solitary, usually in axillary receptacles. Fruit a syncarp.

USEFUL PARTS AND THEIR CURATIVE PROPERTIES

Seeds	:	Possesses acholine activity
Leaves	:	Estrogenic, ulcers, skin diseases
Seed	:	Lectin extraction potent and selective stimulation of distinct human T and B cell function
Latex	:	Bacteriolytic, pus forming wounds
Bark	:	Severe headache
Tender shoots	:	Leprosy
Unripen fruits	:	Dysentery, tuberculosis, antiamoebic, aphrodisiac

69. *Arundo donax* L.

Family : Poaceae
Common names : S: Dhamana H: Bara nal E: Spanish cane
Description : Tall, stout, perennial shrubs. Leaves broad flat. Panicles large. Spikelets 2-8 flowered, glumes 2, persistent. Lemmas lanceolate, stamens 3, grain oblong.

USEFUL PARTS AND THEIR CURATIVE PROPERTIES

Rhizome : Hypotensive, bufotenidine – possesses antiacetyl choline effect histamine release activity and uterine stimulant

70. *Asclepias curassavica* L.

Family : Asclepiadaceae
Common names : S: Kakatundi H: Kaura dodi E: Blood flower
Description : Erect herb to 1 m; latex milky. Leaves decussate or whorled, lanceolate, acute at both ends. Flowers red in sub-terminal umbels. Follicles tapering at both ends.

USEFUL PARTS AND THEIR CURATIVE PROPERTIES

Leaf juice : Cuts, wounds
Root bark : Gonorrhoea and piles

71. *Asparagus gonocladus* Baker

Family : Liliaceae
Common names : S: Satavari H: Shatavir E: Wild carrot
Description : Much branched, scandent armed undershrub. Leaves spurred at base with hard spines. Cladodes flat, falcate, acute or acuminate. Raceme often fascicled.Flowers white. Berry globose.

USEFUL PARTS AND THEIR CURATIVE PROPERTIES

Tuber : Increase potency, skin diseases, diabetes

72. *Asparagus racemosus* Willd.

Family : Liliaceae
Common names : S: Satavari H: Shatavir E: Wild Asparagus
Description : Armed vine. Spines erect, leaves scaly, triangular, stiff, acuminate. Cladodes 2-6, linear, narrow, entire, apex acuminate. Raceme solitary or 3 in a cluster. Peduncle much reduced. Flowers white, fragrant. Berry globose, ripening red.3-6, globose.

USEFUL PARTS AND THEIR CURATIVE PROPERTIES

Aerial part : Spasmolytic, antiarrhythmic, epilepsy
Bark : Antibacterial, antifungal
Root : Urinary troubles, in delivery as a tonic, leucorrhoea, diabetes, gonorrhoea, galacta-gogue, nephro-calcinosis and ureteral stones, stomach ulcers, fever, lactation, menstrual disorders, strength, liver problems, diarrhoea, dysentery, haemorrhages, hypertension, jaundice, aphrodisiac Shatavarin- IV- antioxytocic

Tuber : Burning micturition, excess of heat, menstrual disorders, reduces breast milk, stomach pains, weakness, excess menstrual flow, hepatic stimulant, snake bite, diarrhoea, dysentery, cough, tuberculosis, arthritis, cuts, wounds, cooling, dehydration, diabetes

Root paste : Joint pain, malaria, blood dysentery, excessive menstruation, diarrhoea Root juice dropped in mouth or nose to stop bleeding, galactagogue

Leaf paste : Scabies, urinary troubles, blood pressure

73. *Atalantia monophylla* (Roxb.) Corr.

Family : Rutaceae

Common names : S: Atavi-jambira

Description : Densely foliaceous armed tree. Spines 1 or 2, axillary on branches. Leaves glabrous, simple, lanceolate, obtuse or cuneate, entire, emarginate. Flowers creamish in axillary racemes. Berries globose, seeds 4, ovoid.

USEFUL PARTS AND THEIR CURATIVE PROPERTIES

Leaf paste : Scorpion sting

Root bark : Skin diseases

Fruit oil : Rheumatism, paralysis

74. *Atropa acuminata* Royle ex Lindley

Family : Solanaceae

Common names : H: Sag-angur E: Indian Belladona

Description : An erect, branched perennial herb. Leaves brownish green. Flowers in axils of leaves, bell-shaped, yellowish brown. Berry round, purple-black.

USEFUL PARTS AND THEIR CURATIVE PROPERTIES

Roots : Narcotic, sedative, diuretic and anodyne

Leaves : Decreases secretion of sweat and salivary and gastric glands, asthma, antispasmodic, whooping cough, rheumatism, neuralgia, inflammations.

75. *Atropa belladonna* L.

Family : Solanaceae

Common names : H: Saganur E: Deadly nightshade

USEFUL PARTS AND THEIR CURATIVE PROPERTIES

Leaves : Atropine – sedative, antispasmodic, anodyne, cough, gout, mydriative in diseases of the eye, whooping cough, night-sweat, rheumatic inflammation

Roots / leaves : Narcotic, diuretic, sedative, mydriatic, spermatorrhoea.

76. *Atylosia scarabaeoides* (L.) Benth.

Family : Papilionaceae

Description : A slender twining shrub, flowers yellow, calyx densely pubescent, pods linear, seeds 4-6.

USEFUL PARTS AND THEIR CURATIVE PROPERTIES

Plant decoction : Tonic after delivery, burning sensation, diarrhoea, gastric disorders.
Leaf paste : Swellings of leg, prevents labour pains
Root paste : Checks hair fall or cures baldness, rheumatism
Root : Gastric trouble, stomachache

77. *Averrhoa carambola* L.

Family : Oxalidaceae
Common names : S: Karmarangah H: Kamarakh E: Carambola apple
Description : Small handsome evergreen tree. Leaves compound, alternate, glabrous. Flowers variegated in short racemes, axillary. Fruits ovoid. Seeds arillate.

USEFUL PARTS AND THEIR CURATIVE PROPERTIES

Leaves : Antipruritic, antipyretic, anthelmintic, scabies, poisoning, intermittent fevers, intestinal worms
Fruits : Thermogenic, constipating, febrifuge, antipyretic, antiscorbutic, tonic, diarrhoea, vomiting, hyperdypsia, haemorrhoids, general debility

78. *Azadirachta indica* A. Juss.

Family : Meliaceae
Common names : S: Nimba H: Neem E: Margosa tree
Description : Large tree upto 20 m, leaves unipinnate, crowded near the ends of Leaflets 5-6 pairs, ovate-lanceolate, subopposite, glaucous, oblique, crenate-serrate, apex acute to acuminate. Flowers white, axillary panicles. Drupe oblong to globose, yellow when ripe.

USEFUL PARTS AND THEIR CURATIVE PROPERTIES

Leaf aqueous : Antiviral, nimbidin and sodium nimbidinate, extract effective against furunculosis, arsenical dermatitis, ulcer, scabies, dermatitis, bleeding gums, pyorrhoea, reduction in blood pressure, spermicidal and diuretic, nimbidiol – estrogenic, antipyretic, diabetes
Neem oil : Antibacterial, antitubercular, insecticidal, dandruff
Leaves : In gingivitis, periodontitis, chicken-pox, eczema, diarrhoea, dysentery, piles, anthelmintic, measles, ulcer, wounds, skin diseases, cough, liver diseases, malaria, allergies, contraceptive, earache, eye diseases, fevers, piles, post patrum treatment, smallpox. Bark - bitter tonic, astringent and antiperiodic. It is useful in fevers, breaks the periodic sequence of fevers (like malaria), diabetes, leucorrhoea, menorrhagia, scabies
Young buds : Measles, chicken pox, small pox
Tender shoots : Diabetes
Fruit : Helminthiasis
Flowers : Jaundice, diabetes
Seed : Diabetes, abortion, rat bite, skin diseases, kills lice, psoriasis
Gum : Diarrhoea, nephroprotector

79. *Bacopa monnieri* (L.) Penn.

Family : Scrophulariaceae
Common names : S: Saumyalata H: Brahmi E: Brahmi
Description : Prostrate, fleshy herb. Leaves opposite, sessile. Flowers blue or purple, solitary. capsule ovoid, glabrous. Seeds oblong, striate.

USEFUL PARTS AND THEIR CURATIVE PROPERTIES

Whole plant : Nervous debility, brain tonic, memory development, malarial fever
Leaf juice : Catarrh, bronchitis, diarrhoea, stammering, diabetes, fever

80. *Baliospermum montanum* (Willd.) Muell-Arg.

Family : Euphorbiaceae
Common names : S: Danti H: Dantt E: Wild castor
Description : Stout herb to 1m, leaves variavle, lower ovate, upper lanceolate, angled or lobed, glabrescent, acute, sinuate-toothed, base rounded; flowers yellowish axillary racemes. Capsule ovoid.

USEFUL PARTS AND THEIR CURATIVE PROPERTIES

Plant : Effect on respiration, CVS active, anticancer
Root : Jaundice, rib muscle pain, stomach pain
Seed paste : Rheumatism, purgative, snake bite
Leaf juice : Eye diseases, cooling

81. *Bambusa arundinacea* (Retz.) Willd.

Family : Poaceae
Common names : S: Venu H: Kantabams E: Thorny bamboo
Description : Shrubs or trees, often very large, culms form a thick rhizome. Culm sheaths usually broad. Leaves small to moderately large. Inflorescence compound panicle with spikelets in heads. Glumes 1-3, lodicules 3. stamens 6. grain oblong.

USEFUL PARTS AND THEIR CURATIVE PROPERTIES

Whole plant : Estrogenic and antidiabetic
Culms : Haematuria, headache, wounds
Stem bark : Snake bite
Root : Eye diseases
Leaf : Abortion, anthelmintic, sterilization

82. *Barleria cristata* L.

Family : Acanthaceae
Common names : S: Jhinti H: Tadrelu E: Crested purple
Description : Herbaceous hairy undershrub to 1 m, leaves elliptic-oblong, pubescent, cuneate, ciliate, apex acute. Flowers 1-4, in axillary or terminal racemes, subsessile. Corolla purplish pink, violet or white.

USEFUL PARTS AND THEIR CURATIVE PROPERTIES

Leaf	:	Asthma and scorpion sting
Root	:	Body swellings, snake bite

83. *Barleria prionitis* L.

Family	:	Acanthaceae
Common names	:	S: Kantakuranta H: Kat-sareya E: Thornnail dye
Description	:	Armed undershrub to 1 m; spines 2-4, white, young shoots pubescent. Leaves ovate-obovate, coriaceous, sparsely hirsute below, apex obtuse or apiculate. Flowers subsessile, solitary or in cymose clusters in lower axils. Corolla golden yellow to orange.

USEFUL PARTS AND THEIR CURATIVE PROPERTIES

Root	:	Bronchitis, leucorrhoea, infected teeth
Leaf	:	Malaria, foot cracks, cuts and wounds, catarrh, spermatorrhoea, bleeding gums, asthma with cough, skin diseases, boils, toothache, phlegm, headache
Flowers	:	Painful menstruation
Whole plant	:	Stomachache, gastric troubles, oedema, inflammation.

84. *Barringtonia acutangula* (L.) Gaertn.

Family	:	Barringtoniaceae
Common names	:	S: Hijjala H: Ijal E: Indian oak
Description	:	Tree upto 10 m, leaves obovate, crenate acute or acuminate, cuneate, lateral veins 10-12 pairs. Inflorescence pendulous. Flowers pedicelled; calyx lobes distinct in buds; filaments pink. Fruits fibrous, quadrangular.

USEFUL PARTS AND THEIR CURATIVE PROPERTIES

Root / stem bark	:	CNS active
Root	:	Hypoglycaemic
Stem bark	:	Antiprotozoal
Leaf juice	:	Headache
Bark decoction	:	Toothache, gum trouble, rheumatism
Seeds	:	Enlarged abdomen, headache, diarrhoea, eye diseases, liver complaints

85. *Basella alba* L.

Family	:	Basellaceae
Common names	:	S: Potaki H: Poi E: Indian spinach
Description	:	Succulent glabrous climbing perennial herb. Stems twining to the right. Leaves fleshy, broadly ovate, pointed at the apex. Flowers borne in spicate inflorescence. Fruits violet when ripe.

USEFUL PARTS AND THEIR CURATIVE PROPERTIES

Leaf	:	Constipation in children, wounds.

86. *Bauhinia purpurea* L.

Family : Caesalpiniaceae
Common names : S: Kanchan H: Lal kachnar E: Pink Bauhinia
Description : Moderate-sized, evergreen, bushy tree; bark ash coloured to dark brown. Leaves oblong,leaflets connate about half way,subcordate, entire, apex obtuse to subacute. Inflorescence terminal or axillary of racemes. Flowers rose to purple, petals similar; seeds ovoid.

USEFUL PARTS AND THEIR CURATIVE PROPERTIES

Stem bark : Boils, body pains and fever, diarrhoea, headache, sores of small pox, general weakness after child birth
Flower paste : Constipation, diarrhoea
Bark paste : Dissolving cancerous growth in stomach, anasarca, dysentery, diarrhoea, dyspepsia, skin diseases
Leaf paste : Jaundice
Root : Snake bite, astringent, sore throat, ulcers, tympanic gland trouble, arthritis, piles, haemostatic agent.

87. *Bauhinia racemosa* Lam.

Family : Caesalpiniaceae
Common names : S: Swetakanchan H: Ashta
Description : Medium sized deciduous tree; bark blackish, very rough, with deep vertical cracks. Leaves broader than long, connation two-thirds of their length, 7-9 nerved, cordate, entire, apex obtuse, mucronate. Racemes terminal and leaf-opposed. Flowers white or yellow on short pedicles. Calyx tube turbinate, deeply 5-lobed. Pod oblong, twisted or falcate, 10-20 seeded.

USEFUL PARTS AND THEIR CURATIVE PROPERTIES

Seed : Antibacterial
Stem bark : CVS and CNS active, hypothermic, anticancer, fertility, amenorrhoea, dysentery, paralysis, wounds, ulcers, epilepsy, throat pain, astringent, spermatorrhoea
Roots : Rheumatic pains, diarrhoea
Fruits : Indigestion, constipation
Leaf : Malaria, ophthalmic infections

88. *Bauhinia vahlii* Wt. & Arn.

Family : Caesalpiniaceae
Common names : S: Murva H: Mahul E: Camel's foot climber
Description : Liane, stems woody, tendrils opposite, circinate. Leaves broader than long, deeply cordate at base, glabrous or sparsely puberulous above, tomentose beneath. Flowers white in terminal corymbs. Pods flattened, oblong, rusty tomentose,woody.

USEFUL PARTS AND THEIR CURATIVE PROPERTIES

Stem : CVS active, antiarrhythmic, spasmolytic, inflammation, dysentery
Seeds : Expel worms from stomach, general debility, dysentery
Root paste : Bone fracture, dysentery, syphilis, stomach-ache
Stem / leaves : Wounds
Bark : Excessive bleeding, thirst, pains, tumours, ulcers

89. *Bauhinia variegata* L.

Family : Caesalpiniaceae
Common names : S: Kanchana H: Barial E: Variegated bauhinia
Description : Moderate-sized deciduous tree, bark grey, with vertical cracks. Leaves deeply cordate at base, connate for about two-thirds, coriaceous, 10-13 nerved, entire, apex obtuse, panicles terminal. Flowers large, fragrant, sessile or shortly pedicelled, in few flowered corymbs. Petals light pink, upper one dark, variegated. Pod oblong, base and apex narrow, horned.

USEFUL PARTS AND THEIR CURATIVE PROPERTIES

Flower paste : Asthma, diarrhoea
Root decoction : Stomachache, snake bite, astringent, sore throat, ulcers, tympanic gland trouble, arthritis
Bark : Anthelmintic, astringent, ulcers, cutaneous troubles, diarrhoea, dysentery, dyspepsia, skin diseases, laxative, menorrhagia
Buds : tumours

90. *Benkera malabarica* (Lam.) Tirv.

Family : Rubiaceae
Description : Spinescent shrub. Leaves decussate or whorled, coriaceous, oblanceolate, cuneate, entire, apex apiculate. Flowers axillary in corymbose cymes, white. Berry globose, small. Seeds conical, not embedded in pulp.

USEFUL PARTS AND THEIR CURATIVE PROPERTIES

Stem bark : Asthma
Roots : Cough

91. *Benincasa hispida* (Thunb.) Cogn.

Family : Cucurbitaceae
Common names : S: Kusmandah H: Petha E: Ash gourd
Description : Vine; branchlets hirsute. Leaves broadly ovate, 7-lobed, lobes ovate-lanceolate, hirsute, cordate, irregularly dentate, apex acute; tendrils 2 or 3 branched. Flower monoecious, axillary, solitary, yellow.

USEFUL PARTS AND THEIR CURATIVE PROPERTIES

Fruit : Burning micturition, scorpion sting, control bleeding, epilepsy, piles, constipation, dyspepsia
Seed : Increase potency

92. *Beta vulgaris* L.

Family : Chenopodiaceae

Common names : S: Palakya H: Cukkandar E: Beet root

Description : Annual or biennial tuberous herb with condensed stem. Leaves simple, cauline, ovate. Flowers in a cluster or solitary on spike.

USEFUL PARTS AND THEIR CURATIVE PROPERTIES

Roots : Expectorant, tonic, psychopathy, cough, infammation, general debility

Leaves : Diuretic, anodyne, tonic, purgative, cuts and burns, strangury, paralysis, liver and spleen disorders

Seeds : Diuretic, aphrodisiac, carminative, emmanogogue, cough ,asthma, flatulence, anorexia

93. *Betula utilis* D. Don

Family : Betulaceae

Common names : S: Bhurjah H: Bhojpatra E: Himalayan silver birch

Description : Medium sized deciduous tree. Leaves silky, acute, serrate. Flowers in catkins. Fruits narrower than the bracts.

USEFUL PARTS AND THEIR CURATIVE PROPERTIES

Bark : Astringent, thermogenic, alexeteric, deodorant, antibacterial, anticonvulsant, haemostatic, expectorant, carminative, tonic, hysteria, epilepsy, bacterial infections, wounds, diarrhoea, dysentery, haemorrhages, cough, bronchitis, bilious fever, leprosy, skin diseases, general debility

94. *Biophytum sensitivum* (L.) DC.

Family : Oxalidaceae

Common names : S: Amlika H: Lajjalu

Description : Erect herb. Leaflets 7-15 pairs, terminal pair largest, obovate, curved. Umbels 5-10, each 6-10 flowered. Flowers yellow or brick red. Capsule glandular pubescent along septa, 5 valved.

USEFUL PARTS AND THEIR CURATIVE PROPERTIES

Root decoction : Gonorrhoea, impotency

Leaf paste : Wounds, headache, giddiness and fever, rheumatism, hydrocele

Whole plant : Aphrodisiac, malaria, rheumatism

95. *Bixa orellana* L.

Family : Bixaceae

Common names : S: Sinduri H:Sindhuriyan E: Annatto plant

Description : Small evergreen tree. Leaves large cordate acuminate, glabrous on both surfaces. Flowers white or pink in terminal panicles. Fruits reddish brown or green, capsules clothed with soft bristles. Seeds trigonous covered with red pulp.

USEFUL PARTS AND THEIR CURATIVE PROPERTIES

Seed pulp	:	Dysentery, cancer, antipyretic, gonorrhoea
Stem bark	:	Intermittent fever, hypoglycaemic
Root bark	:	Fever, antiperiodic

96. *Blumea eriantha* DC.

Family	:	Asteraceae
Common names	:	S: Kukundara
Description	:	Erect herbs, leaves membranous, heads 0.3 inch broad, bisexual flowers pubescent. Achenes angled, sparsely hairy.

USEFUL PARTS AND THEIR CURATIVE PROPERTIES

Essential oil from leaves	:	Insecticidal, antibacterial, antifungal

97. *Boerhaavia diffusa* L.

Family	:	Nyctaginaceae
Common names	:	S: Sophaghni H: Punura E: Spreading hog weed
Description	:	Perennial creeping herb, branches diffuse, leaves opposite. Flowers pink, red or white, borne in small umbels. Fruit brownish.

USEFUL PARTS AND THEIR CURATIVE PROPERTIES

Root and plant	:	Spasmolytic
Root	:	Antiarrhythmic, antiviral, anticonvulsant, analgesic, asthma, paralysis, epilepsy, jaundice, deworming, eye diseases, diarrhoea, piles, blood dysentery, fever, stomach pain
Whole plant	:	oedema, elephantiasis,dislocated joints, fevers, jaundice
Leaf	:	Fever, kala-azar, diuretic and anti-inflammatory, leprosy, cuts, wounds, leucorrhoea, spermatorrhoea, jaundice

98. *Bombax ceiba* L.

Family	:	Bombacaceae
Common names	:	S: Moca H: Semal E: Red silk cotton tree
Description	:	Large deciduous tree; bark grey, conical sharp, prickles when young. Leaves digitate, leaflets 5-7, lanceolate, oblanceolate, glabrous, acuminate. Flowers fleshy, cup-shaped scarlets, calyx inside silky tomentose, leathery. Capsule 5-angled. Seeds obovate, smooth, surrouded by white silky hairs.

USEFUL PARTS AND THEIR CURATIVE PROPERTIES

Seeds	:	Oxytocic, musculotropic, cardiac stimulant, chicken pox and small pox
Stem bark	:	Red leucorrhoea, cooling tonic, giddiness, diarrhoea, dysentery, menorrhoea, blisters, ulcers
Petals paste	:	Conjunctivitis in infants
Flowers paste	:	Boils, sores, itches, leucorrhoea, chicken pox, contraception, piles, urinary complaints, dysentery

Leaf : Strangury, gonorrhoea, piles
Fruit : Venereal diseases
Root : Urinary troubles, menstrual disorders, impotency, spermatorrhoea, vigour, vitality, sex tonic, aphrodisiac

99. *Borassus flabellifer* L.

Family : Arecaceae
Common names : S: Talah H: Tar E: Palmyrah palm
Description : Tall palm with crown of leaves. Leaves palmately fan shaped, coriaceous. Flowers unisexual. Fruits sub-globose, drupes.

USEFUL PARTS AND THEIR CURATIVE PROPERTIES

Roots : Cooling, restorative, diuretic, stimulant, hyperdypsia, burning sensation, inflammation
Ash of roots : Antacid, antiperiodic, hyperacidity, bilious fever, inflorescence spleno - megaly, skin diseases
Fruits : Cooling, laxative, sedative, anthelmintic, depurative, styptic, stomachic, aphrodisiac, hyperdypsia, general debility

100. *Boswellia serrata* Roxb. ex Colebr.

Family : Burseraceae
Common names : S: Sallaki H: Salai E: The Indian olibanum tree
Description : Large tree upto 20 m; bark scaly. Leaves crowded towards the ends of branches, imparipinnate, leaflets 10-15 pairs, oblong to lanceolate, glabrous, rusty below, cuneate, dentate-serrate, apex acute. Flowers white or pale pink in axillary panicles. Drupes trigonous, greenish-yellow, pyrenes 3, each 1-seeded; seed heart shaped.

USEFUL PARTS AND THEIR CURATIVE PROPERTIES

Root : Anticancer
Stem and fruit : Hypoglycaemic
Root and fruit : CNS active
Gum-resin : Sedative, analgesic, anti-inflammatory, antitumour, scorpion sting, skin eruptions, hypolipidaemic, fever
Stem Bark : Backache, headache, dysuria, traumatic pain, gastric pain, rheumatism, toothache, pus formation in mouth, eye inflammation, skin diseases, diabetes
Whole plant : Cough
Leaf : Scorpion sting

101. *Brassica nigra* Koch

Family : Brassicaceae
Common names : H: Banarasi rai E: Mustard
Description : A glabrous annual plant. Leaves long, broadly ovate, persistent. Flowers yellow in racemes. Fruits siliqua, seeds attached to the replum.

USEFUL PARTS AND THEIR CURATIVE PROPERTIES

Seeds : Acrid, bitter, anodyne, carminative, dyspepsia, flatulence, inflammations, tonic, sudorific, skin diseases, splenomegaly, dengue fever

102. *Bridelia retusa* (L.) Spreng

Family : Euphorbiaceae

Common names : S: Ekavira H: Kattian E: Feather foil

Description : Large deciduous tree with thorns on the bark when young. Bark grey or brown, rough with longitudinal cracks and exfoliating in long irregular plates. Leaves rigidly coriaceous, elliptic-oblong, ovate or obovate, rounded at base, slightly crenulate. Flowers in clusters axillary and terminal spikes. Drupe globose, scaled on the hardly enlarged calyx.

USEFUL PARTS AND THEIR CURATIVE PROPERTIES

Bark : Antiviral, anticancer, effect on respiration and nictitating membrane, fertility, jaundice, fever, chest pain, rheumatism, insect sting

Stem bark : Asthma, dysentery, vomitings

103. *Buchanania lanzan* Spreng

Family : Anacardiaceae

Common names : S: Chara H: Piyala E: Almondi tree

Description : Moderate-sized tree; branchlets with prominent leaf scars. Leaves broadly ovate, round, entire, apex obtuse-retuse. Panicles shorter than leaves. Petals cream. Drupe ovoid-oblong, black when ripe.

USEFUL PARTS AND THEIR CURATIVE PROPERTIES

Aerial plant : Effect on respiration, CVS active, anticancer

Gum : Backache, rheumatic pains, bone fracture, heart complaints, sprains, chest pain

Stem bark : General weakness, diarrhoea, chest pain, boils, ulcers

104. *Bursera delpechiana* L.

Family : Burseraceae

Common names : E: Indian Lavender tree

Description : Large deciduous tree. Inflorescence paniculate cyme with a pubescent axis.It contains 40-50 staminate flowers. Ovary is hairy and surrounded by crenate disc. Fruit is a fleshy berry, pericarp contains resiniferous ducts.

USEFUL PARTS AND THEIR CURATIVE PROPERTIES

Uses : Cosmetics, flavouring food and beverages, perfumery

105. *Butea monosperma* (Lamk.) Taub.

Family : Papilionanceae

Common names : S: Palashah H: Palas E: Bastard teak

Description : Deciduous tree. Leaves trifoliate, coriaceous, glabrous above, cuneate, entire, apex obtuse, retuse. Flowers yellowish red coloured in panicles. Pod flat.

USEFUL PARTS AND THEIR CURATIVE PROPERTIES

Seeds : Anthelmintic and used in treating skin diseases, ringworm and dhobi's itch, whooping cough, amenorrhoea, deworming, abortion, leucoderma, contraceptive, vermicide

Seeds / flowers : Antifertility, fever, asthma, conjunctivitis, anthelmintic

Root bark : Blood pressure, increase potency. The gum called Bengal kino or Butea gum is used for the treatment of diarrhoea, post delivery backache and weakness, gonorrhoea, astringent, dysentery. Leaves and fruits are cathartic and are useful in habitual constipation, fertility, diabetes, diarrhoea, helminthiasis, pimples.

Stem bark : Fracture, antifertility, snake bite, diarrhoea, piles, dysentery, jaundice

Latex : Jaundice

Root decoction : Urinary troubles, congested lungs, goitre

Flower : Nephrocalcinosis, ureteral stones, diarrhoea, gonorrhoea, asthma, sunstroke, constipation, diabetes

Bark decoction : Loose motions

106. *Byttneria herbacea* Roxb.

Family : Sterculiaceae

Description : Ascending herb. Leaves ovate or lanceolate, a linear gland at base, puberulous above, glabrous below, dentate, apex acuminate. Cymes umbellate, flowers purple. Capsule globose, prickled; seeds 5, ovoid, angular.

USEFUL PARTS AND THEIR CURATIVE PROPERTIES

Leaf paste : cuts, wounds

Root paste : Maggot infested sores, cuts by iron tools

Whole plant : Leprosy

107. *Cadaba fruticosa* (L.) Druce

Family : Capparaceae

Common names : H: Kodhab

Description : Unarmed, straggling shrub. Leaves simple, elliptic-oblong, cuneate, entire, apex obtuse to apiculate. Flowers greenish-white or pale yellow in one sided racemes; the upper ones corymbose. Berry cylindrical, red, irregularly torulose; seed striate, clothed by a red aril.

USEFUL PARTS AND THEIR CURATIVE PROPERTIES

Leaf : Gout, boils, laxative, indigestion, purgative, anthelmintic, antispasmodic, uterine obstructions, skin diseases

Root : Intestinal worms, chronic fever decoction

108. *Caesalpinia bonduc* (L.) Roxb.

Family : Caesalpiniaceae

Common names : S: Kuberaksi H: Karanju E: Fever nut

Description : Scandent armed shrub. Stipules foliaceous, leaflets 6-10 pairs, ovate, oblong, obtuse or acute. Racemes often panicled, flowers yellow. Pod obovoid, with wiry prickles, 1-2 seeded.

USEFUL PARTS AND THEIR CURATIVE PROPERTIES

Seed : Antifertility, abortion, malaria, snake bite, emollient, scorpion sting
Nut : Diarrhoea, bodyache
Root and stem : Antiviral
Oil : Paralysis
Leaves : Hernea, trypanosomiasis, malarial fever, hydrocele, skin infection, prevents abortion, anthelminthic, fever
Root bark : Epilepsy, eczema, emmenagogue, anthelmintic, febrifuge

109. *Calamus rotang* L.

Family : Arecaceae
Common names : S: Vetrah H: Bet E: Commom rattan
Description : A slender shrub. Leaflets trigonous, numerous, equidistant. Flowers unisexual. Fruits seated on minute perianth, subglobose, mucronate.

USEFUL PARTS AND THEIR CURATIVE PROPERTIES

Roots : Astringent, expectorant, alexeteric, antidysenteric, hypotensive, tonic, depurative, anti-inflammatory, febrifuge, hyperdypsia, bronchitis
Leaves : Astringent, laxative, leprosy, pruritis
Seeds : Expectorant, depurative, laxative

110. *Callicarpa macrophylla* Vahl

Family : Verbenaceae
Common names : S: Priyangu H: Priyamgu
Description : Erect shrub. Leaves simple, opposite, ovate. Flowers rose coloured in axillary peduncled globose cymes. Fruits white drupes.

USEFUL PARTS AND THEIR CURATIVE PROPERTIES

Flowers / fruits : Astringent, cooling, anodyne, deodorant, digestive, constipating,styptic, alexeteric, febrifuge, rheumatoid arthritis, burning sensation, fever, cephalalgia, diaphoresis, haemoptysis, poisonous bites, diabetes, vomiting
Leaves : Gout, arthralgia

111. *Calophyllum inophyllum* L.

Family : Clusiaceae
Common names : S: Punnagah H: Sultan campa E: Alexadrian laurel
Description : Medium sized tree. Leaves elliptic with emarginate apex. Flowers pure white, fragrant, racemes. Fruits globose, drupes, pulp scanty. Seeds ovoid.

USEFUL PARTS AND THEIR CURATIVE PROPERTIES

Bark : Astringent, emollient, anodyne, purgative, resolvant, wounds, strangury, pruritis, haemorrhages

Leaves : Vertigo, migraine

Seed oil : Anodyne, demulscent, gout, gonorrhoea, scabies, leprosy, strangury

112. *Calotropis gigantea* (L.) R. Br. ex Ait.

Family : Asclepiadaceae

Common names : S: Arkah H:Mudar E: Gigantic milk weed

Description : Large bushy shrub to 3 m, covered with white soft wool. Leaves elliptic to oblong, coriaceous, auriculate, apex acute, subsessile. Inflorescence umbellate,extraaxillary panicle. Corolla white or purple, lobes spreading. Follicles oblong, inflated.

USEFUL PARTS AND THEIR CURATIVE PROPERTIES

Latex : Antispasmodic, hypotensive, purgative, ear pain, skin diseases especially of ringworms, sprains, whitlow, leucoderma, toothache, conjunctivitis, epilepsy, menstrual pains, scorpion sting, leprosy, scabies, asthma, abortion, cough, rabies, snake bite, muscular swellings

Root : Spasmolytic, antiarrhythmic, stomach pain, rheumatism, arthritis, fever, abortion, constipation, inflammations, swellings, pneumonia, fertility, leprosy, cough, asthma, snake bite

Seed : Asthma with cough

Leaf and root : Anticancer and rheumatic pains, diarrhoea, paralysis, arthritis, swellings

Flowers : Hydrophobia, preventive from rabies after dog bite, mental disorders, ante-partum treatment, cough, asthma, tuberculosis, whooping cough, joint pains, insomnia, bronchitis, healing wounds, cold

Leaves : Burn injury or swelling, body pain and fractures, elephantiasis, deworming, skin diseases, migraine

Root bark : Dysentery, stomachache, snake bite, filariasis, epilepsy

113. *Calotropis procera* (Aiton) R. Br.

Family : Asclepiadaceae

Common names : S: Arka H: Safed E: Swallow wort

Description : Large bushy shrub to 3 m, leaves decussate, obovate, coriaceous, auriculate, apex acute, subsessile. Inflorescence extra axillary umbellate panicle. Corolla purple, lobes erect.

USEFUL PARTS AND THEIR CURATIVE PROPERTIES

Root bark : Snake bite and intermittent fever, diarrhoea, emetic, diaphoretic, dysentery, asthma, leprosy, scorpion sting

Latex : Scorpion sting, body pains, arthritis, conjunctivitis, irritant, purgative

Flowers : Gonorrhoea, fever, malaria, migraine, digestive, stomachic, tonic

Leaves : Antidote for snake bite, sinus fistula, rheumatism, mumps

Stem : Diarrhoea, skin diseases, ringworms

Stigmas : Cholera

114. *Calycopteris floribunda* (Roxb.) Poir.

Family	:	Combretaceae
Common names	:	S: Susavi H: Kokaray
Description	:	Scandent shrub; branches drooping, rusty brown-puberulous; leaves spiral- sub-opposite, oblong or elliptic-oblanceolate, 9-11 nerved, glabrous above, tomentose below, punctate, obtuse or cuneate, entire, apex acuminate. Panicles terminal and axillary; calyx tubular at base. Fruit ovoid-ellipsoid, 5-ribbed; seed solitary.

USEFUL PARTS AND THEIR CURATIVE PROPERTIES

Tender shoots	:	Malarial fever
Leaf paste	:	Wounds, kill intestinal worms
Root bark	:	Ulcerous wounds, boils

115. *Camellia sinensis* (L.) O. Kuntz.

Family	:	Theaceae
Common names	:	S: Syamaparni H: Cay E: Tea plant
Description	:	An evergreen shrub. Leaves simple, alternate, elliptic-ovate, glabrous. Flowers white, fragrant, solitary. Fruits depressed capsules.

USEFUL PARTS AND THEIR CURATIVE PROPERTIES

Leaves	:	Astringent, thermogenic, appetizer, digestive, carminative, diuretic, nervine tonic, haemorrhoids, inflammations, abdominal disorders, fever, strangury, fatigue, hemicrania

116. *Cananga odorata* (Lam.) Hook.

Family	:	Annonaceae
Common names	:	E: Ylang-ylang
Description	:	A medium sized tree. Leaves evergreen, alternate, entire, glabrous. Flowers aromatic, in fascicles, light yellow. Calyx 3, corolla 3, stamens many.

USEFUL PARTS AND THEIR CURATIVE PROPERTIES

Uses	:	Oil in expensive perfumery and blended particularly in 'Oriental' odours

117. *Cannabis sativa* L.

Family	:	Cannabaceae
Common names	:	S: Bhanga H: Bhang, Charas E: Indian hemp
Description	:	A large aromatic resinous herb. Leaves opposite and alternate. Flowers dioecious, perianth 5 sepalous in males, reduced in females. Stamens 5, ovary 1-celled, stigmas 2, fruit achene, seed pendulous. Embryo curved or spiral. Resin produces inhibitory action on respiratory system, musculotropic action, produces initial excitement followed by depression and increases hexobarnital sleeping time, psychotomimetic effect. Alkali insoluble fraction of the plant shows narcotic property

USEFUL PARTS AND THEIR CURATIVE PROPERTIES

Leaf	:	Inflammed eyes, piles
Plant	:	CVS and CNS active, spasmolytic, analgesic, stomach pain, malaria

118. *Canscora decussata* (Roxb.) Schult.

Family	:	Gentianaceae
Common names	:	S: Sankhini H: Samkhaphuli E: Canscora
Description	:	Erect annual herb. Leaves simple, ovate or lanceolate. Flowers white, dichasial cymes. Fruits cylindrical, septicidal capsule. Seeds small, brown, reticulate.

USEFUL PARTS AND THEIR CURATIVE PROPERTIES

Whole plant	:	Astringent, thermogenic, laxative, vulnerary, alexeteric, antihelmintic, appetizer, aphrodisiac, depuerative, rejuvenating, tonic, insanity, epilepsy, nervous debility, leucoderma, tuberculosis, ulcers

119. *Canthium parviflorum* Lam.

Family	:	Rubiaceae
Common names	:	S: Gangeruki H: Kirma E: Carray cheddie
Description	:	Armed shrub; spines supra-axillary. Leaves elliptic-ovate, glabrous; stipules linear. Flowers in axillary cymes, greenish white. Drupe globose.

USEFUL PARTS AND THEIR CURATIVE PROPERTIES

Unriped fruits	:	Dysentery
Stem bark	:	Poisonous bites decoction
Leaf	:	Fever
Root bark	:	Dysentery in infants

120. *Capparis grandis* L. f.

Family	:	Capparaceae
Common names	:	S: Puchaonda H: Karil E: Caper plant
Description	:	Trees or shrubs. Leaves simple, usually velvety on both sides. Flowers in umbels or corymbs. Fruit globose. Seeds numerous.

USEFUL PARTS AND THEIR CURATIVE PROPERTIES

Aerial part	:	Spasmolytic, anticancer, diuretic
Stem bark	:	Wounds, ulcers
Leaves	:	Skin diseases, insect bite
Root	:	Diarrhoea, dysentery

121. *Capparis sepiaria* L.

Family	:	Capparaceae
Common names	:	S: Kakadani H: Kanthari E: Indian caper
Description	:	Thorny erect or climbing shrub. Leaves oblong-elliptic or obovate, obtuse, emarginate, stipules spinous. Flowers white or rose in dense umbels. Fruit globose, smooth, black when dry.

USEFUL PARTS AND THEIR CURATIVE PROPERTIES

Root : Earache, fever, gout

122. *Capparis spinosa* L.

Family : Capparaceae

Common names : E: Capers

Description : Evergreen shrub which is thorny. Leaves ovate, entire, lanceolate, apex acute, glabrous. Flowers in corymbs. Fruit globose.

USEFUL PARTS AND THEIR CURATIVE PROPERTIES

Uses : Flavouring agents, cosmetics, perfumes

123. *Capparis zeylanica* L.

Family : Capparaceae

Common names : S: Ahimsra H: Ardanda E; Caper plant

Description : Large climbing shrub with hooked spines; stems woody, rough, brown tomentose. Leaves ovate or elliptic-oblong, rusty tomentose when young, glabrous at maturity, cuneate, entire, apex mucronate. Flowers white, turning pink. Berries ripe red, globose.

USEFUL PARTS AND THEIR CURATIVE PROPERTIES

Root : Fever, mouth ulcers, rib muscle pain

Leaf : Piles, syphilis

Whole plant : Arthritis, knee swellings, piles, rheumatism

Root bark : Earache and pus formation, aphrodisiac, tuberculosis, paralysis

124. *Cardiospermum halicacabum* L.

Family : Sapindaceae

Common names : S: Parvatagni H: Kanphuti E: Blister creeper

Description : Climbing herb. Branches slender, leaves biternate, leaflets ovate, pubescent, acuminate, narrow. Flowers white, in a few flowered umbellate cymes, peduncles bearing 2 tendrils arranged oppositely. Capsules trigonous shortly stalked, 3-valved.Seeds smooth, black.

USEFUL PARTS AND THEIR CURATIVE PROPERTIES

Root : Arthritis, leucorrhoea, menstrual disorders, diarrhoea

Leaves : Swellings, burns, tumours, earache, vomiting, giddiness

Whole plant : Rheumatism, earache, gonorrhoea, swellings

125. *Careya arborea* Roxb.

Family : Barringtoniaceae

Common names : S: Kumbhi H: Kamba E: Patana oak

Description : Deciduous tree; leaves obovate, slightly acuminate, base cuneate. Inflorescence in a short spike. Flowers sessile, yellowish-white. Berry green.

USEFUL PARTS AND THEIR CURATIVE PROPERTIES

Stem bark	:	Cold, cough and fever, oedema, swellings, diarrhoea, chest pain, ulcers, blood dysentery, skin diseases, stomachache
Root	:	Snake bite
Flower	:	Tonic after child birth
Leaf	:	Diarrhoea, fever

126. *Carica papaya* L.

Family	:	Caricaceae
Common names	:	S: Brahmairandah H: Pappita E: Papaya
Description	:	Soft wooded tree with palmately lobed leaves. Flowers greenish white, solitary or in cymes, sepals and petals in alternating whorls, fruit 1-celled.

USEFUL PARTS AND THEIR CURATIVE PROPERTIES

Latex	:	Amoebic dysentery, piles, fistula, skin diseases, ringworm
Fruits	:	Constipation, diabetes, abortion, nutritive, helmithiasis, bronchitis, lactation
Seeds	:	Sterility, vermifuge
Root bark	:	Galactagogue, conception, piles
Stem bark	:	Dental caries
Leaf	:	Inflammations, jaundice

127. *Carissa spinarum* L.

Family	:	Apocynaceae
Common names	:	S: Karamadika H: Karaunda E: Karanda
Description	:	Bushy evergreen shrub with rigid, spreading branches; bark grey-white. Leaves broad, ovate-elliptic or suborbicular. Flowers white, sometimes tinged with pink, scented, in axillary and terminal corymbose cymes. Berries dark purple when mature.

USEFUL PARTS AND THEIR CURATIVE PROPERTIES

Root	:	Insect bite, maggot infested sores, acute pain, fever, wounds, jaundice
Seed	:	Toothache
Flowers	:	Opacity of the cornea
Fruits	:	Cough
Leaves	:	Intermittent fevers

128. *Carthamus tinctorius* L.

Family	:	Asteraceae
Common names	:	S: Kusumbah H: Kusum E: Safflower
Description	:	Erect annual herb. Leaves oblong, sessile, spinosely serrate. Flowers yellowish or orange red in large terminal heads. Fruits obovoid, achenes.

USEFUL PARTS AND THEIR CURATIVE PROPERTIES

Leaves	:	Laxative, appetizer, diuretic, ophthalmopathy

Flowers : Liver tonic, laxative, sedative, emmenagogue, expectorant, strangury, leprosy, boils, ring worm, leucoderma, bronchitis,.

Seeds : Purgative, carminative, aphrodisiac, arthritis, constipation, foul ulcers

129. *Carum copticum* L.

Family : Apiaceae

Common names : E: Caraway

Description : Annual or biennial herb. Stem aerial, erect, green and aromatic. Leaves pinnate or decompound, aromatic. Inflorescence compound umbel. Involucre of bracts, petals 5, stamens 5, ovary inferior, fruit cremocarp.

USEFUL PARTS AND THEIR CURATIVE PROPERTIES

Whole plant : Aromatic stimulant, stomachic, flatulence, tonic, indigestion, diarrhoea, cholera, dyspepsia, dipsomania

Uses : Seeds - culinary purposes, flavouring bread, biscuits, cakes, cheeses, apple sauces, cookies

: Seed oil -flavouring meat, canned food, perfumes, mouth preparations, soaps

130. *Caryota urens* L.

Family : Arecaceae

Common names : S: Madyadruma H: Ban-Khajur E: Fish tail palm

Description : Tree, stem annulate, shining. Leaves subopposite, curved, leaflets clustered or spiral, base cuneate, oblique, irregularly serrate. Flowers many, monoecious, solitary or in threes. Fruit globose, seeds 1 or 2.

USEFUL PARTS AND THEIR CURATIVE PROPERTIES

Plant toddy : Indigestion, general debility, urinary disorders, aphrodisiac

Seed : Dandruff

131. *Cascabela thevetia* (L.) Lippold

Family : Apocynaceae

Common names : H: Pilakger E: Yellow oleander

Description : Evergreen, leafy shrub. Leaves spiral, linear-lanceolate, sub coriaceous, cuneate, recurved, apex acute, lateral nerves 15-20 pairs. Inflorescence a terminal cyme. Corolla yellow. Drupe broadly turbinate, compressed laterally.

USEFUL PARTS AND THEIR CURATIVE PROPERTIES

Latex : Maggot infested sores, rib muscle pain,sprains

Flowers : Asthma

Fruit : Venereal disease

Stem bark : Fever

132. *Casearia elliptica* Willd.

Family : Flacourtiaceae

Common names : S: Kampillika H: Chilla

Description : Bushy shrub or small tree; branchlets warty, densely downy pubescent. Leaves spiral, oblong-lanceolate to elliptic, coriaceous, pubescent, cuneate or oblique, serrulate to entire, acute to obtuse, petiole reddish. Flowers in dense axillary clusters. Capsule globose, ribbed, 3-valved.

USEFUL PARTS AND THEIR CURATIVE PROPERTIES

Tender shoots : Whitlow
Fruits /stem bark : Chest pain
Root bark : Enlarged scrotum in children, dysentery
Stem bark : Chest pain, rib muscle pain, stomach pain, wounds, ulcers
Leaf : Skin diseases

133. *Cassia absus* L.

Family : Caesalpiniaceae
Common names : S: Kulatthika H: Chaksu
Description : Erect herb with viscid glandular hairs. Rachis with a gland between the lowest pairs of leaflets. Leaflets elliptic- obovate, oblique, subacute, mucronate, glabrous above, pubescent beneath. Raceme short, terminal or axillary. Petals reddish - yellow. Pod oblique, covered with stiff glandular hairs, 5-7 seeded; seeds black, ovoid.

USEFUL PARTS AND THEIR CURATIVE PROPERTIES

Seed paste : Constipation, skin diseases
Leaves : Bone fractures

134. *Cassia angustifolia* Vahl.

Family : Caesalpiniaceae
Common names : E: Senna
Description : Erect shrub, leaves pinnate with narrow acute lanceolate and glabrous leaflets. Flowers yellow, racemose inflorescence. Pods flat, thin, 5-7 dark brown seeds.

USEFUL PARTS AND THEIR CURATIVE PROPERTIES

Leaves : Purgative in habitual constipation, skin diseases, pinworms, laxative

135. *Cassia auriculata* L.

Family : Caesalpiniaceae
Common names : S: Avarttaki H: Tarval E: The Tanner's Cassia
Description : Shrub to 2 m, branchlets finely pubescent. Leaves long, leaflets 8-12 pairs, elliptic-oblong, obtuse and minutely apiculate, glands between leaflets, subulate. Corymbs axillary and terminal, often panicled. Petals yellow, veined. Pod flat, dehiscent, obtuse.

USEFUL PARTS AND THEIR CURATIVE PROPERTIES

Aerial part / root : Antiviral, spasmolytic and antidiabetic
Flower paste : Aphrodisiac, diabetes, conjunctivitis, stops excessive menstrual flow, hyper diuresis

Shoot paste : Diabetes
Anthers : Dysentery
Seed : Inflammations, diarrhoea, fertility, fever, migraine, night blindness, scorpion sting, ulcers and fissures in mouth, asthma
Root bark : Leucorrhoea, controls frequent urination
Stem bark : Stomachache
Stem : Earache
Root : Nephroprotector, rheumatism, menorrhoea
Leaves : Giddiness, skin diseases, ophthalmic diseases, fractures, diabetes, burns, sun stroke, scorpion sting

136. *Cassia fistula* L.

Family : Caesalpiniaceae
Common names : S: Aragvadha H:Amaltas E: Indian laburnum
Description : Moderate-sized tree upto 8 m, branches glabrous, bark deep fissured. Leaves opposite, oblong, broadly ovate, coriaceous, pubescent below, entire, apex gradually tapering, emarginate. Flowers bright to golden-yellow. Podscylindric, indehiscent, dark blackish-brown. Seeds orbicular, flattened.

USEFUL PARTS AND THEIR CURATIVE PROPERTIES

Pod : Antiviral, hypoglycaemic, anticancer, rheumatism,
Stem bark : leucoderma, leprosy, skin diseases, high fever, pneumonia, filariasis, chest pain, malaria, burns, backache
Fruit pulp : Constipation, intestinal worms in children, asthma, diabetes, whooping cough, jaundice, tongue sore, inflammation
Root paste : Inflammation, antinarcotic, breast diseases, constipation, asthma.
Root bark and leaves : Laxative, liver complaints, spleen enlargement, black fever
Young leaves : Amenorrhoea, scorpion sting, constipation, ringworm, diabetes, blood motions, skin infections, pains, mad dog bite
Seeds : Eye diseases, gout, rheumatism, thirst, jaundice

137. *Cassia italica* (Miller) Lam. ex Andrews

Family : Caesalpiniaceae
Common names : S: Bhumyahuli
Description : Herb, leaves eglandular; leaflets 4-6 pairs, obovate-oblong, obtuse, mucronate at apex. Flowers pale yellow in axillary racemes. Pod flat, falcate, papery, seeds 8-12.

USEFUL PARTS AND THEIR CURATIVE PROPERTIES

Leaves : Constipation, gout

138. *Cassia occidentalis* L.

Family : Caesalpiniaceae

Common names : S: Kasamandah H: Kasondi E: Negro coffee

Description : Undershrub. Branchlets glabrous, petiole glandular. Leaves elliptic-ovate, acuminate, rounded or cuneate. Raceme 2-6 flowered. Pod linear, turgid but compressed, brown with yellow.

USEFUL PARTS AND THEIR CURATIVE PROPERTIES

Root : Diuretic, rotten teeth, scorpion sting, stomach ache, purification of milk in nursing women, whooping cough, filariasis, anthelmintic, paralysis, chest pain, body swellings, antiemetic, jaundice, boils, burns, eye infection, snake bite

Seed, root / leaf : Antibacterial and antidiabetic, cough,urinary troubles, skin diseases, cold, constipation, itch, scabies, headache

Whole plant : Laxative

Leaf paste : Swelling due to clotting, diabetes, diarrhoea, hepatic stimulant, boils and wounds, leucoderma, cough, asthma, jaundice, paralysis, fever, mental disorders, eczema

139. *Cassia tora* L.

Family : Caesalpiniaceae

Common names : S: Chakramardah H: Chakunda E: Foetid cassia

Description : Annual herb or undershrub. Leaves with subulate glands between the leaflets 3-5 pairs, obovate-oblong, obtuse, apiculate at apex. Flowers in axillary pairs. Pod apiculate, subtetragonal.

USEFUL PARTS AND THEIR CURATIVE PROPERTIES

Plant : Antiviral, spasmolytic.

Seeds : Diabetes, cough, headache and fever, malarial fever

Leaf juice : Earache, waist pain, measles, eye diseases

Stem and seeds : Antiasthmatic

140. *Cassytha filiformis* L.

Family : Lauraceae

Common names : S: Akasvalli H: Amarbeli E: Sita's Yarn

Description : Leafless twiner; spikes terminal or axillary; flowers subsessile, tepals yellowish. Drupe globose, enclosed within inflated perianth. Seed 1, globose.

USEFUL PARTS AND THEIR CURATIVE PROPERTIES

Whole plant : Ephemeral fever, hair tonic, chronic ulcers, red eyes, hydrocele, syphilis

Stem paste : Sprains, rheumatism, relieves heat

141. *Catharanthus roseus* (L.) G. Don.

Family : Apocynaceae

Common names : S: Nityakalyani H: Sadabahar E: Madagascar periwinkle
Description : Undershrub to 1 m, leaves elliptic-obovate to oblong. Flowers white and pink in axillary pairs, corolla white or pink. Follicles long.

USEFUL PARTS AND THEIR CURATIVE PROPERTIES

Catharanthine : Diuretic activity
Ajmalicine : Antidiuretic and antihypertensive Alkaloids mostly act as CNS depressants
Vinvalencobler-tine vincristine : Antitumour agents.
Leaf juice : Conjunctivitis and menorrhagia, haemorrhage, diarrhoea, diabetes, allergy, red bleeding, blood cancer, malaria, insect bites, skin diseases, abortion, wounds
Root : Diabetes
Whole plant : Diabetes, blood cancer, insect sting
Latex : Leucoderma

142. *Catunaregam spinosa* (Thunb.) Tirv.

Family : Rubiaceae
Common names : S: Madana H: Mainphal E: Common emetic nut
Description : Thorny shrub. Leaves elliptic or obovate, attenuate, entire, apex obtuse, densely pubescent below. Flowers in axillary corymbs, greenish. Berry globose or oblong-ellipsoid, hairy.

USEFUL PARTS AND THEIR CURATIVE PROPERTIES

Stem bark paste : Cuts by iron tools, wounds, abortion, fever
Leaf paste : Dandruff
Fruit paste : Swellings, anasarca, fever, hysteria, cataract, dandruff, diarrhoea, dysentery
Roots : Ulcers in intestine and stomach, post delivery pains

143. *Cayratia carnosa* (Wall. ex Wight) Gagnep.

Family : Vitaceae
Common names : S: Gandirah H: Amalbel E: Fox-grape
Description : Fleshy climbing shrub. Leaves trifoliate, pubescent. Flowers in branched long peduncled cymes. Fruits fleshy berries. Seeds pyriform, rounded.

USEFUL PARTS AND THEIR CURATIVE PROPERTIES

Whole plant : Astringent, diuretic, tumours, fever, neuralgia, splenopathy, blood purification, hepatopathy, cardiac disorders, ulcers, wounds, dropsy, haemorrhoids, strangury

144. *Celastrus paniculatus* Willd.

Family : Celastraceae
Common names : S: Pitataila H: Jamrasi E: Climbing staff plant

Description : Climbing deciduous shrub; leaves spiral, crenulate or serrate. Flowers in terminal pendent panicle. Fruit yellow, seeds brown, enclosed in a scarlet aril.

USEFUL PARTS AND THEIR CURATIVE PROPERTIES

Aerial part : Antiviral
Leaf : Fever
Seed oil : Hypotensive, spasmolytic, healing wounds, beri-beri, intestinal ulcers, allergy, pneumonia, bodyache, tuberculosis, eczema, hair tonic, brain tonic, stimulant, skin diseases, paralysis, cough, rheumatism, mental disorders
Seed powder : Increases memory power, cough, cold, fever, psoriasis
Stem bark : Snake bite, termination of foetus
Root : Piles and urinary inflammation, spermatorr-hoea, leucorrhoea, amenorrhoea, pneumonia, cancerous tumour, paralysis, ulcers, helminthic infection, eye diseases, diarrhoea, kidney troubles

145. *Celosia argentea* L.

Family : Amaranthaceae
Common names : S: Pothura H: Safed murgha E: Cox comb plant
Description : Erect herb to 1.5 m. Leaves elliptic, ovate below and linear lanceolate above, base cuneate to attenuate, entire, acute, glabrous. Inflorescence axillary and terminal; dense, stout imbricate spikes; flowers white.

USEFUL PARTS AND THEIR CURATIVE PROPERTIES

Seed paste : Aphrodisiac, diarrhoea
Leaf paste : Wasp and scorpion stings
Tender shoots : Galactagogue
Leaf juice : Eye diseases
Whole plant : Blood dysentery, uterine bleeding, haemorrhoids

146. *Centella asiatica* (L.) Urban

Family : Apiaceae
Common names : S: Mandukaparni H: Brahmi E: Indian pennywort
Description : Creeping herb; rooting at nodes. Leaves orbicular-reniform, pubiscent, base cordate, crenate; petioles pink, sheathing at base. Flowers pink or red in axillary fasciculate umbels; central flowers sessile, laterals pedicellate, bracteate. Fruits indehiscent, broadly ovoid, laterally compressed, ridged.

USEFUL PARTS AND THEIR CURATIVE PROPERTIES

Whole plant : Antiprotozoal, spasmolytic, dysentery, boils and tumours, cough, fertility, brain tonic, mouth ulcers, jaundice, leprosy, skin diseases, diarrhoea, liver, spleen, gastric problems, blood purifier, diuretic, nervousness, hair tonic, enhances memory power, syphilis, herpes, heart diseases

Root decoction : Throat clearance

Leaves : Clear voice, increasing memory power, stammering, leprosy, mental disorder, nervous and blood diseases, dysentery, anaemia, hyperacidity, appetite, constipation, jaundice, excessive vomiting, reduce body heat, eczema, scabies, wounds, skin diseases, diabetes, weakness

147. *Cephaelis ipecacuanha* A. Rich.

Family : Rubiaceae

Common names : E: Ipecac

Description : A small trailing herb. Roots slender, moniliform, in bunches. Leaves in opposite pairs, tips pointed. Flowers white, small, in bunches.

USEFUL PARTS AND THEIR CURATIVE PROPERTIES

Root : Emetic, antidysenteric, used in piles and gonorrhoea. It is also used in cold, cough and asthma. In small doses (1/4 g) it is a gastric stimulant. It is also diaphoretic and combined with opium (Dover's powder) used as sedative; expectorant in colds, sore throat and mild rheumatic attacks. It is also used as a direct chologogue

148. *Certaria islandica* (L.) Ach.

Family : Parmeliaceae

Common names : E: Iceland Moss (lichen)

USEFUL PARTS AND THEIR CURATIVE PROPERTIES

Root : Minimizes thrusting

Uses : Internally in the form of an infusion or in herbal teas in the treatment of catarrh of the upper respiratory passages and as a supplementary medicine in lung diseases

149. *Chamaesyce hirta* L.

Family : Euphorbiaceae

Common names : S: Dugdhika H: Lal dudhi

Description : Erect or decumbent herb to 50 cm. Leaves ovate, oblique at base, serrulate- serrate, subacute-acute. Flowers greenish, in axillary-cymose cyathia. Capsule pubescent, seeds angled, shallowly furrowed.

USEFUL PARTS AND THEIR CURATIVE PROPERTIES

Leaves : Constipation, excess of heat, stomach pain

Whole plant : Boils, blisters

150. *Chamaesyce thymifolia* (L.) Millsp.

Family : Euphorbiaceae

Common names : S: Dugdhika

Description : Softly hispid, prostrate herb. Leaves opposite, stipulate, serrulate, apex obtuse, subsessile. Cyathia in axillary clusters. Capsules appressed hairy; seed 4 angular, minutely tuberculate.

USEFUL PARTS AND THEIR CURATIVE PROPERTIES

Whole plant paste : Fever, painful menstruations

151. *Chlorophytum tuberosum* (Roxb.) Baker

Family : Liliaceae

Common names : S: Musili H: Safed musili

Description : Herb, roots tuberous. Leaves flat, coriaceous, narrow, undulate, apex gradually tapering, acuminate. Scape solitary. Pedicels cluster, jointed at or middle. Flowers white, anthers yellow. Capsule oblong, glabrous. Seeds irregularly pitted.

USEFUL PARTS AND THEIR CURATIVE PROPERTIES

Tuber : Increase potency, minimizes excess of heat

152. *Chloroxylon swietenia* DC.

Family : Flindersiaceae

Common names : S: Bhillotaka E: Satin wood

Description : Tree to 10 m; bark rough, corky. Leaves pinnate; leaflets numerous, oblong-lanceolate, gland dotted, oblique, entire, apex obtuse. Flowers white in terminal or axillary panicles. Capsule glabrous, oblong, dark brown, loculicidally 3-valved; seeds compressed, 5 angular, winged above.

USEFUL PARTS AND THEIR CURATIVE PROPERTIES

Stem bark / leaf : Spasmolytic, headache, chest pain, inflammation antiseptic, general tonic, labour pain, boils, blisters, astringent, cuts

Gum : Antidiabetic, urinary disorders

Stem bark : Asthma in children, eye injuries, rheumatic pains, snake bite and other poisonous bites, yoke gall, epilepsy, fever, jaundice, scorpion sting

Root bark : Impotency

153. *Chonemorpha fragrans* (Moon) Alston

Family : Apocynaceae

Common names : S: Murva H: Garbhedaro

Description : A stout laticiferous shrub. Leaves simple, opposite, large, orbicular. Flowers large, whitish, fragrant, in terminal cymose panicles. Fruits long, straight, follicular mericarps. Seeds many, flat, with silky white coma.

USEFUL PARTS AND THEIR CURATIVE PROPERTIES

Roots : Astringent, laxative, thermogenic, depurative, carminative, anthelmintic, digestive, sudorific, anodyne, expectorant, febrifuge, leprosy, colic, constipation, dyspepsia, flatulence, hyperacidity, cough, bronchitis, intermittent fevers, cardiac debility, diabetes, jaundice, hyperdypsia

154. *Cichorium intybus* L.

Family : Asteraceae

Common names : S: Kasani H: Kasni E: Chicory

Description : Erect perennial milky herb. Leaves radical, small, alternate, entire. Flowers bright blue in ligulate heads. Fruits smooth angled achenes.

USEFUL PARTS AND THEIR CURATIVE PROPERTIES

Whole plant : Thermogenic, anti-inflammatory, appetizer, digestive, stomachic, liver tonic, cardiotonic, depurative, diuretic, febrifuge, flatulence, gout, colic, insomnia, jaundice, leprosy, splenomegaly, vomiting, diarrhoea, lumbago, asthma, general debility, strangury

155. *Cinchona calisaya* Wedd.

Family : Rubiaceae

Common names : E: Cinchona

Description : Evergreen perennial tree. Stem branched and woody. Leaves simple, obovate or elliptic. Flowers panicle or dichasial cyme, purple. Fruit ovoid, capsule.

USEFUL PARTS AND THEIR CURATIVE PROPERTIES

Bark : Whooping cough, hay-fever, enlargement of spleen; hemicrania and other neuralgic infections, small pox, septic fevers, pneumonia, acute rheumatism, acute tonsillitis, acute nasal catarrh, pyaemia, abscesses, cavities, ulcers, sore throat, intermittent fevers, tonic in small doses 1 to 3 grains in dyspepsia, gastric catarrh, adynamia, malaria. Indiscriminate use of quinine for a long time weakens the heart.

156. *Cinnamomum camphora* Nees & Eberm.

Family : Lauraceae

Common names : S: Karpura E: Camphor cinnamon

Description : Profusely branched evergreen tree. Leaves simple, alternate, shiny, aromatic, ovate or oblong, flowers yellowish white, in axillary panicles. Fruits ovoid or globose, dark green.

USEFUL PARTS AND THEIR CURATIVE PROPERTIES

Plant : Sedative, anodyne, antispasmodic, diaphoretic, anthelmintic, diarrhoeas, colds, crills, inflammations, bruises, sprains

Leaves : Inflammation

Stem bark : Anthelmintic

Oil : Chemical industry, photographic films, smokeless gum powder, incense sticks

157. *Cinnamomum cassia* (Nees) Nees ex. Blume

Family : Lauraceae

Common names : E: Cassia

USEFUL PARTS AND THEIR CURATIVE PROPERTIES

Uses : Perfumes, cosmetics, dentifrice

158. *Cinnamomum zeylanicum* Wees

Family : Lauraceae

Common names : S: Darushila H: Dalchini E: Cinnamon

Description : A moderate - sized tree. Leaves 3-5 ribbed, shining above. Panicles long. Flowers many, perianth 6 lobes. Stamens 9, ovary sessile. Fruit berry.

USEFUL PARTS AND THEIR CURATIVE PROPERTIES

Uses : Medicine, dentrifices, perfumes, manufacture of cinnamon quills

159. *Cissampelos pareira* L.

Family : Menispermaceae

Common names : S: Patha H: Akanadi E: Velvet-leaf

Description : Climbing, undershrub; leaves peltate, more or less cordate or triangular, softly pubescent on both sides. Flowers small, unisexual, greenish-white. Drupes pubescent, scarlet.

USEFUL PARTS AND THEIR CURATIVE PROPERTIES

Stem and root : CNS depressant; hayatin methioide – power muscle relaxant, antidiabetic, labour pains

Root : Bleeding piles, constipation in children, diarrhoea, indigestion, pains in stomach, snake bite, jaundice, malaria, fever, leprosy, piles, chest pain, deworming, rheumatism, typhoid, urinary troubles, dyspepsia, bowel complaints, menstruation, abortion

Leaf paste : Scabies, peptic ulcers, snake bite, diphtheria, jaundice, toothache, itches, intestinal worms

Tuber : Chest pain, stomach pain

Plant paste : Blisters, fever, urinary diseases, kidney stones, antidote to poison, heart diseases, jaundice, stomach pains

160. *Cissus quadrangularis* L.

Family : Vitaceae

Common names : S: Vajravalli H: Hadjora E: The edible stemmed vine

Description : Climbing, glabrous plant with fibrous roots. Stem 4-angled. Leaves simple, ovate or reniform, thick and fleshy, tendril leaf opposed, highly coiled. Flowers white; fruit globose, reddish brown, 1-seeded.

USEFUL PARTS AND THEIR CURATIVE PROPERTIES

Aerial part : Analgesic; Coloside A possesses smooth muscle relaxant and cardiovascular effect, CVS active, fractures, asthma

Stem : Oxytocic, diuretic, bone fracture, fever, mad dog bite, expel tape worms, headache, fractured bones, asthma, anorexia, insect bite, appetite, burns, wounds, cough, dyspepsia

161. *Citrullus colocynthis* (L.) Schrad

Family	:	Cucurbitaceae
Common names	:	S: Indra varuni H: Indrayan E: Bitter cucumber
Description	:	Perennial trailing herb; branchlets hairy, tendrils 2-3 fid. Leaves variable, deeply lobed. Flowers solitary yellow in colour. Calyx tube broadly campanulate, petals 5, stamens 3, fruit globose, indehiscent, seeds much compressed, pale green.

USEFUL PARTS AND THEIR CURATIVE PROPERTIES

Fruit	:	Expels worms in stomach, dropsy, jaundice, diabetes
Root	:	Termination of foetus, enlargement of abdomen, ante-partum treatment,intermittent fever
Seed oil	:	Premature greying of hair
Whole plant	:	Leprosy and eczema

162. *Citrus aurantium* L.

Family	:	Rutaceae
Common names	:	S: Nimbuphala H: Khatta E: Seville Orange
Description	:	Small tree, leaves alternate, petioles often winged, flowers white, in axillary fascicled cymes. Hesperidium globose, yellow.

USEFUL PARTS AND THEIR CURATIVE PROPERTIES

Aerial part	:	CNS active, diuretic
Rind	:	Chronic bronchitis, nausea, fainting
Leaves	:	Arthritis
Stem bark	:	Tuberculosis
Fruit	:	Whitlow
Oil	:	Extender, ingredient in synthetic perfumes

163. *Citrus bergamia* Risso.

Family	:	Rutaceae
Common names	:	E: Basil
Description	:	A medium sized tree. Leaves compound, alternate, entire. Petiole winged. Flowers white, racemes. Fruit hesperidium, seeds many.

USEFUL PARTS AND THEIR CURATIVE PROPERTIES

Uses	:	Greenish oil from the rind or fruits – scenting toilet soaps

164. *Citrus limon* (L.) Burm. f.

Family	:	Rutaceae
Common names	:	S: Jambirah H: Jamiri nimbu E: lemon
Description	:	Much branched thorny shrub. Leaves unifoliately compound. Flowers white in short racemes. Fruits large, globose, berries. Seeds many, testa coriaceous.

USEFUL PARTS AND THEIR CURATIVE PROPERTIES

Fruit : Thermogenic, digestive, carminative, stomachic, laxative, anthelmintic, stimulant, dyspepsia, flatulence, colic, constipation, anorexia, scabies, fatigue, hemicrania, cough, bronchitis, heartburn

165. *Citrus paradisii* Macf.

Family : Rutaceae

Common names : E: Grape fruit

Description : Evergreen tree. Leaves alternate, petiole winged. Flowers white, fragrant. Fruit hesperidium. Seeds many.

USEFUL PARTS AND THEIR CURATIVE PROPERTIES

Uses : Perfumes, cosmetics

166. *Citrus reticulata* Blanco

Family : Rutaceae

Common names : S: Narangah H: Santara E: Loose-skinned orange

Description : Evergreen moderate sized tree. Leaves unifoliate, petioles short, wingless. Flowers white, fragrant. Fruits globose or subglobose. Seeds many, white.

USEFUL PARTS AND THEIR CURATIVE PROPERTIES

Flowers : Stimulant, diuretic, anodyne, sedative, febrifuge, tonic, catarrh, strangury, haemorrhoids, fever, general debility

167. *Citrus sinensis* (L.) Osbeck

Family : Rutaceae

Common names : E: Orange

Description : Evergreen moderate tree. Leaves unifoliate, petioles winged. Flowers white, fragrant, white. Fruits hesperidium. Seeds numerous.

USEFUL PARTS AND THEIR CURATIVE PROPERTIES

Uses : Perfumes, cosmetics, flavouring soaps

168. *Claviceps purpurea* (Fr.) Tul.

Family : Hypocreaceae

Common names : E: Ergot

USEFUL PARTS AND THEIR CURATIVE PROPERTIES

Ergot alkaloids : Ergot alkaloids affect smooth muscles and some have action on nervous system They are used in obstetrics and gynaecology to check uterine haemorrhage during birth, block pain and eradicate inflammations of nervous origin; and in recent years used in psychiatry

169. *Cleistanthus collinus* (Roxb.) Benth. ex Hook.f.

Family : Euphorbiaceae

Common names : S: Indrayava H: Garrar E: Rafter wood

Description : Small tree to 8 m; branchlets terete, glabrous. Bark black, rough with numerous cracks; wood scarlet. Leaves elliptic-ovate, glabrous, lip often retuse at apex; flowers pale green in axillary clusters; capsule depressed, globose. Seeds globose, smooth.

USEFUL PARTS AND THEIR CURATIVE PROPERTIES

Stem bark : Wounds, sores
Root bark : Ring worm

170. *Cleome gynandra* L.

Family : Cleomaceae
Common names : S: Ajagandha H: Karalia
Description : Erect, glandular, pubescent showy herb. Leaves 3-5 foliate, flowers white, purple or violet, borne in corymbose racemes. Capsule terete, striate, glandular; seeds many, concentrically ridged and transversely crested.

USEFUL PARTS AND THEIR CURATIVE PROPERTIES

Leaf : Acute stomach pain, boils, ulcers, insect bites, migraine, headache, anthelmintic, earache, high blood pressure, wounds, muscular pains
Root decoction : Fever
Whole plant : Peptic ulcer, easy delivery

171. *Cleome monophylla* L.

Family : Cleomaceae
Description : Erect herb; branchlets glandular pubescent; leaves simple, oblong or lanceolate, truncate, ciliate, apex acute; flowers pink; capsule strongly ribbed, ribs glandular, beak flat, seeds ridged.

USEFUL PARTS AND THEIR CURATIVE PROPERTIES

Leaf : Insect bite, breast ulcers

172. *Cleome viscosa* L.

Family : Cleomaceae
Common names : S: Adityabhakta H: Hulhul E: Sticky cleome Viscid herb.
Description : Leaves softly pubescent. Flowers yellow and white. Capsule terete, ribs oblique, glandular hairy, dehiscing from above; seeds glabrous, transverse ridges prominent, concentric ones faint.

USEFUL PARTS AND THEIR CURATIVE PROPERTIES

Leaf : Body pains, earache, fever, wounds, boils, dental caries, cuts, deafness, headache
Seed : Lice killer, maggot infested sores
Fruit juice : Intermittent fever
Root : Earache

173. *Clerodendrum phlomides* L. f.

Family : Verbenaceae
Common names : S: Agni mantha H: Urni E: Wind killer

Description : Foetid shrub. Leaves deltoid-ovate, glabrescent to thinly pubescent, truncate to acute, entire to serrate, apex acute. Panicles axillary and terminal. Corolla cream. Drupe obovoid.

USEFUL PARTS AND THEIR CURATIVE PROPERTIES

Root powder : Body swellings, gonorrhoea
Leaf : chest pain, gonorrhoea, scabies, syphilis, ophthalmic diseases
Whole plant : Joint pains

174. *Clerodendrum serratum* (L.) Mo.

Family : Verbenaceae
Common names : S: Bharangi H:Barangi E: Beetle killer
Description : Perennial shrub. Stem 4-angular. Leaves sessile. Flowering branches form a sub-pyramid. Corolla blue. Drupe 4-lobed.

USEFUL PARTS AND THEIR CURATIVE PROPERTIES

Aerial part : Spermicidal, CNS active and antidiabetic, irregular menstruation
Leaf : Asthma, leprosy, scorpion sting, backache, inflammation
Root decoction : Bronchitis and malaria, stomachache, common fever, analgesic, asthma, cholera, paralysis, menstrual disorders

175. *Clerodendrum viscosum* Vent.

Family : Verbenaceae
Common names : S: Bhandirah H: Titabhant
Description : Gregarious undershrub, leaves ovate, acuminate at base, flowers white, long, terminal, panicles. Drupes bluish-black.

USEFUL PARTS AND THEIR CURATIVE PROPERTIES

Leaf : Cholagogue, anthelmintic, catarrhal colds
Root paste : Blood dysentery, chest pain, menstrual problems, anthelmintic, asthma
Root bark : Ear infections

176. *Clitoria ternatea* L.

Family : Papilionanceae
Common names : S: Aparajita H: Aparjit E: Clitoria
Description : Perennial climbing herb. Leaves imparipinnate; leaflets 2-3 pairs, opposite, ovate, base and apex obtuse, entire. Flower axillary, deep blue or white. Pod linear-oblong, apically beaked. Seeds reniform.

USEFUL PARTS AND THEIR CURATIVE PROPERTIES

Seed powder : Memory power, vermifuge, syphilis, constipation
Flower juice : Diabetes
Root paste : Insect bite, gonorrhoea, swollen joints, bronchitis
Root bark : Diuretic, laxative, swollen joints

177. *Coccinia grandis* (L.) Voigt

Family : Cucurbitaceae
Common names : S: Bimbi H: Kanduri E: Ivy gourd

Description	:	Large climber from a woody base. Leaves 5-angled to entire, glabrous, denticulate, apex obtuse, mucronate, tendril simple. Flowers solitary, corolla white; fruit oblong, blood red when ripe; seeds ovoid, compressed.

USEFUL PARTS AND THEIR CURATIVE PROPERTIES

Root	:	Antiprotozoal, hypoglycaemic, diabetes, fertility, bodyaches, rheumatism, headache
Fruit	:	Mouth ulcers, diabetes, diarrhoea
Leaf paste	:	Wounds, eye sores, diabetes, conjunctivitis, galactagogue, jaundice, diarrhoea, stomach worms
Whole plant juice	:	Checks bleeding

178. *Cocculus hirsutus* (L.) Diels

Family	:	Menispermaceae
Common names	:	S: Vanatiktika H: Jamti-ki-bel E: Broom creeper
Description	:	Climbing, evergreen, undershrub. Leaves variable in shape and size, tomentose, rounded or cuneate, apex mucronate. Staminate flowers in short, slender panicles, pistillate flowers in cluster. Drupe reddish black.

USEFUL PARTS AND THEIR CURATIVE PROPERTIES

Stem and root	:	Sedative, hypotensive, bradycardiac, cardiotonic, spasmolytic, anticonvulsant, rheumatism
Whole plant	:	Diuretic, snake bite, liver disorder, menstruation
Leaf	:	Eczema, itches, gonorrhoea, cooling, blood dysentery, chronic syphilis, leucorrhoea, menorrhagia, diabetes, corns, spermatorrhoea, red bleeding, venereal diseases, skin diseases, wounds, postnatal pains
Root	:	Asthma, venereal diseases, urine burning, strength, cooling effect

179. *Cochlospermum religiosum* (L.) Alston

Family	:	Cochlospermaceae
Common names	:	S: Girisalmalika H: Gabdi E: Yellow flowered cotton tree
Description	:	A small deciduous tree. Leaves palmately 5-lobed. Flowers large, golden yellow in terminal panicles. Fruits large, pear shaped, 3-5 valved capsules.

USEFUL PARTS AND THEIR CURATIVE PROPERTIES

Dried leaves and flowers	:	stimulant, cooling Gum – thermogenic, anodyne, sedative, cough, diarrhoea, dysentery, gonorrhoea, syphilis, trachoma, pharyngitis.

180. *Coix lacryma-jobi* L.

Family	:	Poaceae
Common names	:	S: Gavedhukah H: Gurlu E: Job's tears

Description : An erect perennial grass. Leaves linear-lanceolate, membranous, racemes drooping from long peduncles carrying male and female spikelets. Fruit subglobose.

USEFUL PARTS AND THEIR CURATIVE PROPERTIES

Roots : Menstrual disorders, strangury
Seeds : Tonic, diuretic, cathartic, depurative, pneumonosis

181. *Coldenia procumbens* L.

Family : Boraginaceae
Common names : S: Trepakashe H: Tripungki E:
Description : A prostrate, scabrid herb, branches radially spreading, leaves obovate-oblong, flowers white, axillary, solitary, ovary puberulous, drupes ovoid, 4-lobed.

USEFUL PARTS AND THEIR CURATIVE PROPERTIES

Leaves : Psoriasis, leucoderma, scorpion sting, rheumatic swellings
Root paste : Epilepsy
Whole plant : Eczema, white patches, allergy and other skin diseases

182. *Coleus ambonicus* Lour.

Family : Lamiaceae
Common names : S: Pashanbhedi E: Indian Borage
Description : Much branched herb. Leaves orbicular, thick, pubescent, margin serrate, aromatic. Small pale purple flowers.

USEFUL PARTS AND THEIR CURATIVE PROPERTIES

Root : Cardiovascular effect, spasmolytic, CNS active, hypothermic, diuretic
Coleonol : Hypotensive, CNS depressant
Forskolin : Bronchodilator stimulates adenylate cyclase activity
Whole plant : Nephrocalcinosis, ureteral stones
Leaf juice : Cough, asthmatic effects, nephrocalcinosis, ureteral stones

183. *Colocasia esculenta* (L.) Schott

Family : Araceae
Common names : S: Kachwi H: Arvi E: Taro
Description : Tall tuberous herb. Petiole sheathing at the base, lamina peltate. Inflorescence with peduncle shorter than petiole. Spathe yellow. Berry ovoid.

USEFUL PARTS AND THEIR CURATIVE PROPERTIES

Corm paste : Insect bite, laxative, demulcent, anodyne, haemorrhoids, congestion
Leaves : Kidney stones, styptic, stimulant, rubefacient, haemorrhages

184. *Commelina attenuata* Koen. ex Vahl

Family : Commelinaceae

Description : Spreading herb. Leaves linear or lanceolate, obtuse, abruptly jointed to sheath, apex tapering, acuminate. Spathes narrowly lanceolate. Flowers blue. Capsule oblong. Seeds 4, whitish appendaged at the ends.

USEFUL PARTS AND THEIR CURATIVE PROPERTIES

Leaf juice : Maggot infested sores

Root paste : Diarrhoea

185. *Commelina benghalensis* L.

Family : Commelinaceae

Common names : S: Kancata H: Kanchera

Description : Spreading herb. Root stock with cleistogamous flowers. Leaves ovate, membranous, subtruncate, apex acute-obtuse. Flowers blue. Capsule ellipsoid. Seeds pitted.

USEFUL PARTS AND THEIR CURATIVE PROPERTIES

Leaf paste : Pimples, skin eruptions

Whole plant : Body and foot sores

Stem : Eyelid infection

186. *Commelina diffusa* Burm.f.

Family : Commelinaceae

Common names : S: Katsapriya H: Kanshura

Description : Diffuse herb. Leaves lanceolate, subcordate, entire, apex acuminate. Spathes complicate, oblong-lanceolate. Petals blue or purple. Capsule oblong, apex beaked. Seeds tuberculate.

USEFUL PARTS AND THEIR CURATIVE PROPERTIES

Leaves : Body swellings, dysentery

187. *Commiphora mukul* (Hook. ex Stocks) Engl.

Family : Burseraceae

Common names : S: Gugguluh H: Gugal E: Indian bdellium tree

Description : A small armed tree. Leaves alternate, obovate. Flowers small, brownish red, polygamous in fascicles. Fruits ovoid drupes, red when ripe.

USEFUL PARTS AND THEIR CURATIVE PROPERTIES

Gum : Astringent, thermogenic, aromatic, expectorant, digestive, anthelmintic, anodyne, depurative, nervine tonic, aphrodisiac, liver tonic, gout, scrofula, facial paralysis, leprosy, leucoderma, epilepsy, fever, strangury, wounds, haemorrhoids, amenorrhoea, ulcers, anaemia, diabetes

188. *Coptis teeta* Wall.

Family : Ranunculaceae

Common names : S: Supita H: Pitmula haldiya bachag E: Golden thread root

Description : Rhizomatous, perennial herb. Leaves ternatisect, pinnatifid. Flowers small, white. Fruits seeded follicles, black.

USEFUL PARTS AND THEIR CURATIVE PROPERTIES

Whole plant : Antidiabetic, bitter tonic, carminative, expectorant, febrifuge, ophthalmic and stomachic. Useful in nervous diseases, eye troubles, atonic dyspepsia, asthma and cough, appetizer, constipation, indigestion, debility after fever, jaundice, flatulence, mild form of intermittent fevers and visceral obstruction

189. *Corchorus aestuans* L.

Family : Tiliaceae

Common names : S: Cancu

Description : Erect herb. Leaves oblong, lanceolate, glabrous, apex acute. Flowers in cymes. Fruits capsules.

USEFUL PARTS AND THEIR CURATIVE PROPERTIES

Plant : Anticancer, CVS active, impotency

190. *Corchorus trilocularis* L.

Family : Tiliaceae

Common names : S: Kaunti

Description : Erect herb. Branchlets glabrescent. Leaves oblong-ovate, lanceolate, glabrous, cuneate, serrate or crenate, apex acute. Cymes leaf opposed, 2-4 flowered, yellow. Capsule 3 in a cluster, angular, 3 or 4 valved. Seeds truncate.

USEFUL PARTS AND THEIR CURATIVE PROPERTIES

Root paste : Eczema, scabies, gonorrhoea

191. *Cordia dichotoma* Forst. f.

Family : Boraginaceae

Common names : S: Bahuvarah H: Lasura E: Sebesten plum

Description : A medium sized tree. Leaves simple, entire, dentate, rounded. Flowers white, small in terminal or axillary cymes. Fruits drupes, yellowish brown.

USEFUL PARTS AND THEIR CURATIVE PROPERTIES

Bark : Astringent, constipating, anthelmintic, depurative, dyspepsia, leprosy, skin diseases, diarrhoea, fever

Leaves : Aphrodisiac, gonorrhoea

Fruits : Cooling, emollient, purgative, diuretic, dry cough, bronchitis, ulcers, expectorant, hyperdypsia, strangury

192. *Coriandrum sativum* L.

Family : Apiaceae

Common names : S: Dhanyakam H: Dhaniyam E: Coriander

Description : Erect herb, leaves ternately lobed ,ovate, base cuneate, apex obtuse. Flowers white, in umbels, fruits sub-globose, mericarps hollow within.

USEFUL PARTS AND THEIR CURATIVE PROPERTIES

Seed extract	:	Antimicrobial, nausea Et.OH (50 %) extract fungitoxic against Helminthosporium oryzae.
Whole plant	:	Sore-throat, haemorrhoids
Fruits	:	Carminative, diuretic, tonic, stomachic, aphrodisiac

193. *Costus speciosus* (J. Koen.) Smith

Family	:	Costaceae
Common names	:	S: Canda H: Kemuk E: Spiral ginger
Description	:	Erect herb with rhizome. Stem spiral, slightly woody at base. Flowers bluish white in dense spikes. Seeds black, angular with white aril.

USEFUL PARTS AND THEIR CURATIVE PROPERTIES

Saponin	:	Hypotensive, spasmolytic from seeds
Rhizome	:	Possesses antifertility, anticholinesterase and anti-inflammatory activities, cooling, relieves headache, allay body heat and burning sensation in the eyes, giddiness, earache, expel intestinal worms, contraception, abortion, lactation, snake bite, rheumatism, conception, backache, fever, aphrodisiac, skin diseases, gastric trouble, wounds, chicken pox
Tuber	:	Earache, female sterility, joint pains, ulcers, piles, fever, overheat, snake bite, helminthiasis, aphrodisiac, urinary troubles
Root	:	Checks tumour formation
Plant	:	Anthelmintic, ophthalmic

194. *Crataeva magna* (Lour.) DC.

Family	:	Capparaceae
Common names	:	S: Varunah H: Barun E: Three leaves caper
Description	:	Medium sized deciduous tree. Leaves digitately trilobed. Flowers large, greenish white, polygamous, terminal corymbs, stamens longer than petals. Fruit fleshy, ovoid berry. Seeds brown, embedded in pulp.

USEFUL PARTS AND THEIR CURATIVE PROPERTIES

Whole plant powder	:	Cholinergic in smooth muscles including urinary bladder and antidiabetic
Stem bark	:	Diphtheria, urinary troubles, gastric irritation, fever, kidney stones
Leaves	:	Spongy gums and toothache
Root bark	:	Gastric trouble

195. *Cressa cretica* L.

Family	:	Convolvulaceae
Common names	:	S: Rudantika H: Rudravanti
Description	:	An erect, small, dwarf shrub. Leaves simple, numerous, subsessile, ovate, acute. Flowers white, corolla lobes reflexed. Fruit ovoid capsules. seeds solitary.

USEFUL PARTS AND THEIR CURATIVE PROPERTIES

Whole plant : Thermogenic, alterant, anthelmintic, expectorant, carminative, digestive, stomachic, aphrodisiac, tonic, asthma, colic, anorexia, anaemia, diabetes, leprosy, general debility

196. *Crocus sativus* L.

Family : Iridaceae

Common names : S: Kesaram H: Kesar E: Saffron

Description : Small bulbous perennial plant. Leaves narrowly linear, radical, leaf sheaths reticulate. Flowers blue, scented, perianth bearded, anthers yellow. Ovary 3-celled. Fruits loculicidal capsules.

USEFUL PARTS AND THEIR CURATIVE PROPERTIES

Dried stigmas : Bitter, acrid, stimulant, tonic, stomachic, aphrodisiac, anodyne, emmenagogue, diuretic, laxative, galactagogue, bronchitis, vomiting, fever, epilepsy, skin diseases

197. *Crotalaria alata* Ham.

Family : Papilionaceae

Description : Herbs or shrubs, leaves simple, obovate, flowers in racemes, many flowered. Flowers 0.5 inches long. Pods 1.2 inches long.

USEFUL PARTS AND THEIR CURATIVE PROPERTIES

Whole plant paste : Joint and muscular pains.

Root decoction : Scorpion sting and snake bite

198. *Crotalaria laburnifolia* L.

Family : Papilionanceae

Common names : S: Muna

Description : Erect, much branched shrub. Leaves trifoliate, ovate-elliptic, appressed pubescent beneath, subacute to cuneate, entire, apex mucronate. Flowers yellow in elongated racemes. Pods glabrous, stipitate.

USEFUL PARTS AND THEIR CURATIVE PROPERTIES

Crotalaburnine : Anti-inflammatory, antispasmodic and CNS depressant

Flower paste : Insect bite

Leaves : Ulcers in mouth, sore-throat, scorpion sting, allergy, pains, swellings, fits

199. *Crotalaria verrucosa* L.

Family : Papilionanceae

Common names : S: Sharnapushpi E: Wild jute

Description : Undershrub; branches angled. Leaves simple, ovate to deltoid, pubescent, attenuate, entire, apex obtuse. Racemes terminal but become lateral. Flowers white or blue. Pod oblong-terete, pubescent.

USEFUL PARTS AND THEIR CURATIVE PROPERTIES

Et. OH (50 %) extract of plant : CNS depressant and diuretic

Root paste	:	Scorpion sting, snake bite
Seed	:	Abortion
Leaf paste	:	Scabies, snake bite, scorpion sting

200. *Croton bonplandianum* Baill.

Family	:	Euphorbiaceae
Description	:	Annual, erect much branched herb to 75 cm. Leaves ovate-lanceolate, glandular, acute, denticulate; flowers yellowish-white in terminal androgynous spikes. Capsules 3-angled, stellately hairy; seed oblong, corniculate.

USEFUL PARTS AND THEIR CURATIVE PROPERTIES

Leaf	:	Cuts, wounds, wasp sting, headache, scurvy
Stem	:	Cough, congestion of nose, chest pain, headache, breathing troubles

201. *Croton roxburghii* L.

Family	:	Euphorbiaceae

USEFUL PARTS AND THEIR CURATIVE PROPERTIES

Root and stem bark paste	:	dysentery, stomach clearance, snake bite, scorpion sting, muscular pain, chest pain, antifertility
Stem juice	:	Cures blindness, cataract
Bark decoction	:	Cholera, diarrhoea, fever
Fruit	:	Antidote to poison

202. *Croton tiglium* L.

Family	:	Euphorbiaceae
Common names	:	S: Jepalah H: Jamalgota E: Purging cotton
Description	:	A small evergreen tree. Leaves oblong, obtuse, acuminate, membranous. Flowers small, unisexual. Fruits ovoid, trigonous capsules. Seeds smooth.

USEFUL PARTS AND THEIR CURATIVE PROPERTIES

Seeds	:	Thermogenic, emollient, drastic purgative, digestive, carminative, vermifuge, anthelmintic, rubefacient, convulsions, leucoderma, anasarca, dropsy, cough, insanity, constipation, dyspepsia

203. *Cryptolepis buchanani* Roem. & Schult.

Family	:	Periplocaceae
Common names	:	S: Krishnasariva
Description	:	Climbing shrubs, leaves elliptic acuminate, obovate. Flowers pale yellow, in cymes, corona clavate, follicles long. Et.OH (50 %) of extract of roots and stem hypotensive, CNS depressant and antiamphetеminic

USEFUL PARTS AND THEIR CURATIVE PROPERTIES

Root	: Rheumatic pain, bite of reptiles, lactation, antinarcotic, joint pains, diarrhoea
Latex	: Cuts

204. *Cucurbita maxima* Duchesne ex Lam.

Family	: Cucurbitaceae
Common names	: S: Gudayogaphala H: Kaddu E: Red pumpkin
Description	: Climbing shrub, tendrils branched. Leaves suborbicular, 5-6 angled, denticulate. Staminate and pistillate flowers axillary, solitary, white. Berries large, variable in shape.

USEFUL PARTS AND THEIR CURATIVE PROPERTIES

Fruit	: Galactagogue
Flower paste	: Scorpion sting

205. *Cuminum cyminum* L.

Family	: Apiaceae
Common names	: S: Jiraka H: Jira E: Cumin
Description	: Small slender glabrous annual herb. Leaves bluish green, filiform. Flowers small, white compound umbels, fruits greyish, compressed laterally with ridges, covered over by papillose hairs.

USEFUL PARTS AND THEIR CURATIVE PROPERTIES

Fruit	: Astringent, digestive, carminative, anodyne, constipating, stomachic, stimulant, diuretic, galactagogue, febrifuge, uterine and nervine stimulant, dyspepsia, colic, flatulence, anorexia, leucorrhoea, piles, chronic diarrhoea, skin diseases, leprosy, leucoderma, fever, gonorrhoea, hiccups, asthma, cough, general debility, ulcers, bronchitis

206. *Cupressus sempervirens* L.

Family	: Cupressaceae
Common names	: E: Cypress

USEFUL PARTS AND THEIR CURATIVE PROPERTIES

Uses	: flavouring, culinary purposes, cosmetics, perfumes

207. *Curculigo orchioides* Gaertn.

Family	: Hypoxidaceae
Common names	: S: Talamuli H:Mushali E: Black muscale
Description	: Small herb without stem. Root stock elongate. Leaves lanceolate, narrow, flowers yellow, solitary. Seeds globose.

USEFUL PARTS AND THEIR CURATIVE PROPERTIES

Plant	: Hypoglycaemic, spasmolytic and anticancer, aphrodisiac, poultice, haemostatic, antiseptic. Root – cuts, wounds, jaundice, hard and large breast for women, increase potency, migraine, stomach trouble and

		dysentery, leucorrhoea, epilepsy, nose bleeding, anaemia, asthma, increases blood content, conjunctivitis, earache, blindness and white spots on the eye ball
Tuber	:	Asthma, leucorrhoea, diarrhoea, general tonic, spleen troubles, chest pain, hiccups, scorpion sting, nervous weakness, aphrodisiac, piles, cuts, dysentery, jaundice, skin diseases, wounds

208. ***Curcuma angustifolia*** **L.**

Family : Zingiberaceae

USEFUL PARTS AND THEIR CURATIVE PROPERTIES

Root : Weakness and rheumatism

Rhizome : Diarrhoea, typhoid, tuberculosis, aphrodisiac

Tuber : Lactogenic, boils

209. ***Curcuma aromatica*** **Sal.**

Family : Zingiberaceae

Common names : S: Aranyaharidra H: Ban-Haridra E: Wild turmeric

Description : Stemless herbs. Root fibres not ending in small tubers. Leaves elliptic, flowers pink, lip yellow. Ovary 3-celled. Fruit capsule. Seeds ovoid.

USEFUL PARTS AND THEIR CURATIVE PROPERTIES

Rhizome : Antibiotic, leprosy, leucoderma, eczema, skin infection, stomach pain, aphrodisiac, sprains, hiccough, bronchitis, cough, appetizer, tonic, carminative, bitter

210. ***Curcuma longa*** **L.**

Family : Zingiberaceae

Common names : S: Haridra H: Haldi E: Turmeric

Description : Rhizomatous plant, leaves elliptic oblong, flowers few yellow. Calyx with few fine hairs, ovary stiffly hairy at the top.

USEFUL PARTS AND THEIR CURATIVE PROPERTIES

Curcumin : Anti-inflammatory

Rhizome : Antiprotozoal, spasmolytic, CNS active, antiparasitic for skin infections, antispasmodic, antibacterial, antiarthritic, psoriasis, bone fracture, skin diseases, cough, cold, deworming, inflammation, diarrhoea, whooping cough

211. ***Curcuma pseudomontana*** **Graham**

Family : Zingiberaceae

Common names : S: Vanaharidra H: Banhaldi E: Wild turmeric

Description : An erect herb; root stock small with almond-like tubers. Leaves lanceolate- oblong, acuminate, tapering towards base. Flowers yellow, in spikes. Capsule globose.

USEFUL PARTS AND THEIR CURATIVE PROPERTIES

Rhizome paste : Swellings due to wounds, insect bite, diabetes, jaundice, body swelling, increase lactation, cough, cold, stomach troubles, overheat, antiseptic, skin infections

Tuber : Hepatic stimulant, jaundice, body swellings, lactation, cooling

Seed : Eczema, ringworm infections

212. *Curcuma zedoaria* Rosc.

Family : Zingiberaceae

Common names : E: Zedoary

Description : Stemless herbs, root stock tuberous. Fleshy fibres, ending in smaller tubers. Leaves oblong, acuminate. Petioles long, flowers yellow. Ovary 3-celled. Fruit capsule.

USEFUL PARTS AND THEIR CURATIVE PROPERTIES

Whole plant : Antiseptic, cooling, insect bite

213. *Cuscuta reflexa* Roxb.

Family : Cuscutaceae

Common names : S: Akasha valli H: Akashabela E: Dodder

Description : Twining, leafless, parasitic herb. Branches fleshy, forming dense, yellow masses on shrubs and trees. Flowers pale white, solitary, clustered or in racemes. Corolla lobes reflexed. Stigmas diverging. Capsules depressed globose.

USEFUL PARTS AND THEIR CURATIVE PROPERTIES

Whole plant : Body swellings, insect bite, fever, eksira, bodyache, rheumatism, spermatorrhoea, haematuria, tongue ulcers, epilepsy, broken bones, gastric troubles, cuts, wounds, fractures, sprains, haemostatic, lower blood pressure

Stem : Unfertility

214. *Cyclamen europaeum* L.

Family : Primulaceae

Common names : E: Cyclamen

USEFUL PARTS AND THEIR CURATIVE PROPERTIES

Uses : Synthetic perfumes, cosmetics

215. *Cyclea peltata* (Lam.) Hook.f. & Thoms.

Family : Menispermaceae

Common names : S: Patha H: Pathi E: Pata root

Description : Twining pubescent herb. Leaves peltate, ovate, coriaceous, entire-wavy, acuminate. Inflorescence a panicle, axillary. Staminate flowers regular, pistillate flowers irregular. Drupe obovoid, style scar sub-basal.

USEFUL PARTS AND THEIR CURATIVE PROPERTIES

Leaf : Insect bite, fractures, fever, reduces body heat

Whole plant : Skin disorders

216. *Cymbopogon citratus* Stapf.

Family : Poaceae

Common names : S: Bhustrnah H: Gandhatrn E: Lemon grass

Description : Perennial aromatic herbs. Leaves flat, often very coarse. Panicles with fertile spikelets, linear. Lodicules 2, stamens 3, grain oblong.

USEFUL PARTS AND THEIR CURATIVE PROPERTIES

Whole plant : Epilepsy, bronchitis, cholera

Uses : Mircin or lemongrass oil – soaps, perfumes, vitamin A extraction from citral, flavouring agent, hair oil, cooling agent, burning feet syndrome, confectionery

217. *Cymbopogon martinii* L.

Family : Poaceae

Common names : S: Rohisah H: Rusa ghas E: Russa grass

Description : Perennial aromatic herbs. Leaves linear-lanceolate, panicles. Fertile spikelets bears a slender awn. Lodicules 2, stamens 3, grain oblong.

USEFUL PARTS AND THEIR CURATIVE PROPERTIES

Uses : Source of palmarosa and ginger-grass oils, substitute of Otto of roses

: Oil - Cosmetics, soap and perfume industries, flavouring agent in tobacco, blends in essential oil

218. *Cymbopogon nardus* (L.) Rendle

Family : Poaceae

Common names : Cucurbitaceae

Description : Perennial, densely tufted, often aromatic herbs. Leaves flat, often very coarse. Lower glume of fertile spikelets lanceolate, acute. Panicles linear-oblong. Lodicules 2, stamens 3, grain oblong.

USEFUL PARTS AND THEIR CURATIVE PROPERTIES

Uses : Oil of Citronella in expensive soaps, perfumes, insect repellant, substitute of Otto of roses

219. *Cymbopogon winterianus* Jowitt

Family : Poaceae

Common names : E: Citronella

Description :

USEFUL PARTS AND THEIR CURATIVE PROPERTIES

Uses : Oil - soaps, incense sticks, mosquito repellants, deodorants, perfumes, cosmetics, flavouring

220. *Cynodon dactylon* (L.) Pers.

Family : Poaceae
Common names : S: Durva H: Hariali E: Conch grass
Description : Perennial, stoloniferous grass. Culms creeping, decumbent, later erect. Leaves linear, rounded, apex acuminate. Spikes 3-4, digitate. Spikelets subsessile. Caryopsis oblong.

USEFUL PARTS AND THEIR CURATIVE PROPERTIES

Plant : Antiviral and antidiabetic, control bleeding and abortion, dog bite, bleeding piles, bleeding from nose, stomach, anus, head reeling, restore vigour, wounds, oedema, phlegm, urinary troubles
Basal stems : Increase potency
Root decoction : Fever, leucorrhoea
Leaves : Dysuria, checks vomiting, fevers

221. *Cyperus rotundus* L.

Family : Cyperaceae
Common names : S: Musta H: Motha E: Nut grass
Description : Stem sparsely tufted. Leaves several, flat, scabrous, sheaths brown. Inflorescence simple or compound. Glumes closely imbricating, ovate. Nut oblong, trigonous, apiculate.

USEFUL PARTS AND THEIR CURATIVE PROPERTIES

Root : Fever, galactagogue, joint pains, white leucorrhoea, increase potency, intermittent fevers, lactation, wounds, sores, ulcers, jaundice, dermatitis
Corm : Abdominal and stomach pains, nausea and vomiting, hyper acidity, dysmenorrhoea, traumatic injuries
Stolons : Diarrhoea, indigestion
Whole plant : Malarial fever

222. *Dalbergia latifolia* Roxb.

Family : Papilionanceae
Common names : S: Simsapa H: Kala shisham E: East Indian Rosewood
Description : Deciduous tree upto 10 m, leaflets elliptic, orbicular, rounded or emarginate, cuneate at base, glabrous, subcoriaceous. Corolla white, stamens 9, monadelphous. Pod oblong, narrowed at both ends, 1 - 4 seeded.

USEFUL PARTS AND THEIR CURATIVE PROPERTIES

Stem bark : Anthelmintic, CVS and CNS active, spasmolytic, paralysis, gout, rheumatic pains, fever, leucoderma, leprosy

223. *Dalbergia sissoo* Roxb.

Family : Papilionaceae
Common names : S: Simsapa H: Shisham E: Sissoo
Description : Tree to 10 m, leaflets 3-5, elliptic, acuminate, glabrous, coriaceous. Corolla white. Stamens monadelphous. Pod oblong, glabrous, obtuse, minutely apiculate.

USEFUL PARTS AND THEIR CURATIVE PROPERTIES

Leaf decoction : Control of vomitings, gonorrhoea, dysentery, diarrhoea
Stem bark : Cuts, wounds, sores

224. *Datura innoxia* Mill.

Family : Solanaceae
Common names : S: Dhattura H: Safed datura E: Thorn apple
Description : Erect undershrub. Stem green, branches glandular, tomentose. Leaves ovate or elliptic, oblique, undulate, apex acute, softly pubescent. Flowers white, solitary, axillary. Capsule globose, covered with long, weak spines.

USEFUL PARTS AND THEIR CURATIVE PROPERTIES

Plant : Effect on respiration, CVS active, antiarrhythmic
Root : Rheumatic pains, fever
Leaves : Headache, asthma, boils, blisters
Seeds : Reddish rashes, pyorrhoea, diabetes
Leaves / fruits : Rheumatic and rib muscle pains

225. *Datura metel* L.

Family : Solanaceae
Common names : S: Dhastura H: Kala Datura E: Thorn apple
Description : Erect, annual-perennial, undershrub. Stems green or purplish, glabrous or short hairy. Leaves oblique at base, acute or acuminate. Flowers white or purple, axillary, solitary. Corolla single or double. Capsule globose, glabrous or hairy with short, blunt, conical spines.

USEFUL PARTS AND THEIR CURATIVE PROPERTIES

Plant and fruit : CVS active, spasmolytic
Plant : Anticancer, anthelmintic, digested in wine the long white corollas form a tincture used as an anaesthetic. A lotion is made from them which reduces eruptions on the face and swellings of the feet. The flowers are used in asthma and the fruits in ear ache. The pounded leaves are applied to swellings, tumours and rheumatic pains. A decoction of the seeds is used for diseases of the eye.
Leaves : Amenorrhoea, dog bite, scabies, fever, potency in males, red rash, asthma, body pain, boils, sores, burns
Root : Permanent sterility, antiseptic
Seeds : Asthma, reddish rashes, diarrhoea, leprosy, sciatica, sprains, insanity, cerebral complaints, skin diseases, snake bite, scorpion sting

226. *Dendrophthoe falcata* (L.f.) Etting

Family : Loranthaceae
Common names : S: Vrkshadani H: Banda E: Mistletoe
Description : Large bushy parasite, bark smooth grey, branches smooth. Leaves opposite, unequal, coriaceous. Flowers single, orange-red or scarlet.

USEFUL PARTS AND THEIR CURATIVE PROPERTIES

Plant : Hypotensive and antiviral, paralysis, leucorrhoea, mumps, bone fracture, blood vomiting due to tuberculosis

Haustoria : Mensruation, antifertility

Stem bark : Wounds, asthma, menstrual troubles.

Flower : Regulating menstrual cycle, malarial fever, chicken pox

Leaf : Earache

227. *Desmodium gangeticum* (L.) DC.

Family : Papilionaceae

Common names : S: Shalaparni H: Shalparni

Description : Erect, ascending undershrub. Branches slightly angled, pubescent. Leaves simple ovate, acuminate. Raceme 20-50 flowered. Flowers 2 per bract, violet. Pod linear, moniliform, reticulate, as long as broad, with hooked hairs.

USEFUL PARTS AND THEIR CURATIVE PROPERTIES

Root : Anti-inflammatory, analgesic, asthma, whooping cough, diarrhoea

Whole plant : Diarrhoea

Leaf : Hyper acidity, boils, blisters

228. *Dianthus caryophyllus* L.

Family : Caryophyllaceae

Common names : E: Carnation

USEFUL PARTS AND THEIR CURATIVE PROPERTIES

Uses : Cosmetics, flavouring agents, perfumery

229. *Dichrostachys cinerea* (L.) Wt. & Arn.

Family : Mimosaceae

Common names : S: Vellantara H: Vurutuli

Description : Shrub to small thorny tree. Leaves bipinnate, leaflets 12-18 pairs. Flowers in spikes. Pods dark brown, linear-oblong, flattened.

USEFUL PARTS AND THEIR CURATIVE PROPERTIES

Stem bark : Gonorrhoea, fever, joint pains, chicken-pox, urinary troubles

Root : White and red leucorrhoea, paralysis, fractured bone, nephrocalcinosis, ureteral stones, rheumatism, menstrual disorders, chicken-pox

Leaf paste : Skin diseases, leucorrhoea, menorrhoea

230. *Digera* muricata (L.) Mart.

Family : Amaranthaceae

Common names : S: Kunanjara H: Lesua

Description : Erect herb to 75 cm. Leaves spiral, elliptic ovate, base truncate, entire, obtuse to acutely apiculate, glabrous. Inflorescence axillary and terminal. Flowers pink. Fruit indehiscent, rugose, not enclosed in perianth. Seed globose.

USEFUL PARTS AND THEIR CURATIVE PROPERTIES

Leaf	:	Wounds and constipation, laxative
Whole plant	:	Indigestion
Flowers	:	Urinary troubles, impotency

231. *Digitalis purpurea* L.

Family	:	Scrophulariaceae
Common names	:	H: Tilpushpi E: Common fox glove
Description	:	Biennial herb. Lower basal leaves hairy, ovate. Flowers white or purple, with ciliate lobes, one-sided bunches. Fruit ovoid.

USEFUL PARTS AND THEIR CURATIVE PROPERTIES

Leaves	:	Cardiac stimulant and tonic. The glycosides of this drug are used in the treatment of heart disease, regulation of heart rate, rhythm, tone, contraction of impulses

232. *Dillenia indica* L.

Family	:	Dilleniaceae
Common names	:	S: Bhavya E: Elephant apple
Description	:	A medium to large sized tree, leaves sharply serrate, flowers creamy, sepals thick, fruit fleshy, seeds compressed, embedded in glutinous pulp.

USEFUL PARTS AND THEIR CURATIVE PROPERTIES

Leaf	:	CNS active and CVS depressant, hypothermic, laxative, abdominal pains. Alcoholic seed extract – antimicrobial
Fruit juice	:	Weakness, kills lice, dandruff, digestive agent

233. *Dillenia pentagyna* Roxb.

Family	:	Dilleniaceae
Common names	:	S: Aksikiphala H: Karmal E: Dog teak
Description	:	Deciduous tree upto 15 m, bark grey or pale brown, smooth with shallow irregular depressions. Leaves obovate, acute, base attenuate. Inflorescence fascicled on short shoots. Flowers white, 2-3 cm across. Fruit pendulous with the enclosed fleshy sepals.

USEFUL PARTS AND THEIR CURATIVE PROPERTIES

Stem bark	:	Paralysis, bone fracture, cough, rheumatic pains, burns, measles
Root	:	Body pain
Fruit	:	Appetizer, tonic, general stamina

234. *Dioscorea bulbifera* L.

Family	:	Dioscoreaceae
Common names	:	S: Brahmaputri H: Bhirvolikanda E: Bulb bearing yam
Description	:	Vine. Tubers solitary or 2-3, large, globose. Stems twining to left. Leaves broadly ovate, sub-orbicular, deeply cordate, entire, apex acuminate. Staminate flowers green or purplish spikes. Pistillate flowers sessile, solitary or fascicled, pendulous spikes. Capsules recurved. Seed winged at the base only.

USEFUL PARTS AND THEIR CURATIVE PROPERTIES

Tuber paste : Cuts, wounds,ulcers, insect bite, leucoderma, stomach pain, lactation

Young rhizome : Precaution against snake bite, indigestion tuberous root cough, cold.

235. *Diospyros melanoxylon* Roxb.

Family : Ebenaceae

Common names : S: Kenduka H: Tendu E: Ebony

Description : Deciduous tree, branches fulvous-tomentose. Leaves elliptic-oblong, obtuse, entire, base acute to rounded, pubescent beneath. Staminate flowers in short cymes, pistillate solitary. Fruit pubescent when young, smooth and yellow when ripe, seeds 4 - 8, compressed.

USEFUL PARTS AND THEIR CURATIVE PROPERTIES

Tender shoots : Dysentery, mouth ulcers, excess of heat, blood motions

Root : Syphilis

Whole plant : Typhoid

Stem bark : Cold, cough, diarrhoea, burning wounds

Fruit : Dysentery, bone fracture, recovery of decayed fingers

Leaf : Diarrhoea

Gum-resin : Typhoid

236. *Dipteracanthus prostratus* (Poir.) Nees

Family : Acanthaceae

Common names : S: Kalighavni

Description : Prostrate herb to 30 cm. Leaves ovate-elliptic to deltoid, strigose, truncate to acute, apex subacute to obtuse. Flowers solitary, axillary. Corolla blue to violet. Capsule slightly pubescent. Seeds orbicular, flattened.

USEFUL PARTS AND THEIR CURATIVE PROPERTIES

Plant : Extract mild hypoglycaemic and anticancer against human epidermoid carcinoma of nasopharynx

Leaf : Cuts and scorpion sting

237. *Dodonaea viscosa* (L.) Jacq.

Family : Sapindaceae

Common names : S: Rasna H: Sanatta E: Jamaica switch sorrel

Description : Evergreen shrub to small tree. Leaves spiral, simple, subsessile, oblanceolate, subacute, shining. Flowers small, greenish, yellow in short few flowered cymes. Capsule compressed, thin, winged, yellowish brown. Seeds black.

USEFUL PARTS AND THEIR CURATIVE PROPERTIES

Leaves : Paralysis, waist pain, backache, epilepsy, bone fracture, wounds, boils, premature greying of hair, dandruff, myalgia, dental diseases, muscle swellings

Whole plant : Eye diseases, vision improvement
Seed : Permanent sterility
Stem bark : Muscle pain

238. *Drimia indica* (Roxb.) Jessop

Family : Amaryllidaceae
Common names : S: Putakanda H: Janglipiyaz E: Indian squill
Description : Herb with tunicate bulb. Leaves appearing after flowers, nearly flat, linear, acute. Scape erect, brittle. Flowers dark brown, very distant, in slender racemes. Capsules ellipsoid, tapering to both ends. Seeds elliptic, flattened, black.

USEFUL PARTS AND THEIR CURATIVE PROPERTIES

Bulb : Headache, rheumatism, scorpion sting

239. *Dryabalanops aromatica* Gaertn. f.

Family : Dipterocarpaceae
Common names : E: Borneo camphor

USEFUL PARTS AND THEIR CURATIVE PROPERTIES

Uses : Cosmetics, perfumes, flavouring soaps

240. *Drypetes roxburghii* (Wall.) Huresawa

Family : Euphorbiaceae
Common names : S: Putrajivah H: Jivputrak
Description : A moderate sized evergreen tree. Leaves simple, alternate, dark green, shiny. Male flowers pedicellate, female flowers 3-celled. Fruits rounded drupes. Seed 1.

USEFUL PARTS AND THEIR CURATIVE PROPERTIES

Leaves : Refrigerant, procreant, catarrh, fever, sterility
Seeds : Procreant, ophthalmic, laxative, anti-inflammatory, aphrodisiac, diuretic, hyperdypsia, constipation, filariasis, strangury, abortion

241. *Echinops echinatus* Roxb.

Family : Asteraceae
Common names : S: Brahma dandi H: Utakanta
Description : Annual erect herb to 50 cm. Leaves lanceolate, pinnatifid, sessile, lobes ovate, spinescent, amplexicaul. Heads many, collected into globose clusters, compound head, solitary, terminal, homogamous, florets white. Involucral bracts spinescent. Achenes elongate, villous.

USEFUL PARTS AND THEIR CURATIVE PROPERTIES

Flowers : Eye diseases
Root paste : Gout, diarrhoea, wounds
Whole plant : Giddiness, appetite, pimples
Leaves : Labour pains, quick delivery, acute fevers

242. *Eclipta prostrata* (L.) Mant.

Family : Asteraceae
Common names : S: Bhringaraja H: Bhangra E: Trailing eclipta
Description : Annual prostrate to erect herb to 70 cm. Leaves opposite with appressed hairs. Flowers white.

USEFUL PARTS AND THEIR CURATIVE PROPERTIES

Plant : Antihepatic, nematicidal, ovicidal, antiviral, CVS active, spasmolytic, gonorrhoea, hair fall, jaundice, cooling effect to brain, tonic, fever, bronchitis, rheumatism, blood purifier, skin diseases
Leaf : Liver complaints, dandruff, eye diseases, cough, cold, asthma, cuts, wounds, eczema, epilepsy, seasonal allergies, hair tonic, headache, migraine, jaundice, body swellings, snake bite
Root : Cataract
Flower buds : Headache
Seed : Burns, hepatitis, conjunctivitis

243. *Eicchornia crassipes* Solms.

Family : Pontederiaceae
Common names : S: Jalakumbhi E: Water hyacinth
Description : Fresh water herb. Leaves floating, parallel-nerved. Petioles enlarged. Flowers bisexual, perianth distinctly tubular. Anthers equal, filaments not horned. Ovary superior, ovules 1-many, fruit capsule, seeds small.

USEFUL PARTS AND THEIR CURATIVE PROPERTIES

Flowers : Antimicrobial Shoot extract showed gibberellin like activity.
Leaves : Cleaning of wounds

244. *Elephantopus scaber* L.

Family : Asteraceae
Common names : S: Gojihva H: Gobhi E: Prickly leaved elephant's foot
Description : A stiff, perennial herb, leaves obovate-oblong, serrate-dentate, heads purple, flat topped inflorescence, achenes 10-ribbed, pappus of 4-5 bristles.

USEFUL PARTS AND THEIR CURATIVE PROPERTIES

Plant : Anticancer, skin diseases, malaria, diarrhoea
Shoot : Antibiotic
Root paste : Toothache, malaria, urinary troubles, pimples in infants, inflammations, eczema, ringworm, diarrhoea, ulcers, stomach pain, antinarcotic, tonsilitis, gonorrhoea, headache, dysentery, leprosy, acidity, anthelmintic
Leaf : Loose motions, ulcers

245. *Elettaria cardamomum* Mat.

Family : Zingiberaceae

Common names : S: Elo H: Chhoti Ilaichi E: Cardamom

Description : Perennial herb. Leaves distichous, flowers in panicles, calyx 3-lobed, corolla tube cylindric, stamen with a short filament, ovary 3-celled, fruit capsule.

USEFUL PARTS AND THEIR CURATIVE PROPERTIES

Uses : Flavouring various preparations of food, confectionery, beverages and liquors.

246. *Elytraria acaulis* (L.f.) Lindau

Family : Acanthaceae

Description : Acaulescent herb to 30 cm. Leaves subradical, in close spirals, obovate to oblanceolate, villous along the nerves below, cuneate, apex obtuse. Spikes scapigerous, 10-25 cm. Corolla white tinged pink. Seeds flattened.

USEFUL PARTS AND THEIR CURATIVE PROPERTIES

Root : Eczema, maggot infested sores, skin diseases, wounds, rotten teeth, snake bite, anasarca, boils and body swellings

Leaf : Wounds, boils, menstrual disorders, cough, venereal diseases

Whole plant : Cold, cough

Tuber : Regulates menstrual cycle

247. *Emilia sonchifolia* (L.) DC.

Family : Asteraceae

Common names : S: Sasasrutih H: Hirankhuri

Description : A weak erect, annual herb. Leaves radical, cauline. Heads purple in terminal corymbs, achenes cylindrical, pappus copious.

USEFUL PARTS AND THEIR CURATIVE PROPERTIES

Leaf : Night blindness, boils, bruises, wounds, breast abscess, sore eyes, inflammation

Root : Diarrhoea, bowel complaints, mouth dryness

248. *Entada pursaetha* DC.

Family : Mimosaceae

Common names : S: Gilla E: Garbee bean

Description : Unarmed lianes upto 30 m long. Leaves alternate, bipinnate, leaflets about 4 pairs, glabrous, base subacute, entire, apex obtuse, retuse. Flowers pale green in panicled spikes. Pod woody, falcate; seeds obtusely orbicular, shining.

USEFUL PARTS AND THEIR CURATIVE PROPERTIES

Aerial part : CVS and CNS active, saponin from seeds – spasmolytic

Seed pulp : Arthritis, skin diseases, snake bite, toothache, intestinal worms, rheumatism

Leaf	:	Rat bite
Pod juice	:	Removes dandruff

249. *Ephedra gerardiana* (Wall.) Stapf.

Family	:	Ephedraceae
Common names	:	H: Asmania E: Ephedra
Description	:	Small shrub. Stems woody, branches whorled. Leaves reduced to minute 2-toothed sheaths. Male flowers in ovate spikes. Female flowers 1-2 in short spikes. Fruits ovoid, red, surrounded by succulent bracts.

USEFUL PARTS AND THEIR CURATIVE PROPERTIES

Whole plant	:	Decoction of the stems and roots is a popular remedy for rheumatism and syphilis and the juice of the berries is given in affection of the respiratory passage. The thin leafless branches are considered diaphoretic and antipyretic.
Root	:	Astringent, alterative, diuretic, stomachic and tonic. Ephedrine has the property of dilating the pupil of the eye. Its liquid extract is used for controlling asthmatic paroxysms.
Tincture	:	Cardiac and circulatory stimulant. It is also used to control bed-wetting (urinating) in children.

250. *Erythrina variegata* L.

Family	:	Papilionanceae
Common names	:	S: Paribhadrah H: Dadap E: Indian Coral tree
Description	:	Small medium sized tree. Leaves 3-foliate, flowers on leafless branches, stout racemes, terminally arranged, corolla bright red, pods greyish.

USEFUL PARTS AND THEIR CURATIVE PROPERTIES

Bark	:	Leucorrhoea, backache, diarrhoea, lactation, joint pains, cough, diabetes
Leaf juice	:	Intestinal worms, joint pains, whooping cough, eczema, mind concentration
Flowers	:	Aphrodisiac

251. *Erythroxylum monogynum* Roxb.

Family	:	Erythroxylaceae
Common names	:	S: Devataru E: Bastard sandal
Description	:	Large shrub; leaves obovate to elliptic, glabrous, cuneate, entire, apex obtuse, emarginate. Flowers axillary, solitary or clustered, white; drupes oblong, 1-seeded, ripening red.

USEFUL PARTS AND THEIR CURATIVE PROPERTIES

Aerial part	:	CNS active, hypothermic
Stem bark	:	Dysentery, mouth ulcers, stomach troubles, itching
Leaf	:	Hepatic stimulant, malaria, intestinal worms, jaundice, wounds, itching

252. *Eucalyptus citriodora* Hook.

Family : Myrtaceae
Common names : E: Lemon scented gum

USEFUL PARTS AND THEIR CURATIVE PROPERTIES

Leaves : The leaves yield a strong pungent essential oil, valued in medicine as an antiseptic, febrifuge, carminative, stimulant, diaphoretic, antimalarial and anthelmintic Eucalyptus oil increases the flow of saliva, gastric and intestinal juices and thus, increases appetite and digestion. It increases the rate of heart beats, lowers arterial tension and quickens respiration. In large doses it is an irritant of the alimentary canal producing eructation, indigestion, nausea, vomiting and purging. In toxic doses it is a narcotic poison. It paralyses the respiratory centre in the medulla. Citridorol isolated from the leaves showed significant anti-tubercular activity.

Uses : Cosmetics, perfumery

253. *Eucalyptus globulus* L.

Family : Myrtaceae
Common names : S: Tailaparnah H: Yukeliptas E: Eucalyptus
Description : Trees. Leaves usually opposite, flowers solitary or in umbels or heads. Petals 5, stamens many, ovary inferior, 3-4 celled, fruit capsule. Seeds small.

USEFUL PARTS AND THEIR CURATIVE PROPERTIES

Oil : Astringent, thermogenic, antiseptic, stimulant, anodyne, carminative, digestive, cardiotonic, diuretic, cephalalgia, tuberculosis, chronic cough, asthma, pneumonia, bronchitis, pyorrhoea, burns, dyspepsia, flatulence, cardiac debility, chronic and intermittent fevers

254. *Euphorbia hirta* L.

Family : Euphorbiaceae
Common names : S: Dugdhika H: Lal dudhi E: Australian asthma weed
Description : Erect or decumbent herb. Leaves elliptic, ovate-oblong, flowers greenish, in axillary, cyathia, capsules pilose.

USEFUL PARTS AND THEIR CURATIVE PROPERTIES

Plant : Anticancer, hypoglycaemic, antiprotozoal, CVS active, boils, spasmolytic, gonorrhoea, carbuncle, body pain, worms, bowel complaints, asthma, fertility
Latex : Warts, headache, conjunctivitis, cough, wounds, leprosy, skin diseases, cuts
Leaves : Leucorrhoea, dysentery, itches, ulcers and fissures in mouth
Fruit juice : Wounds
Flower : Fever
Root : Excessive urination

255. *Euphorbia nivulia* Buch. – Ham.

Family : Euphorbiaceae

Common names : S: Snuhi H: Thor E: Dog's tounge

Description : Succulent tree upto 9 m; branchlets cylindrical, with stipular well-developed divaricate persistent sharp spines, arranged in regular rows. Leaves obovate - oblong to sub-spathulate, deciduous. Cyathia in axillary, subterminal cymes.

USEFUL PARTS AND THEIR CURATIVE PROPERTIES

Latex : Body pains, foot cracks, ulcerous wounds

Stem bark : Bone fracture

Root : Paralysis

Leaf : Cold, headache

256. *Euphorbia tirucalli* L.

Family : Euphorbiaceae

Common names : S: Vajraduma H: Sehund E: Round milk hedge

Description : Succulent shrub or small tree of 5 m, branchlets terete, succulent. Leaves linear to lanceolate, cuneate, apex obtuse to subacute, deciduous. Cyathia a few, usually terminal, sub-sessile. Capsule smooth, seeds carunculate.

USEFUL PARTS AND THEIR CURATIVE PROPERTIES

Leaves : Dry cough

Latex : Toothache, febrifuge, swellings, rheumatism

Stem : Earache, cough, cold

Whole plant : Swellings and rheumatism

257. *Evolvulus alsinoides* (L.) L.

Family : Convolvulaceae

Common names : S: Vishnukrantha H: Syama kantha E: Sankapushpi

Description : Small hairy procumbent, diffused perennial herb with small woody root stock, leaves densely clothed with apprised silky hairs, flowers light blue, solitary or sometimes pairs, jointed near the middle of the peduncle.

USEFUL PARTS AND THEIR CURATIVE PROPERTIES

Plant : Diuretic, antifungal, cold, cough, hiccough, bronchitis, urinary disorder, brain tonic, teeth hardening, spermatorrhoea, hiccups, hysteria, general stamina, longevity of the teeth, earache, asthma

Root : Fever, hiccups, jaundice, whitlow

Leaf : Jaundice, aphrodisiac, ulcers, honey bee and other insect stings, snake bite, scorpion sting

258. *Ficus bengalensis* L.

Family : Moraceae
Common names : S: Bahupada H: Bor E: Banyan tree
Description : Very large, much branched tree. Prop roots arise from branches and support the plant. Leaves spiral, minutely pubescent. Inflorescence hypanthodium. Receptacles globose, red when ripe.

USEFUL PARTS AND THEIR CURATIVE PROPERTIES

Root bark : Diabetes, gonorrhoea, increase potency, rheumatism, bruises, toothache, fever, arthritis, ulcers
Tender root : Female sterility, leucorrhoea
Fruit : Spermatorrhoea, nausea, boils, leprosy
Buds : Diarrhoea
Latex : Kibes, piles, fissures in the feet, boils, blisters, gonorrhoea, impotency, throat pains
Aerial roots : Toothache, bone fracture, diabetes, diarrhoea, quick healing of decayed fingers, increase height
Leaves : Sores, menorrhagia, cuts, wounds, aphrodisiac

259. *Ficus hispida* L. f.

Family : Moraceae
Common names : S: Kakodumaru H: Dagarin E: Devil fig
Description : Small tree. Leaves decussate, broadly oblong, coriaceous, entire to minutely toothed, apex acute. Figs dioecious, on special shoots, depressed, globose, ripening yellow. Achenes lenticular, keeled with prominent hilum.

USEFUL PARTS AND THEIR CURATIVE PROPERTIES

Aerial parts : CNS active, hypothermic
Root : Dog bite, diabetes
Fruit : Galactagogue, ulcers, sores, increase lactation, hepatic hindering
Leaf juice : Leucoderma patches, boils
Stem Bark : Intestinal and stomach ulcers, cuts and wounds, nephroprotector, leucoderma
Watery latex : Tonsils, blood dysentery, diarrhoea, warts

260. *Ficus microcarpa* L. f.

Family : Moraceae
Common names : S: Plaksah H: Kamarup
Description : Small tree, adventitious roots very short, leaves elliptic-ovate, narrowed at base. Syconia white, globoid, glabrous, in axillary pairs.

USEFUL PARTS AND THEIR CURATIVE PROPERTIES

Fruit : Toothache, dental caries
Root : Dental caries, pyorrhoea, wounds
Latex : Rheumatism

261. *Ficus racemosa* L.

Family : Moraceae
Common names : S: Udumbarah H: Gular E: Gular fig
Description : Tree to 10 m, bark whitish brown. Leaves spiral, subcoriaceous, blade glaucous above, rounded to acute, entire. Figs monoecious, cauliflorous, white, pilose, ripening purplish red.

USEFUL PARTS AND THEIR CURATIVE PROPERTIES

Stem bark : Hypoglycaemic, antiprotozoal, menorrhagia, fertility in women, diarrhoea, diabetes, dysentery, unusual and painful menstruation
Flower : Diarrhoea
Latex : Diabetes, fever, gonorrhoea, cuts, muscle pain
Leaf juice : Paralysis, gonorrhoea
Galls : CVS active
Ripen fruits : General debility, leucorrhoea
Root : Prevents abortion

262. *Ficus religiosa* L.

Family : Moraceae
Common names : S: Asvatthah H: Pipal E: Peepal tree
Description : Tree, leaves ovate-rotund, cusp linear, receptacles depressed globose, in axillary pairs.

USEFUL PARTS AND THEIR CURATIVE PROPERTIES

Bark : Hypoglycaemic, gonorrhoea, laxative, burns, skin diseases
Stem bark : Antiprotozoal, anthelmintic, antiviral, black patches on the face, jaundice, swelling due to ulcers, toothache, sores, leucorrhoea, paralysis, gonorrhoea, diarrhoea, snake bite
Whole plant : Diseases of blood, vagina, uterus, region of leucorrhoea, burning sensation, biliousness, ulcers
Ripe fruit : Cooling, alexipharmic, good for burning sensation, foul taste, thirst, diseases of the blood and heart
Root : Gout, malaria, conception
Root bark : Stomatitis, cleanses ulcers, as an astringent, vomiting
Young bark : Bone fractures
Seeds : Urinary discharge
Leaf juice : Earache, cardiotonic

263. *Flacourtia indica* (Burm. f.) Merr.

Family : Flacourtiaceae
Common names : S: Svadukantaka H: Baichi E: Madgascar plum
Description : Small tree; branchlets sparsely armed. Leaves spiral, oblong, orbicular or obovate, coriaceous, tomentose on nerves above, glabrous below, cuneate, crenate, retuse. Flowers creamy. Drupe globose, seeds obovoid.

USEFUL PARTS AND THEIR CURATIVE PROPERTIES

Root : Body pains, bronchial allergy, blood pressure, skin affections, dysentery, expectorant, stomach heat, excess body heat, snake bite

Leaf juice : Jaundice, hepatic stimulant, diarrhoea

Stem bark paste : Rheumatic pains, leucorrhoea, menstrual disorders, chest pain, backache

264. *Flemingia strobilifera* (L.) R. Br. ex Ait.

Family : Papilionaceae

Common names : H: Kanphuti

Description : Erect undershrub. Branches striate and pubescent. Leaves simple, ovate - lanceolate, glabrous, gland-dotted, round, entire, apex acuminate. Flowers white in axillary and terminal racemes. Pods oblong, enclosed by bract, 2-seeded.

USEFUL PARTS AND THEIR CURATIVE PROPERTIES

Root paste : Inducing sleep, stomach flank pains, diarrhoea, constipation

265. *Foeniculum vulgare* Mill.

Family : Apiaceae

Common names : S: Madhurika H: Badhesoppu E: Fennel

Description : Stout erect, aromatic herb. Leaves pinnate, flowers small yellow, fragrant in compound terminal umbels. Fruits oblong, slightly curved.

USEFUL PARTS AND THEIR CURATIVE PROPERTIES

Fruit : Emollient, expectorant, haematinic, ophthalmic, carminative, stomachic, galactagogue, diuretic, febrifuge, aphrodisiac, tonic, cough, bronchitis, anaemia, dyspepsia, flatulence, dysentery, haemorrhoids, dysuria, fever

Uses : Culinary purposes, drugs, flavouring, perfumery

266. *Fritillaria roylei* Hook. f.

Family : Liliaceae

Common names : S: Kakoli H: Kakoli E: Fritillary

Description : A glabrous bulbous unbranched herb. Leaves opposite, linear, hooked. Flowers yellowish green, dull purple. Fruits obovoid, 6-angled capsules. Seeds winged.

USEFUL PARTS AND THEIR CURATIVE PROPERTIES

Bulbs : Refrigerant, galactagogue, expectorant, aphrodisiac, diuretic, tonic, antipyretic, cough, bronchitis, hyperdypsia, intermittent fevers, rheumatalgia

267. *Garcinia gummi-gutta* (L.) Robs.

Family : Clusiaceae

Common names : S: Vrksamlah H: Bilatti-amli

Description : A moderate sized evergreen tree. Leaves simple, opposite, dark green, shining. Flowers tetramerous, polygamous in fascicles. Fruits ovoid, yellow. Seeds 6-8, arillate.

USEFUL PARTS AND THEIR CURATIVE PROPERTIES

Leaves / fruits : Astringent, thermogenic, constipating, digestive, ulcers, colic, diarrhoea, dysentery, flatulence, dyspepsia, hyperdypsia, piles

268. *Gardenia turgida* Roxb.

Family : Rubiaceae

Common names : S: Bharangi H: Thanella

Description : Trees or shrubs, armed. Leaves obovate. flowers dimorphic, males in fascicles, females solitary, calyx lobed or cleft. Corolla 5 or more. Stamens as many as corolla lobes. Ovary 1-celled, ovules numerous. Fruit berry. Seeds many.

USEFUL PARTS AND THEIR CURATIVE PROPERTIES

Extract : Antiviral, hypotensive and anticancer

Root : Spermatorrhoea, induce abortion

Fruit : Conception

269. *Garuga pinnata* Roxb.

Family : Burseraceae

Common names : S: Garngudi H: Khogar E: Garuga

Description : Large tree upto 18 m, leaves crowded towards the ends of branches, spiral, imparipinnate, leaflets 4-8 pairs, opposite, oblong, ovate-lanceolate, puberulous with characteristic fruit-like reddish galls, oblique or cuneate, apex acuminate. Flowers cream or yellow, in large terminal panicles. Drupes oblong, horned, pyrenes 2 or 3. Seed solitary.

USEFUL PARTS AND THEIR CURATIVE PROPERTIES

Leaf : Astringent, asthma, burns and wounds

Bark : Antidiabetic, wounds, stomach pain, fractured bone

270. *Gaultheria fragrantissima* Wall.

Family : Ericaceae

Common names : S: Hemant-harit H: Gandhapur-ka-til E: Winter green

Description : Shrubs, leaves alternate, flowers in racemes or solitary, calyx 5, corolla 5. Stamens 10, ovary 5-celled, fruit 5-celled capsule. Seeds many.

USEFUL PARTS AND THEIR CURATIVE PROPERTIES

Uses : Oil mixed with massaging agents counters irritation, stomach worms, stimulates digestive juices, carminative, flavouring agent in cool drinks, lemon drops, tooth pastes, ingredient in mosquito, houseflies, and other insect repellants.

271. *Gendarussa vulgaris* Nees

Family : Acanthaceae

Common names : S: Krishna nirgundi H: Nili-nargandi E: Black purification plant

Description : Erect undershrub to 2 cm; branchlets dark purple, terete, smooth. Leaves oblong - lanceolate, gradually tapering at ends. Flowers clustered in terminal spikes. Corolla white with purple lines.

USEFUL PARTS AND THEIR CURATIVE PROPERTIES

Leaf : Earache and skin eruptions

272. *Gentiana kurroo* Royle

Family : Gentianaceae

Common names : S: Trayamana H: Trayaman E: Indian gentian

Description : A small perennial decumbent herb. Leaves radical. Flowers blue spotted, racemose clusters. Fruits oblong capsules.

USEFUL PARTS AND THEIR CURATIVE PROPERTIES

Rhizomes : Thermogenic, digestive, carminative, anthelmintic, laxative, diuretic, colic, flatulence, leprosy, cardiac debility, dysmenorrhoea, ulcers, wounds, skin diseases, constipation, helminthiasis

273. *Geodorum densiflorum* (Lam.) Schltr.

Family : Orchidaceae

Description : Stout, terrestrial herb with swollen root stock. Stem short, stout, arising laterally from the underground root stock with tubular sheaths at base. Leaves elliptic, acute. Inflorescence crowded raceme; scape thick arise from the side of the fresh off-shoot, covered by sheaths. Flowers purplish white.

USEFUL PARTS AND THEIR CURATIVE PROPERTIES

Tuber : Ephemeral fever, insect bite

274. *Gloriosa superba* L.

Family : Liliaceae

Common names : S: Langali H: Karkari E: Malabar glory lilly

Description : Herbaceous, annual climber. Root stocks tuberous. Leaves subsessile. Leaf tip modified into tendrils. Flowers orange red, solitary stamens. Fruit capsule. Seeds many, globose, warty.

USEFUL PARTS AND THEIR CURATIVE PROPERTIES

Rhizome : Oxytocic, vermicide, chronic fevers, abortion

Fresh plant juice : Uterine stimulant

Root : Antibiotic, delivery, periodic fever, abortifacient, rheumatism, gonorrhoea, scorpion sting, Pirhi disease, leucoderma

Tuber : Termination of 2-3 months old foetus, gonorrhoea, hernea, rheumatism, leprosy, chicken pox, stomach pain, piles, cough, pinworms, ulcers, arthritis

Leaf juice : Lice eradication, dandruff, skin diseases, gonorrhoea, snake bite
Leaf paste : Asthma in children, scorpion sting, piles

275. *Glycosmis arborea* (Roxb.) DC.

Family : Rutaceae
Common names : S: Kupiluh H: Girgiti
Description : An aromatic shrub. Leaves compound, imparipinnate, alternate, entire. Flowers small, white in axillary panicles. Fruits yellowish white. Seeds globose.

USEFUL PARTS AND THEIR CURATIVE PROPERTIES

Whole plant : Astringent, febrifuge, anti-inflammatory, fever, cough, bronchitis
Roots : Facial inflammations, rheumatism, jaundice, anaemia
Leaves : Fever, hepatopathy, eczema, skin diseases, wounds
Fruits : Cough, bronchitis

276. *Glycyrrhiza glabra* L.

Family : Papilionaceae
Common names : S: Madhuyashti H: Mulethi E: Liquorice
Description : Tall perennial undershrub. Leaves compound. Flowers violet in racemes. Pods oblong to linear, flattened, seeds reniform.

USEFUL PARTS AND THEIR CURATIVE PROPERTIES

Dried roots : Dried roots and underground stems constitute the drug liquorice. This is used in cough, sore throat, bronchitis, abdominal pains, constipation, epilepsy, urination, diuretic, excessive menstruation, jaundice, fever, skin diseases

277. *Gmelina arborea* Roxb.

Family : Verbenaceae
Common names : S: Gamhari H: Gamhar E: Candahar tree
Description : Unarmed, deciduous tree. Tender parts fulvous tomentose. Leaves broadly ovate, cordate, subcoriaceous, apex obtuse to acute. Corolla brownish yellow. Drupe yellow.

USEFUL PARTS AND THEIR CURATIVE PROPERTIES

Stem wood/ bark : Hypoglycaemic
Leaf : Lice eradication, scorpion sting, ulcers
Stem bark : Antiviral, malarial fever, chest pain
Ripen fruits : Increase potency, dysentery, diarrhoea, dandruff
Root decoction : Galactagogue

278. *Gmelina asiatica* L.

Family : Verbenaceae
Common names : H: Badhara E: Small cashmere tree
Description : Armed shrub. Leaves elliptic, ovate, cuneate, apex obtuse to acute, glaucous below. Racemes axillary and terminal. Corolla golden yellow. Drupe yellow.

USEFUL PARTS AND THEIR CURATIVE PROPERTIES

Stem bark paste : Rheumatism
Fruit : Skin eruptions, dandruff, wounds, swellings, inflammations, hair tonic
Root : Toothache

279. *Gnetum ula* Brogn.

Family : Gnetaceae
Common names : S: Kumbal
Description : A large robust climber. Bark thick, brown, rough with scales. Branchlets slender with thickened nodes. Leaves ovate-oblong. Fruit reddish-orange.

USEFUL PARTS AND THEIR CURATIVE PROPERTIES

Aerial parts : Spasmolytic and hypotensive extract
Leaves : Pains, lactogenic
Seed : Stomach pains, fevers

280. *Gossypium herbaceum* L.

Family : Malvaceae
Common names : S: Karpasah H: Kapas E: Indian cotton
Description : Shrub; leaves sub-orbicular, 3-5 lobed; flowers axillary, solitary. Capsules ovoid, acute.

USEFUL PARTS AND THEIR CURATIVE PROPERTIES

Aerial part : Diuretic, oxytocic
Leaf : Antibacterial, earache, intestinal worms
Seed extract : Galactagogue, demulscent, mild laxative, diabetes, abortifacient, nervine tonic

281. *Grangea maderaspatana* Poir.

Family : Asteraceae
Common names : S: Mustaru H: Mukhatari E: Madras warm weed
Description : Herbs. Villous, leaves alternate, heterogamous heads, corollas of female flowers filiform. Bisexual flowers campanulate. Anthers produced at apex. Fruit achene.

USEFUL PARTS AND THEIR CURATIVE PROPERTIES

Plant extract : Spasmol, antifertility and hypotension
Roots : Galactagogue, appetizer
Leaf : Earache

282. *Grewia tiliifolia* Vahl

Family : Tiliaceae
Common names : S: Dhanvangah H: Dhamni E: Dhaman
Description : A medium sized tree. Leaves simple, alternate, ovate. Flowers yellow. Fruits globose drupes, black. Seeds 1-2.

USEFUL PARTS AND THEIR CURATIVE PROPERTIES

Bark	:	Astringent, expectorant, constipating, emetic, styptic, tonic, aphrodisiac, burning sensation, cough, skin diseases, wounds, ulcers, diarrhoea
Fruits	:	Cooling, general debility

283. *Gymnema sylvestre* (Retz.) R. Br. ex Schultes

Family	:	Asclepiadaceae
Common names	:	S: Meshasringi H: Meshasingi E: Periploca of the woods
Description	:	Large woody climber running over the tops of small trees. Leaves elliptic to obovate, pubescent along nerves below, obtuse, apex abruptly acute. Flowers dull yellow in axillary cymes.

USEFUL PARTS AND THEIR CURATIVE PROPERTIES

Leaf	:	Antidiabetic, insulinotropic, chronic fever, bone fracture, asthma, corneal opacity, regularization of menstruation, snake bite, malaria, liver and spleen infections, laxative, diuretic, scorpion sting, cataract, jaundice
Whole plant	:	Parkinsonism
Root extract	:	Eye diseases, snake bites, galactagogue, lactagogue, scorpion sting
Fruits	:	Diabetes, labour pains

284. *Habenaria edgeworthii* Hook. f. ex Collett.

Family	:	Orchidaceae
Common names	:	S: Rddhi H: Rddhi
Description	:	A tuberous herb. Leaves sheathing, ovate. Flowers yellowish green, spur longer than ovary. Ovary glabrous, twisted.

USEFUL PARTS AND THEIR CURATIVE PROPERTIES

Tubers	:	Refrigerant, emollient, aphrodisiac, depurative, appetizer, anthelmintic, hyperdypsia, fever, cough, asthma, insanity, leprosy, skin diseases, gout, general debility, anorexia

285. *Hedyotis corymbosa* (L.) Lam.

Family	:	Rubiaceae
Common names	:	S: Parpata H: Daman pappar
Description	:	Diffuse herb upto 30 cm. Leaves decussate, linear-lanceolate, revolute, apex acute. Flowers generally 3, often in stalked pairs. Corolla white to pinkish. Capsule loculicidal.

USEFUL PARTS AND THEIR CURATIVE PROPERTIES

Whole plant	:	Dysentery, trypanosomiasis

286. *Helicteres isora* L.

Family	:	Sterculiaceae
Common names	:	S: Avaratam H: Maraphali E: East Indian Screw Tree
Description	:	Shrub or small tree with grey bark and red flowers, turning pale blue when red. Fruits 5 spirally twisted follicles, pubescent.

USEFUL PARTS AND THEIR CURATIVE PROPERTIES

Fruit : Mild uterine stimulant, roundworms in children, earache, stomach pain, cough, diarrhoea, dysentery, malnutrition, polio, astringent, colic, flatulence, scabies, diabetes, ulcers, vermifuge

Aerial part : Spasmolytic

Stem bark : Cold, cough, fever in children, headache, retained placenta in women in child birth, antidote for snake bite, wounds

Seed paste : Ulcers in ear, snake bite, dysentery, stomach pain

Root : Diabetes, infantile diarrhoea, dysentery, snake bite, dog bite, chest pain, cholera, asthma, cough, sciatica, wounds, fractures, postnatal pains

287. *Heliotropium indicum* L.

Family : Boraginaceae

Common names : S: Srihastini H: Siriyari E: Heliotrope

Description : Herb with woody base; branches hirsute. Leaves broadly elliptic ovate, truncate to attenuate, undulate, apex acute. Lateral nerves 6 pairs spikes terminal or leaf–opposed. Corolla white to bluish. Nutlets combined in pairs, angled, beaked above.

USEFUL PARTS AND THEIR CURATIVE PROPERTIES

Leaf : Anticancer, antifungal, cuts, scorpion and insect stings, ulcerous wounds

Seed : Snake bite

288. *Heliotropium subulatum* (DC.) Vatke

Family : Boraginaceae

Description : Erect herb. Leaves linear- lanceolate, cuneate, revolute, apex acute, 1-nerved; racemes axillary or terminal, profusely branched; flowers white or blue. Nutlets sparsely hairy.

USEFUL PARTS AND THEIR CURATIVE PROPERTIES

Leaf paste : Cuts, ulcerous wounds, boils, scorpion sting

Seeds : Antidote for snake bite

289. *Hemidesmus indicus* (L.) R. Br.

Family : Asclepiadaceae

Common names : S: Sariva H: Salsa E: Indian Sarsapilla

Description : Twining perennial shrub. Leaves linear to lanceolate, blotched above, pubescent beneath, margin often folded back, obtuse or broadly acute. Flowers yellowish brown in subsessile cymes in the opposite axils.

USEFUL PARTS AND THEIR CURATIVE PROPERTIES

Oil from roots : Antibacterial

Plant : Antiviral

Roots : Fever, skin diseases, loss of appetite, syphilis, leucorrhoea, nephrocalcinosis, stomach pain, diarrhoea, stomach ulcers, lactation,

		menstrual disorders, cholera, galactagogue, carious teeth, dysentery, gonorrhoea, health tonic, malaria, eczema, arthritis, scorpion sting, menorrhagia, excess of heat, foot cracks, urinary disorders, debility, body pains, snake bite, stimulant drink, blood purification, nausea
Tuber	:	Diabetes

290. *Hemigraphis latebrosa* (Heyne ex Roth) Nees

Family	:	Acanthaceae
Description	:	Erect to straggling herb to 50 cm. Stems faintly angled, hairy. Leaves ovate, crenate-serrate, apex acuminate. Flowers pale blue, in axillary, peduncled cymes. Corolla funnel-shaped. Capsules tetragonous, 6-seeded, pubescent.

USEFUL PARTS AND THEIR CURATIVE PROPERTIES

Leaf	:	Heals the cuts caused by iron knives

291. *Heterostemma deccanense* (Talb.) Swarup. & Mangaly

Family	:	Asclepiadaceae
Description	:	Wiry climber; branches pubescent, latex milky. Leaves opposite, thick, obovate to obtuse or rounded, apex acute to acuminate, glabrous, basal nerves 7 pairs, spreading. Flowers small, in subsessile to pedunculate cymes arising between the petioles; calyx lobes ovate, obtuse; corolla ovoid-urceolate, coronal scales rounded. Follicles 2, divergent. Seeds 8-12, imbricated in 2 rows.

USEFUL PARTS AND THEIR CURATIVE PROPERTIES

Root	:	Kidney troubles and stomachache

292. *Hibiscus rosa-sinensis* L.

Family	:	Malvaceae
Common names	:	S: Japa H: Jasum E: Chinese hibiscus
Description	:	Shrub, leaves obovate-lanceolate, flowers crimson, solitary, fruit oblong, but not reaching maturity

USEFUL PARTS AND THEIR CURATIVE PROPERTIES

Aerial part	:	Hypotensive, spasmolytic, CNS depressant, hypothermic
Petals	:	Antiimplantation, asthma, irritable conditions of genito-urinary tract, refrigerant drink in fevers, demulscent in cough, swells, boils
Flower	:	Antiestrogenic, antispermatogenic, abortifacient, hair tonic, jaundice, menorrhagia, impotency, bronchitis, gastroenteritis, mumps, syphilis
Flower / roots	:	Resorptive
Leaf	:	Anti-inflammatory, analgesic, antipyretic, blood tumours on the body, boils, carbuncles, alopecia, dandruff, syphilis
Root	:	Antifungal
Buds	:	Seminal weakness
Stem bark	:	Epilepsy

293. *Hiptage benghalensis* (L.) Kurz

Family : Malphigiaceae

Common names : S: Madhavi H: Madhavilata E: Clustered hiptage

Description : A large woody, evergreen, climbing shrub. Leaves simple, opposite, elliptic, ovate. Flowers yellowish white, fragrant, racemes. Fruits 2-3 winged samara.

USEFUL PARTS AND THEIR CURATIVE PROPERTIES

Bark, leaves : Aromatic, astringent, refrigerant expectorant, and flowers cardiotonic, anti-inflammatory, wounds, ulcers, cough, asthma, leprosy, skin diseases, scabies, rheumatism, hyperdypsia

294. *Holarrhena pubescens* Wall. ex G. Don.

Family : Apocynaceae

Common names : S: Kutajah H: Karchi E: Kurchi tree

Description : Large shrub to small tree to 6 m; bark brown, rough. Leaves elliptic-oblong, glabrous, broadly rounded, apex shortly acuminate. Cymes paniculate or corymbose, terminal and axillary. Corolla white. Follicles paired.

USEFUL PARTS AND THEIR CURATIVE PROPERTIES

Conessine : Antitubercular, amoebicidal

Conkurchine hydrochloride : Hypotensive, vasodilator

Fruit : Spasmolytic, muscular pain, hepatic stimulant

Stem bark : CVS active, tonic, febrifuge, anti-dysenteric, expectorant, digestive, cures piles, trouble of biles, leprosy, arthritis, fever, asthma, body swellings, diarrhoea, malaria, headache, astringent, liver tonic, amoebic dysentery, boils, cough, cold

Seed oil : Antifungal

Seeds : Antidote against poison, relieves pain and swelling in snake-bites, fever, intestinal worms, dysentery, antitetanic, stomachic, carminative, diarrhoea, kidney stones

Root : Acute stomach pain, leucorrhoea, anthelmintic, ulcers, stomach disorders, easy delivery, rheumatism, gout, paralysis, stomach ulcers

Leaf : Joint pains, piles, arthritis, lactagogue, haemorrhages, dental caries

Latex : Cuts, wounds, eczema, skin diseases, ringworm

Flower : Leucoderma

295. *Holoptelea integrifolia* (Roxb.) Planch.

Family : Ulmaceae

Common names : S: Cirabilvah H: Papri/Kanju E: Indian elm

Description : Large deciduous tree, tender parts pubescent. Leaves distichous, elliptic, ovate, apex acute, flattened above. Fruit dry winged.

USEFUL PARTS AND THEIR CURATIVE PROPERTIES

Whole plant : Antidiabetic and antiobesity
Stem bark : Piles, rheumatic swellings, scabies, asthma, juice dysmenorrhoea, remove pus from boils, fractured bone, fertility
Leaves : Wounds, boils, jaundice, puerperal fever, blisters
Bark : Hydrocele, abortion, oxytocic, scabies, ringworm, rheumatism.

296. *Holostemma ada-kodien* Schult.

Family : Asclepiadaceae
Common names : S: Jivanti H: Chirvel
Description : A laticiferous twining shrub. Leaves simple, opposite, cordate. Flowers purple in axillary umbellate cymes. Fruits thick follicles.

USEFUL PARTS AND THEIR CURATIVE PROPERTIES

Roots : Refrigerant, ophthalmic, emollient, alterant, tonic, stimulant, aphrodisiac, cough, fever, stomachalgia, burning sensation

297. *Hugonia mystax* L.

Family : Linaceae
Common names : S: Kamsamarah E: Climbing flax
Description : A rambling scandent shrub. Leaves simple, alternate, elliptic. Flowers yellow, pedicels short. Fruits globose fleshy drupes. Seeds 2 or 3 compressed.

USEFUL PARTS AND THEIR CURATIVE PROPERTIES

Roots : Astringent, febrifuge, anthelmintic, fevers, verminosis, inflammations

298. *Humulus lupulus* L.

Family : Cannabinaceae
Common names : E: Hops

USEFUL PARTS AND THEIR CURATIVE PROPERTIES

Uses : Oil for flavouring, clarifying, giving sparkle to beer, tobacco flavours, used in mineral waters

299. *Hybanthus enneaspermus* (L.) F. v. Muell

Family : Violaceae
Common names : S: Charati H: Ratan purus
Description : Small perennial erect herb. Leaves simple, linear-ovate, attenuate, serrate, apex acute. Flowers pink, axillary, solitary; the lowest petal largest with spurred claw and broad limb. Capsule 8-12 seeded.
Description :
Root : Diuretic, reduces body heat, fever, obesity
Leaves : Demulscent, snake bite
Whole plant : Increase potency, gastric disorders, antidote for (powder) snake bite, sex tonic, aphrodisiac, stomach pain, leucoderma
Seed : Snake bite

300. ***Hydnocarpus laurifolia*** **(Dennst.) Sleumer**

Family : Flacourtiaceae

Common names : S: Tuvarakah H: Calmogara E: Marothi tree

Description : Medium sized evergreen tree. Leaves simple, alternate, ovate, oblong, serrate. Flowers small, greenish white, racemes. Fruits globose berries.

USEFUL PARTS AND THEIR CURATIVE PROPERTIES

Seeds : Astringent, thermogenic, emollient, anodyne, purgative, leucoderma, skin diseases, pruritis, chronic ulcers, dyspepsia, colic, flatulence, diabetes, wounds, verminosis, eczema, haematinic

301. ***Hygrophila schulli*** **(Ham.) Almeida & Almeida**

Family : Acanthaceae

Common names : S: Kokilaksha H: Gokula-kanta E: Long-leaved barleria

Description : Erect armed, strigose-hispid herb to 70 cm, generally with three whorls of 8 leaves and 4 long and 2 small thorns at each node. Outer pair larger, lanceolate, cuneate, apex acute, subsessile. Flowers in axillary whorls. Corolla pink or bluish - purple. Seeds orbicular, hygroscopic.

USEFUL PARTS AND THEIR CURATIVE PROPERTIES

Leaf : Spasmol, hypotensive, rheumatism, gonorrhoea, chronic piles, jaundice

Root : Fever, swelling of face and entire body, jaundice

Seed : Gonorrhoea, spermatorrhoea, jaundice

302. ***Hyoscyamus niger*** **L.**

Family : Solanaceae

Common names : S: Parasikayavani H: Khurasani ajavayan E: Henbane

Description : An erect, foetid, annual herb. Leaves small, sessile, ovate. Flowers yellowish green. Fruits capsules, globose. Seeds numerous, minute, kidney shaped.

USEFUL PARTS AND THEIR CURATIVE PROPERTIES

Leaves / seeds : Thermogenic, anodyne, anthelmintic, expectorant, scabies, rheumatoid arthritis, epilepsy, whooping cough, fever, insomnia, catarrh, spermatorrhoea, dysmenorrhoea, dental caries

303. ***Hyptis suaveolens*** **(L.) Poit.**

Family : Lamiaceae

Common names : S: Bhustrna H: Vilaiti-Tulsi E: Hyptis

Description : Aromatic, erect, undershrub to 3 m; branches terete to tetragonous, ovate, strigose, base obliquely truncate to acute, irregularly serrulate, acute. Flowers in verticils or in short, stalked cymes of 6 flowers, corolla blue. Nutlets 2, ovoid or oblong.

USEFUL PARTS AND THEIR CURATIVE PROPERTIES

Leaf : Cuts by iron tools, wounds and tumours due to excess of heat

Seeds : Gonorrhoea, ulcers

Root paste : Fever

304. ***Ichnocarpus frutescens*** **(L.) R. Br.**

Family : Apocynaceae

Common names : S: Shariva H: Siama-lota E: Black creeper

Description : Evergreen, climbing shrub. Leaves variable, elliptic, oblong, ovate. Inflorescence rusty villous. Flowers greenish white.

USEFUL PARTS AND THEIR CURATIVE PROPERTIES

Root : Aphrodisiac, blood purifier and minimises excess of heat, fever, epilepsy, dysentery

Whole plant : Bone fractures

Leaf : Diabetes, sprain or local pain

305. ***Illicium verum*** **Hook. f.**

Family : Magnoliaceae

Common names : S: Takkolakam H: Anasphal E: Star anise of China

Description : An evergreen tree. Leaves simple, entire, oblanceolate. Flowers white or red. Fruit star shaped, 8-carpels. Seeds ovoid, compressed, shiny.

USEFUL PARTS AND THEIR CURATIVE PROPERTIES

Fruits : Aromatic, carminative, digestive, stomachic, expectorant, deodorant, dyspepsia, flatulence, dysentery, cough, asthma, rheumarthritis, paralysis

306. ***Indigofera cassioides*** **Rottb. ex DC.**

Family : Papilionaceae

Description : Deciduous, grey-pubescent shrub. Leaflets 13-23, opposite, rarely spiral, elliptic-oblong, obtuse, emarginate. Raceme 15-20 flowered. Pod straight, cylindric, 10-12 seeded.

USEFUL PARTS AND THEIR CURATIVE PROPERTIES

Extract of root : Antiviral and spasmol, stomachache, preventing conception, haematuria, asthma

307. ***Indigofera tinctoria*** **L.**

Family : Papilionaceae

Common names : S: Nilini H: Nil E: Indian Indigo

Description : Shrub. Leaves with 7-13 leaflets, tender branches bluish red in colour, flowers red or pink. Fruit cylindrical. Pods greenish grey when young and dark brown on ripening. Seeds 10-12.

USEFUL PARTS AND THEIR CURATIVE PROPERTIES

Alcoholic : Useful in liver damage extract

Aerial part : Hypoglycaemic, CNS depressant

Root : Jaundice, scorpion sting, urinary complaints, wounds infested with worms and on foul ulcers, asthma, bronchitis, antidote to arsenic poisoning

Leaf paste : Rabies, severe toothache

308. *Inula racemosa* Hook. f.

Family : Asteraceae

Common names : S: Pauskaram H: Pohakarmul

Description : A stout herb with grooved stem. Leaves simple, alternate, leathery, hairy. Flowers yellow, heads, tips triangular. Fruits slender achenes with pappus.

USEFUL PARTS AND THEIR CURATIVE PROPERTIES

Roots : Thermogenic, aromatic, stimulant, antiseptic, deodorant, anodyne, expectorant, aphrodisiac, emmenagogue, hiccough, cough, skin diseases, febrifuge, tonic, flatulence, cardiac debility, amenorrhoea.

309. *Ipomaea aquatica* Forsk.

Family : Convolvulaceae

Common names : S: Kalambi H: Kalmisag E: Water spinach

Description : Large prostrate herb; rooting at nodes, branchlets usually floating. Leaves lanceolate to hastate, apex acuminate, basal nodes triangular acute or obtuse. Flower solitary or in cymes, pink.

USEFUL PARTS AND THEIR CURATIVE PROPERTIES

Leaf : Increase potency, skin disorders

310. *Ipomaea obscura* (L.) Ker. – Gowl.

Family : Convolvulaceae

Common names : S: Laksmana

Description : Slender twining herb. Leaves cordate, glabrescent above, villous below, acuminate, often with reddish scars. Flowers pale yellow with purple base, axillary, solitary or in sub umbellate cymes.

USEFUL PARTS AND THEIR CURATIVE PROPERTIES

Leaf : Aphrodisiac, bone fracture

311. *Jasminum arborescens* Roxb.

Family : Oleaceae

Common names : S: Nagamalli H: Cameli E: Tree jasmine

Description : A large suberect shrub. Leaves simple, opposite, acuminate. Flowers white, fragrant, in pubescent panicles. Fruit single, ellipsoid, black, berry.

USEFUL PARTS AND THEIR CURATIVE PROPERTIES

Leaves : Astringent, refrigerant, stomachic, emetic, tonic, menstrual disorders, colic, flatulence, cough and general debility

Uses : Cosmetics, flavouring, perfumery

312. *Jasminum auriculatum* Vahl

Family : Oleaceae

Common names : S: Magadhi H: Juhi E: Needle flower jasmine

Description : A scandent pubescent shrub. Leaves trifoliate, acuminate or rounded. Petioles very short. Flowers white, sweet scented, in paniculate cymes. Fruits globose.

USEFUL PARTS AND THEIR CURATIVE PROPERTIES

Root : Skin diseases especially ringworm

Flowers : Refrigerant, astringent, cardiotonic, diuretic, depurative, ulcers, strangury, dermatopathy, hyperdypsia

Uses : Cosmetics, flavouring, perfumery

313. *Jasminum grandiflorum* L.

Family : Oleaceae

Common names : S: Mallika H: Juhi E: Jasmine

Description : A large glabrous, evergreen shrub. Leaves imparipinnately compound, opposite, acute or acuminate. Flowers very fragrant, white in axillary cymes. Fruits elliptic, globose, berries.

USEFUL PARTS AND THEIR CURATIVE PROPERTIES

Flowers : Perfume oil, cosmetics, flavouring, perfumery

Plant : Astringent, thermogenic, aphrodisiac, antiseptic, anodyne, diuretic, tonic

Roots : Cephalalgia, paralysis, mental debility, chronic constipation, flatulence, sterility, dysmenorrhoea, amenorrhoea, leprosy, giddiness

Leaves : Stomatitis, skin diseases, otalgia, strangury, ulcers, wounds and corns

Flowers : Refrigerant, pruritus, stomatopathy, ophthalmic, dysmenorrhoea

314. *Jasminum multiflorum* (Burm. f.) Andr.

Family : Oleaceae

Common names : S: Kundah H: Kundphul E: Downy jasmine

Description : Large scandent shrub. Leaves simple, opposite, ovate, petioles villous. Flowers white, slightly fragrant, sessile in capitate cymes. Fruits black, globose berries.

USEFUL PARTS AND THEIR CURATIVE PROPERTIES

Leaves : Indolent ulcers.

Flowers : Refrigerant, laxative, cardiotonic, digestive, inflammations, cephalalgia, rheumatism

Uses : Cosmetics, flavouring, perfumery

315. *Jasminum sambac* (L.) Ait.

Family : Oleaceae

Common names : S: Mallika H: Moghra E: Arabian jasmine

Description : Suberect or climbing shrub. Leaves simple, opposite, elliptic, acute. Flowers white, very fragrant, solitary or in cymes, calyx lobes curved. Fruits berries, black when ripe.

USEFUL PARTS AND THEIR CURATIVE PROPERTIES

Roots : Ophthalmopathy
Leaves : Skin diseases, ulcers, fever
Flowers : Refrigerant, ophthalmic, purgative, cephalalgia, leprosy, ulcers, fever, vomiting, hiccough, insanity, galactorrhoea
Uses : Cosmetics, flavouring, perfumery

316. *Jatropha curcas* L.

Family : Euphorbiaceae
Common names : S: Dravanti H: Safed-arnad E: Purging nut
Description : Deciduous shrub to small tree of 3 m, bark smooth, whitish green, peeling of thin flakes, leaves orbicular. Flowers unisexual, yellowish-green in axillary cymes. Pedicels and peduncles tomentose; outer petals equal in staminate flowers and unequal in pistillate flowers.

USEFUL PARTS AND THEIR CURATIVE PROPERTIES

Seed : Highly toxic, muscular pains, body swellings, purgative, helminthiasis, piles, abortion
Root : Toothache, sore throat, intestinal ulcers, wounds
Aerial part : CNS depressant, diuretic
Latex : Acute headache, blisters, earache, rotting of teeth, dysentery, lymph gland swelling, measles, burns, eczema, diarrhoea
Tender stem : Toothache, hardens the gums, dysentery, ulcers, wounds, dermatitis
Leaves : Inflammations, dysentery, eczema
Bark : Leprosy, rheumatism, sprains, cough

317. *Jatropha gossypifolia* L.

Family : Euphorbiaceae
Common names : S: Raktaeramada H: Bherenda E: Tua-tua
Description : Shrub to 1.5 m; branchlets glandular hairy. Leaves in close spirals, deeply 3-5 lobed, subcordate, lobes obovate, glandular hairy, apex acute. Flowers in axillary cymes. Capsules 3-lobed, seeds oblong, carunculate.

USEFUL PARTS AND THEIR CURATIVE PROPERTIES

Plant : Hypothermic, CNS depressant, toothache, tonsilitis, tongue inflammation
Leaves : Boils, itches, skin diseases
Latex : Honorrhoea, leucorrhoea, piles, boils, burns, toothache, body pain, syphilis, wounds
Seed : Insecticidal, antileukaemic
Root paste : Menstrual pain
Stem bark : Blood dysentery, diarrhoea

318. *Juglans regia* L.

Family : Juglandaceae
Common names : S: Aksotah H: Akhor E: Common walnut

Description : Large deciduous tree. Leaves alternate, imparipinnate. Leaflets aromatic. Flowers small, yellowish green, in slender catkins. Fruits drupes.

USEFUL PARTS AND THEIR CURATIVE PROPERTIES

Leaves : Astringent, tonic, anthelmintic, herpes, eczema, scrofula, syphilis
Fruits : Emollient, ther mogenic, aphrodisiac, tonic, carminative, rheumatism
Kernels : Colic and dysentery

319. *Juniperus communis* L.

Family : Coniferae
Common names : E: Juniper

USEFUL PARTS AND THEIR CURATIVE PROPERTIES

Diterpene phenol : Totarol isolated from bark
Uses : Cosmetics, perfumery, flavouring

320. *Justicia adhatoda* L.

Family : Acanthaceae
Common names : S: Vasaka H: Arusha E: Vasaca
Description : Large evergreen shrub to 2 m. Leaves oblanceolate, coriaceous, acute to attenuate, entire to minutely crenate, apex acuminate. Spike dense, leafy, axillary. Corolla white. Capsule basally beaked. Seeds 4.

USEFUL PARTS AND THEIR CURATIVE PROPERTIES

Root : Antiviral
Root and leaf : Hypoglycaemic
Alkaloid vasicine : Hypotensive, bronchodilator, respiratory and uterine stimulator, uterotonic, abortifacient
Leaf : Antispasmodic, asthma, cough, cold, psoriasis, dysuria, rheumatism, tuberculosis, bleeding, inflammation, body pain
Inflorescence : Asthma
Shoot : Cough, asthma, bronchitis

321. *Justicia betonica* L.

Family : Acanthaceae
Common names : S: Sahacarah E: Rose-spotted white-flowered justice wort
Description : Erect shrub upto 2 m. Leaves ovate-lanceolate, base acute to attenuate, apex acuminate. Flowers in terminal spikes, bracts and bracteoles with green nerves. corolla greenish-white. Capsule long, clavate, pubescent.

USEFUL PARTS AND THEIR CURATIVE PROPERTIES

Leaf : Cuts, wounds and insect bite
Root : Muscle pains

322. *Kaempferia galanga* L.

Family : Scitamineae
Common names : E: Spiked Ginger Lily
Description : Herbs, stemless, leaves 2. Flowers spikate, calyx as long as outer bracts. Corolla tube obovate. Anthers 2. ovary 3-celled. Fruit capsule.

USEFUL PARTS AND THEIR CURATIVE PROPERTIES

Uses : Tuber - Ayurvedic medicines, expectorant, diuretic, carminative
Rhizome : Aromatic, bitter, stomachache, appetizer, flatulence, hair growth, perfumery

323. *Kalanchoe lanceolata* (Forsk.) Pers.

Family : Crassulaceae
Description : Erect succulent herb, leaves simple, crenate, flowers yellowish white, in dense paniculate cymes, follicles oblong-ellipsoid.

USEFUL PARTS AND THEIR CURATIVE PROPERTIES

Leaves : Stomachache, purgative, diuretic, rheumatism, sprains, antiseptic, wounds, cuts, boils, ulcers, piles, scorpion sting, body swellings
Plant : Siuretic, purgative
Root : Malarial fever

324. *Kalanchoe pinnata* (Lam.) Pers.

Family : Crassulaceae
Common names : S: Asthibhaksha H: Zakhmhaiyat
Description : Subsucculent glabrous herb to 1 m, leaves decussate, crowded in young shoots, distant in adult ones, often 3-5 foliate, oblong or ovate-elliptic, coriaceous, glabrous, greenish, oblique, crenate-dentate, apex obtuse-subacute. Cymes panicled. Corolla 8 folded, reddish.

USEFUL PARTS AND THEIR CURATIVE PROPERTIES

Leaf : Insect bite, cuts and injuries as haemostatic, stomach ache, diarrhoea, wounds, boils, cough, antiseptic, dysentery, cold, small pox, diabetes, reduce pus formation, abscess, ulcers, eye sores
Latex : Cuts, wounds, cough, diarrhoea, eye sores, boils, insect bites

325. *Kyllinga nemoralis* (Forster) Dandy. ex Hutch

Family : Cyperaceae
Common names : S: Svetanirvisa H: Nirbisi
Description : An erect creeping rhizome. Tubers aromatic. Leaves simple, linear, acute. Flowers minute in spikes. Fruits obovoid, compressed nuts, pale reddish brown.

USEFUL PARTS AND THEIR CURATIVE PROPERTIES

Tubers : Fragrant, aromatic, astringent, febrifuge, diuretic, anthelmintic, sudorofic, tonic, demulcent, expectorant, fever, diarrhoea, strangury, cough, tumours, fistula, diabetes, colonopathy

326. ***Lagasca mollis*** **Cav.**

Family	:	Asteraceae
Description	:	Annual slender erect herb to 50 cm. Branches terete, striate, pubescent. Leaves elliptic to ovate, rhomboid, acuminate, serrate, apex acuminate. Head white, a compound capitulum, subtended by leafy bracts. Achenes obovate, 3-angled.

USEFUL PARTS AND THEIR CURATIVE PROPERTIES

Leaf	:	Cuts, wounds, scorpion sting, wasp sting

327. ***Lagerstroemia parviflora*** **Roxb.**

Family	:	Lythraceae
Description	:	Tree, leaves elliptic-obtuse, coriaceous, flowers white, terminal and axillary panicles, petals obovate.

USEFUL PARTS AND THEIR CURATIVE PROPERTIES

Leaves	:	Anthelmintic, dysentery, stomach pain
Root bark	:	Fever
Stem bark	:	Rheumatism

328. ***Lannea coromandelica*** **(Houtt.) Merr.**

Family	:	Anacardiaceae
Common names	:	S: Jhingini H: Jingan E: Wodier
Description	:	Tree, leaves crowded at ends of branches, flowers pale yellow, in branched racemes, drupes oblique, compressed.

USEFUL PARTS AND THEIR CURATIVE PROPERTIES

Plant	:	Antibacterial
Stem bark	:	Anticancer, CNS and CVS active, hypothermic, and leaf bleeding, bone fracture, cuts by iron tools, stomach pain, tumours, chest pain, muscle pain, gastric troubles, fever, expectorant, burns, wounds, headache
Fruits	:	Cold and cough
Gum	:	Diarrhoea, dysentery
Seed	:	Dandruff

329. ***Lantana camara*** **L. (L.) Mold.**

Family	:	Verbenaceae
Common names	:	S: Caturangi H: Lantana E: Wild sage
Description	:	Straggling armed shrub. Leaves crenate-serrate, rugose, hispid above. Flowers pink or orange, in axillary capitate spikes. Drupes ripe in black, globose.

USEFUL PARTS AND THEIR CURATIVE PROPERTIES

Alkaloids	:	Lowered blood pressure, accelerated respiration
Shoot	:	Antibacterial, rheumatism Lantadenes A and B cause toxicity, jaundice, photosensitization, kidney and liver lesions

Lancamarone : Cardioactive
Flower : Giddiness
Leaf juice : Cuts, wounds, tuberculosis, mouth ulcers, fever
Seeds : Antidote for poisoning

330. *Lavendula vera* DC.

Family : Lamiaceae
Common names : H: Lavender E: Lavender
Description : Perennial bushy lower leafless plant. Leaves opposite, long, narrow, lanceolate. Flowers densely packed in whorls. Calyx 5-lobed. Corolla bilabiate.

USEFUL PARTS AND THEIR CURATIVE PROPERTIES

Uses : Cosmetics, perfumery, disinfectants

331. *Lawsonia inermis* L.

Family : Lythraceae
Common names : S: Nakharanjani H:Mehndi E: Henna
Description : Medium-sized, much branched shrub, branches, 4-angled. Flowers greenish white, very fragrant. Seeds many angular, brown.

USEFUL PARTS AND THEIR CURATIVE PROPERTIES

Leaf : Antibacterial, anti-inflammatory and possesses antihyaluronidase-activity, cuts between toes especially during monsoon, gynaecological diseases, leucoderma, burning feet, jaundice, gonorrhoea, syphilis, piles fissures, loose motions, hepatic stimulant, headache, conjunctivitis, debility, hair tonic, spermatorrhoea, pimples
Seed paste : Diarrhoea with blood
Root : Diarrhoea
Bark : Jaundice, enlargement of spleen

332. *Lens culinaris* Medikus

Family : Papilionaceae
Common names : S: Masurah H: Masur E: Lentil
Description : A small erect pubescent herb. Leaves compound, sessile. Flowers white, solitary in racemes. Fruits smooth, compressed, oblong pods. Seeds 2, smooth.

USEFUL PARTS AND THEIR CURATIVE PROPERTIES

Seeds : Refrigerant, astringent, constipating, diuretic, tonic, dysentery, strangury, ulcers, skin diseases, anaemia, general debility

333. *Leonotis nepetaefolia* (L.) R. Br.

Family : Lamiaceae
Common names : S: Granthi H: Hejurchei
Description : Annual erect herb to 2 m; branchlets pubescent. Leaves ovate, base truncate to cuneate, deeply crenate to serrate, acute. Verticils axillary, dense flowered; calyx tubular, spinescent. Corolla orange, bilabiate.

USEFUL PARTS AND THEIR CURATIVE PROPERTIES

Leaf : Crying of infants, leucoderma, diarrhoea
Plant ash : Paralysis
Flowers : Burns, post natal breast pain, skin diseases, sores, wounds
Seed : Malaria

334. *Lepidagathis cristata* Willd.

Family : Acanthaceae
Common names : S: Bhuiteradu
Description : Herbs or undershrubs. Leaves entire. Flowers sessile. Heads. Calyx lobes with dense soft silky hairs. Stamens 4, didynamous. Ovary 2-celled.

USEFUL PARTS AND THEIR CURATIVE PROPERTIES

Leaf juice : Cuts and wounds
Plant : Pus - oozing wounds, controls bleeding, measles, antiallergic, febrifuge, fevers, sores, itches
Tuber paste : Scorpion sting

335. *Lepidium sativum* L.

Family : Brassicaceae
Common names : S: Asalika H: Candsur E: Garden cress
Description : An erect annual herb. Leaves entire, sessile. Flowers white, small, in racemes. Fruits obovate, small pods, 2 seeds per pod.

USEFUL PARTS AND THEIR CURATIVE PROPERTIES

Roots : Secondary syphilis
Leaves : Stimulant, diuretic, hepatopathy, antibacterial
Seeds : Thermogenic, depurative, galactagogue, tonic, aphrodisiac, dysentery, diarrhoea, splenomegaly, leucorrhoea, asthma, cough, hiccough

336. *Leptadenia reticulata* (Retz.) Wt. & Arn.

Family : Asclepiadaceae
Common names : S: Jivanti E: Meda
Description : Twining shrub with watery latex. Leaves elliptic-oblong or lanceolate, chartaceous, base truncate, obtuse or rounded, apex acute; umbellate cymes axillary or terminal. Flowers yellow. Follicles paired, cylindric, bluntly acute at both ends.

USEFUL PARTS AND THEIR CURATIVE PROPERTIES

Stigmasterol and lipoid fraction of the plant : Estrogenomimetic effects
Latex : Scorpion sting, cold
Leaf : Galactagogue, earache, cold, paralysis, joint pains, abortifacient, skin infections

337. *Leucas aspera* (Willd.) Link

Family : Lamiaceae

Common names : S: Drona pushpi H: Chhota-italkusa

Description : Erect or diffuse herb to 50 cm, leaves lanceolate, puberulous, cuneate, entire to serrate, apex acute, verticels terminal and axillary, corolla bilipped, lower lip twice as long as upper lip. Nutlets oblong, smooth, brown.

USEFUL PARTS AND THEIR CURATIVE PROPERTIES

Leaf : Aphrodisiac, eye diseases, headache, malaria, cold, cough, ringworms, urinary disorder, antiemetic, epilepsy, snake bite, skin diseases, rheumatic swellings, sinusitis

Whole plant decoction : Jaundice, bronchitis, fever, antipyretic

Root : Hemicrania

Flower : Asthma, bowel complaints

338. *Leucas cephalotes* (Roth) Spreng

Family : Lamiaceae

Common names : S: Drona pushpi H: Goma

Description : Erect herb upto 40 cm, leaves ovate to lanceolate, membranous, pubescent, crenate-serrate, apex acute. Flowers sessile in large, globose, dense, terminal whorls. Bracts foliaceous, green, lanceolate, acute, awned, corolla bilipped, lower lip not much longer than the upper (bearded) lip. Nutlets dark brown.

USEFUL PARTS AND THEIR CURATIVE PROPERTIES

Leaf : Headache, skin eruptions, migraine, piles, boils on head

Flower seed paste : Pus formation in ears, cold, cough

Whole plant : Malaria

339. *Limnophila aromatica* (L.) Merr.

Family : Scrophulariaceae

Common names : S: Amragandhah H: Kutra

Description : A much branched aromatic herb. Leaves sessile, opposite, serrate. Flowers purplish in axillary and terminal racemes. Fruits small, obovoid.

USEFUL PARTS AND THEIR CURATIVE PROPERTIES

Whole plant : Refrigerant, emollient, antiseptic, galactagogue, appetizer, anthelmintic, carminative, digestive, foul ulcers, constipation, strangury, inflammations, anorexia, dyspepsia, fever

340. *Limonia acidissima* L.

Family : Rutaceae

Common names : S: Kapitthah H: Kavita E: Elephant apple

Description : Medium sized deciduous spinescent tree. Leaves 3-7 foliate, petiole and rachis winged. Flowers polygamous, white with a pinkish tinge, axillary panicles, berries globose, seeds several, embedded in edible pulp.

USEFUL PARTS AND THEIR CURATIVE PROPERTIES

Leaf : Stomach pain, vomitings
Bark : Fertility in women, syphilis, diabetes
Root bark : Whooping cough
Fruit pulp : Whooping cough
Fruit juice : Blood dysentery, constipation, carminative, diarrhoea
Seed : Mouse bite

341. *Linum usitatissimum* L.

Family : Linaceae
Common names : S: Atasi H: Alsi E: Linseed
Description : An annual herb. Leaves linear-lanceolate. Flowers small, blue, in terminal panicles. Fruits capsular. Seeds compressed, ellipsoid, smooth, dark brown.

USEFUL PARTS AND THEIR CURATIVE PROPERTIES

Flowers : Cardiotonic
Seeds : Emollient, thermogenic, expectorant, diuretic, astringent, laxative, boils, local inflammations, carbuncles, ulcers

342. *Litsea glutinosa* (Lour.) C.B. Robinson

Family : Lauraceae
Common names : S: Medasaka H: Garbijaur E: Vasa
Description : Evergreen tree upto 20 m, branches and peduncles softly pubescent; bark somewhat corky, brownish grey; leaves aromatic, elliptic-ovate or oblong- lanceolate, pubescent. Flowers white or yellowish, borne in umbellate heads.

USEFUL PARTS AND THEIR CURATIVE PROPERTIES

Essential oil : Antibacterial
Oil from bark : Anthelmintic, antifungal
Aerial part : Antispasmodic
Stem bark : Bone fracture, poisonous bites, rheumatic pains, sprains, bruises, wounds, leucorrhoea, chest pain, dysentery
Root decoction : Emmenagogue
Root powder : Blood purification

343. *Litsea monopetala* (Roxb.) Pers.

Family : Lauraceae
Common names : S: Gajapippali

USEFUL PARTS AND THEIR CURATIVE PROPERTIES

Stem bark : Effect on respiration, CVS and CNS active, effect on nictitating membrane, spasmolytic
Leaves : Boils
Root bark : Bone fracture, giddiness

344. *Lodoicea maldivica* (Poir.) Pers.

Family : Arecaceae
Common names : S: Arkaragah H: Dariya-ka-nariyal E: Double coconut palm
Description : A tall palm with smooth annulated trunk bearing a crown of large fan shaped leaves. The palm is dioecious and its fruits are large, 1 seeded.

USEFUL PARTS AND THEIR CURATIVE PROPERTIES

Husk : Diabetes
Kernel : Refrigerant, digestive, carminative, febrifuge, tonic, cholera, oedema, Aconite poisoning, cardiotonic, hyperdypsia

345. *Ludwigia octovalvis* (Jacq.) Raven

Family : Onagraceae
Common names : S: Bhulavangah H: Banlumga E: Primrose willow
Description : An erect perennial undershrub. Leaves alternate, sessile, acute. Flowers yellow, tetramerous. Fruits truncate, 8-ribbed capsules. Seeds numerous, minute.

USEFUL PARTS AND THEIR CURATIVE PROPERTIES

Whole plant : Astringent, carminative, vermifuge, laxative, diuretic, expectorant, strangury, dropsy, cough, asthma, neuropathy, diarrhoea, fever, leucorrhoea, cephalalgia, dysentery

346. *Lygodium flexuosum* (L.) Sw.

Family : Lygodiaceae
Description : Pinnae arising in pairs from the ends of short spurs of twining rachis, margin finely serrate, surface slightly hairy.

USEFUL PARTS AND THEIR CURATIVE PROPERTIES

Rhizome : Body inflammation, earache, leucorrhoea extract
Root : Regaining health, loss of appetite, cholera, indigestion, dysmenorrhoea, anaemia, diarrhoea, stomach pain, cuts, wounds, scabies, ringworms, eczema, spermatorrhoea, diabetes, blood purifier
Leaf : Jaundice
Whole plant : Antifertility

347. *Madhuca indica* J. Gmel.

Family : Sapotaceae
Common names : S: Madhuka H: Mowa E: Indian butter tree
Description : Deciduous tree. Leaves elliptic, coriaceous when old, rounded, apex apiculate. Flowers creamish-white in axillary panicles. Stamens in 3 series. Berry ovoid, pedicel stout. Seeds 2.

USEFUL PARTS AND THEIR CURATIVE PROPERTIES

Stem bark	:	Acute stomach pain, skin diseases, fevers
Latex	:	Conjunctivitis
Flowers/fruits	:	Dengue fever, cough, piles, leprosy
Seed	:	Snake bite
Leaves	:	Earache

348. *Madhuca longifolia* (Koen.) Macb.

Family	:	Sapotaceae
Common names	:	S: Madhukah H: Mohva E: South Indian Mahua
Description	:	A tree, leaves elliptic-acuminate, flowers in terminal panicles,,pedicels brown pubescent. Berries ovoid.

USEFUL PARTS AND THEIR CURATIVE PROPERTIES

Root	:	Abdominal pain, scorpion bite, lactation
Stem bark	:	Snake bite, easy delivery, jaundice, toothache, galactagogue, cholera
Flowers	:	Aching muscles, deworming
Seeds	:	Snake bite, joint pains, sprains
Oil	:	Cold, chest pain, pneumonia

349. *Maerua oblongifolia* (Forsk.) A. Rich.

Family	:	Capparaceae
Common names	:	S: Murahari
Description	:	Unarmed straggler; branchlets glabrous. Leaves ovate to lanceolate, base and apex obtuse, entire; racemes corymbose, flowers greenish white, anthers green. Berry moniliform twisted. Seeds globose, tuberculate

USEFUL PARTS AND THEIR CURATIVE PROPERTIES

Root bark	:	Aphrodisiac
Tubers	:	General debility

350. *Majorana hortensis* Moench.

Family	:	Lamiaceae
Common names	:	H: Murwa E: Marjoram sweet
Description	:	Perennial, bushy annual plant. Leaves round, soft, green, sweet smell. Flowers sessile, bisexual. Calyx 5, corolla 5, stamens 4, epipetalous. Ovary superior. Fruit 1-4 seeded nutlets within the persistent calyx.

USEFUL PARTS AND THEIR CURATIVE PROPERTIES

Uses	:	Confectionery, cooking, drugs, flavouring, perfumery, potpourri

351. *Malaxis muscifera* (Lindley) Kuntz.

Family	:	Orchidaceae
Common names	:	S: Rsabhakah H: Rsabhak E: Risabak
Description	:	A terrestrial herb. Leaves 3-5 unequal, oblong. Flowers pale yellowish green in terminal racemes, lip fleshy, apex acuminated.

USEFUL PARTS AND THEIR CURATIVE PROPERTIES

Stem : Refrigerant, aphrodisiac, styptic, antidysentric, febrifuge, tonic, sterility, seminal weakness, general debility, haemorrhages, fever

352. *Mallotus philippensis* (Lam.) Muell-Arg.

Family : Euphorbiaceae
Common names : S: Kampillaka H: Kamala E: Kamela
Description : Evergreen tree to 8 m, leaves spiral, ovate-lanceolate, stellate pubescent below, base acute to rounded, entirely or sparsely serrate, apex to acuminate, lateral nerves 5-7 pairs, basal pair prominent. Staminate flowers in long spikes and pistillate flowers in short spikes. Capsule smooth, red glandular seeds subglobose, black.

USEFUL PARTS AND THEIR CURATIVE PROPERTIES

Hair of capsule : Pregnancy inhibition ascribes to rottlerin
Fruit : Antibacterial, hypoglycaemic, spasmolytic, anticancer, eruptions of leprous skin, anthelmintic, cathartic, styptic, purgative
Seed decociton : Constipation
Stem bark paste : Chest pain, jaundice
Leaf : Bruises, cuts, wounds, eye diseases, skin diseases
Root : Anthelmintic

353. *Mangifera indica* L.

Family : Anacardiaceae
Common names : S: Amrah H: Aam E: Mango
Description : Large evergreen tree. Leaves oblong or elliptic, lanceolate, coriaceous, cuneate - subacute, entire-wavy, apex acuminate. Panicles terminal. Flowers polygamous; drupe ovoid-oblong.

USEFUL PARTS AND THEIR CURATIVE PROPERTIES

Stem bark : Syphilis, diarrhoea, contraceptive, menorrhagia, gonorrhoea, rheumatism, Mahua disease
Leaves : Dysuria, dysentery, hiccups, jaundice, diarrhoea, excessive urination, antidiabetic
Gum : Cuts, boils
Resin : Black patches on face, scorpion sting
Buds : Jaundice
Flower bark : Diarrhoea, dysentery, rheumatism

354. *Manilkara hexandra* (Roxb.) Dubard

Family : Sapotaceae
Common names : S: Rajadani H: Khair E: Milk tree
Description : Medium sized tree. Leaves broadly ovate, cuneate to rounded, apex obtuse, flowers few in leaf axils. Corolla white, brownish when dry. Berry ellipsoid, slightly curved, oblong, beaked with persistent style when young. Seed 1.

USEFUL PARTS AND THEIR CURATIVE PROPERTIES

Stem bark : Dysentery, piles decoction
Fruits : To increase potency, digestion
Root : Headache, eye sight

355. *Manilkara zapota* (L.) P. Royen

Family : Sapotaceae
Common names : H: Sapota E: Sapota
Description : Small to medium sized tree. Leaves elliptic-oblong or oblong-lanceolate, acute at ends. Flowers white axillary, solitary. Berry globose, seeds 3-5.

USEFUL PARTS AND THEIR CURATIVE PROPERTIES

Latex : Wounds
Unripe fruits : Dysentery, diarrhoea

356. *Maranta arundinacea* L.

Family : Marantaceae
Common names : S: Tavaksiri H: Tikhor E: Arrowroot
Description : An erect branched herb. Leaves ovate-oblong, tip acute. Flowers white in clusters, fertile stamen with appendage. Ovary 1-celled, I-ovuled.

USEFUL PARTS AND THEIR CURATIVE PROPERTIES

Starch from rhizome : Astringent, refrigerant, tonic, aphrodisiac, emollient, expectorant, febrifuge, rubefacient, dysentery, diarrhoea, dyspepsia, bronchitis, cough

357. *Marsilea quadrifolia* L.

Family : Marsileaceae
Common names : S: Sunisannah H: Caupatiya
Description : A creeping herbaceous perennial plant. Leaves quadrifoliate, circinate when young, petioles long. Sporocarps bean shaped.

USEFUL PARTS AND THEIR CURATIVE PROPERTIES

Whole plant : Astringent, refrigerant, emollient, anodyne, diuretic, expectorant, aphrodisiac, depurative, febrifuge, diarrhoea, cough, leprosy, skin diseases, fever, insomnia, dyspepsia, haemorrhoids

358. *Martynia annua* L.

Family : Pedaliaceae
Common names : S: Kakanasa H: Hatha-jori E: Tiger's claw
Description : Undershrub upto 1m, stem purplish green, glandular-hairy, sticky. Leaves opposite, palmate, cordate, sinuate, apex acute. Flowers in axillary racemes. Corolla purple with yellow throat. Drupe ovoid with 2 apical, curved beaks dehiscing into 2-valves.

USEFUL PARTS AND THEIR CURATIVE PROPERTIES

Leaf : Blood purifier, scorpion sting, epilepsy, wounds
Root : Bronchial disorders, cold, painful urination

359. *Maytenus emarginata* (Willd.) Ding- Hu.

Family : Celastraceae
Common names : S: Vikantaki H: Vingar
Description : A shrub to small tree. Leaves ovate, obovate, coriaceous. Flowers in axillary dichotomous cymes. Capsule subglobose, 3-loculed.

USEFUL PARTS AND THEIR CURATIVE PROPERTIES

Whole plant : Cytotoxic and antidiabetic
Leaf : Wounds, ulcers, kills lice, dandruff, fertility, dental caries
Stem bark : Dandruff
Stem : Toothache

360. *Melastoma malabathricum* L.

Family : Melastomaceae
Common names : S: Tinisah H: Phutki E: Indian Rhododendron
Description : Evergreen shrub to 2 m; branches 4-angled, densely strigose. Leaves elliptic- lanceolate-oblong, rounded, entire, apex acute, strigose above with appressed thick hairs, tomentose beneath, 3-5 nerved. Flowers bright purple in terminal corymbose, 1-5 flowered panicles. Fruit broadly ovoid, seeds numerous.

USEFUL PARTS AND THEIR CURATIVE PROPERTIES

Leaves : Blood motions, piles, scabies, haemorrhages, wounds

361. *Melia azedarach* L.

Family : Meliaceae
Common names : S: Mahanimbah H: Mahanimb E: Persian lilac
Description : Medium sized tree with dark grey bark. Leaves imparipinnate, leaflets opposite, elliptic, glabrous, oblique, cuneate, serrate, apex acuminate. Flowers lilac, in panicles. Drupes globose, fleshy, yellow.

USEFUL PARTS AND THEIR CURATIVE PROPERTIES

Fruit powder : Insecticidal dust of fruit
Leaf extract : Antihelmintic, bronchitis in children, chest pain, boils, wounds
Seed oil : Antibacterial, CNS depressant and mild analgesic
Stem bark : Antiviral, spasmolytic, anticancer, fever, stomach disorders, dysentery, diarrhoea, malarial fever, paralysis, dermatitis

362. *Memecylon umbellatum* Burm. f.

Family : Melastomaceae
Common names : S: Anjani H: Nirasa

Description : Small tree to 4 m; branches terete, glaucous. Leaves elliptic, coriaceous, glabrous, obtuse, attenuate, apex emarginate. Flowers reddish-purple in umbellate cymes. Berries globose, reddish tinged, ripening black.

USEFUL PARTS AND THEIR CURATIVE PROPERTIES

Leaf : Leucorrhoea, wounds.
Stem bark : Anti-inflammatory, anasarca
Root bark : Leucorrhoea

363. *Mentha arvensis* DC.

Family : Lamiaceae
Common names : S: Pudina H: Pudina E: Japanese Mint
Description : An erect aromatic herb with suckers. Leaves simple, opposite, shortly petioled, oblong, crenate. Flowers in distinct whorls. Fruits nutlets, smooth.

USEFUL PARTS AND THEIR CURATIVE PROPERTIES

Whole plant : Aromatic oil, flavouring agent in food, medicine and drinks
Leaves : Stimulant, anodyne, anthelmintic, carminative, cardiotonic, expectorant, diuretic, emmenagogue, febrifuge, contraceptive, wounds, ulcers, cuts, dyspepsia, flatulence, peptic ulcers, diarrhoea, cough, asthma, bronchitis, skin diseases, amenorrhoea, dysmenorrhoea, dental caries, jaundice

364. *Mentha piperata* L.

Family : Lamiaceae
Common names : E: Peppermint

USEFUL PARTS AND THEIR CURATIVE PROPERTIES

Volatile oil : Antiseptic, stimulant, carminative, stomachic, confectionery, perfumes, liquors, tooth pastes, flavouring pickles
Seed : Spice, allaying nausea, flatulence, sickness and vomiting Bruised fresh leaves if applied will relieve local pains and headache. Hot infusion taken as tea soothes stomachache, allays sickness, and stops diarrhoea. This will also subdue menstrual colic.

365. *Mentha spicata* L.

Family : Lamiaceae
Common names : E: Spearmint

USEFUL PARTS AND THEIR CURATIVE PROPERTIES

Uses : Digestive, perfumes, cosmetics, flavouring agents

366. *Mesua nagassarium* (Burm. f.) Kosterm.

Family : Clusiaceae
Common names : S: Nagapuspah H: Nagakesar E: Mesua
Description : A medium sized evergreen tree. Leaves simple, opposite, thick, lanceolate, red when young. Flowers white very fragrant. Fruits ovoid. Seeds 1-4, smooth.

USEFUL PARTS AND THEIR CURATIVE PROPERTIES

Flowers : Astringent, anodyne, sudorific, digestive, carminative, constipating, anthelmintic, diuretic, expectorant, stomachic, haemostatic, aphrodisiac, febrifuge, cardiotonic, asthma, cough, hiccough, leprosy, scabies, ulcers, leucorrhoea, dypsia, haemorrhoids, burning sensation

367. *Michelia champaca* L.

Family : Magnoliaceae

Common names : S: Campakah H: Champa E: Champaca

Description : Trees. Leaves evergreen, flowers solitary, yellow. Sepals and petals similar, 9-15 or more. Stamens numerous. Seeds pendulous.

USEFUL PARTS AND THEIR CURATIVE PROPERTIES

Root/root bark : Purgative, emmenagogue, abscesses, inflammation, constipation, amenorrhoea, dysmenorrhoea

Stem bark : Astringent, febrifuge, diuretic, fever, cough, bronchitis, cardiac debility

Flowers/fruits : Dyspepsia, nausea, pruritus, leprosy, wounds, ulcers, colic, cephalalgia, cough, bronchitis, dysmenorrhoea, malarial fever

Flowers : Perfumes

368. *Miliusa tomentosa* (Roxb.) Sinclair

Family : Annonaceae

Common names : H: Hoom

Description : Large deciduous tree upto 20 m, bark blackish-brown, longitudinally deeply fissured. Leaves elliptic to ovate-lanceolate, coriaceous, tomentose beneath, rounded, entire, apex acute. Flowers axillary, terminal, solitary or in leaf-opposed or terminal cymes. Fruit a ring of subglobose stalked carpels.

USEFUL PARTS AND THEIR CURATIVE PROPERTIES

Stem bark : Stomachache, trypanosomiasis

369. *Mimosa intsia* L.

Family : Mimosaceae

Description : Prickly shrub. Leaflets 11-15 pairs, oblong, mucronate at apex, obliquely rounded or truncate at base. Flowers pink. Stamens 8. pod falcate, glabrous, without any prickles.

USEFUL PARTS AND THEIR CURATIVE PROPERTIES

Aerial part : CNS active, hypothermic

Whole plant : Peptic ulcer

Root bark : Bone fracture, chest pain, gastric pain

370. *Mimosa pudica* L.

Family : Mimosaceae

Common names : S: Lajjahah H: Lajwanti E: Sensitive plant

Description : Spreading herb; branchlets hispid; prickles short, erect or curved. Leaflets 15-20 pairs, linear acute at apex. Flowers pale pink. Pods 2-5 jointed and bristly along margins.

USEFUL PARTS AND THEIR CURATIVE PROPERTIES

Plant : Antiviral, spasmolytic, fever
Aerial part : Diuretic
Mimosine : Abortive
Root : Attracting the opposite sex, diarrhoea, malarial fever, dysuria, urinary complaints, whooping cough, conception, rickets
Flowers : Increasing potency
Stem powder : Kidney stones
Leaf : Filariasis, prevents conception, diabetes, filariasis, sores, piles, fistula

371. *Mitragyna parviflora* (Roxb.) Korth.

Family : Rubiaceae
Common names : S: Bhumikedamba H: Kaddam E: Kaime
Description : A tree, leaves oblong-elliptic, obovate, flowers in globose heads, capsules obovoid, slightly angled.

USEFUL PARTS AND THEIR CURATIVE PROPERTIES

Stem Bark : Febrifuge, peptic ulcers, menorrhagia, dysentery, cough, cold, muscular pains
Fruit : Headache
Leaves : Antiseptic, jaundice, hepatic stimulant

372. *Mollugo pentaphylla* L.

Family : Aizoaceae
Description : Ascending annual herb. Radical leaves oblanceolate, spathulate; cauline leaves whorled at each node, obovate-elliptic, cuneate-attenuate, apex subacute. Flowers white in terminal or leaf opposed cymes. Capsules faintly trilobed; seeds, reniform, dark brown.

USEFUL PARTS AND THEIR CURATIVE PROPERTIES

Whole plant : Fever and ulcers

373. *Momordica charantia* L.

Family : Cucurbitaceae
Common names : S: Karavellah H: Kareli E: Bitter gourd
Description : Climbing herb. Leaves orbicular, deeply 5-7 lobed, densely villous below, cordate, dentate-lobulate, apex acuminate. Flowers monoecious, solitary, yellow. Fruit oblong, ribbed, tubercled. Seeds ovoid, compressed.

USEFUL PARTS AND THEIR CURATIVE PROPERTIES

Seed oil : Possesses antifeeding and insecticidal properties inhibitory activity against gram negative bacteria, helminthiasis

Seed/ fruit : Hypoglycaemic, cytotoxic, antifeedant, fever, diabetes, impotency
Leaf : Children diseases, jaundice, high blood pressure, impotency, leucorrhoea, diarrhoea
Root : Peptic ulcer
Whole plant : Stomachache, liver, spleen diseases, rheumatism
Stem : Haemorrhoids

374. *Momordica dioica* Roxb. ex Willd.

Family : Cucurbitaceae
Common names : S: Karkota H: Jangli karela E: Small bitter gourd
Description : Climber. Leaves broadly ovate, deeply 3-5 lobed, glabrous, cordate, denticulate, apex obtuse-acute. Flowers dioecious, solitary, fruits obtuse at ends, not ribbed, softly spinous.

USEFUL PARTS AND THEIR CURATIVE PROPERTIES

Tuber : Spermicidal, anthelmintic, rib muscle pain, dandruff
Roots : Snake bite, diphtheria
Leaf : Skin diseases
Fruit : Diabetes

375. *Morinda pubescens* Sm.

Family : Rubiaceae
Common names : S: Papahnah H: Ach E: Togari wood of Madras
Description : Small tree; apex acumiante; inflorescence a simple head; corolla white. Fruit syncarp. Seeds oblong-ovoid.

USEFUL PARTS AND THEIR CURATIVE PROPERTIES

Stem bark : Asthma in rainy season, heart stroke, acute body pains, stomach pain, jaundice
Root/leaves : Diarrhoea, dysentery
Fruit : Strength

376. *Moringa oleifera* Lam.

Family : Moringaceae
Common names : S: Sigruh H: Soanjna E: Drumstick tree
Description : Small tree upto 8 m, bark thick. Leaves usually 3-pinnate, ultimate leaflets elliptic or obovate. Flowers white in panicles. Capsules cylindric. Seeds winged.

USEFUL PARTS AND THEIR CURATIVE PROPERTIES

Fruit and root : Spasmolytic
Root : Abortifacient, sore throat
Aerial part : Anticancer, anthelmintic, antifertility
Flower stem bark : Hypoglycaemic, sterilization, snake bite
Flower : Hypothermic

Bark : Antibacterial, antifungal, antitubercular, malarial fever, foot sores, warts, cold, cuts, wounds
Leaf : Bacteriostatic, hypotensive, eye diseases, hiccough, rheumatism, high blood pressure, boils, dysmenorrhoea, joint pains, stomach pain during menstrual cycle, warts
Root bark : Antiviral, anti-inflammatory, analgesic, cough
Seed : Agglutinates blood cells
Root bark / gum : Termination of foetus
Fruit : Cold, cough, fever, diabetes

377. *Morus alba* L.

Family : Moraceae
Common names : S: Toola H: Tut E: Mulberry
Description : Small tree. Young shoots pubescent. Leaves broadly ovate, often cordate, spiral, dentate, apex acuminate, thinly pubescent. Flowers monoecious. Fruit white to turning black when ripe.

USEFUL PARTS AND THEIR CURATIVE PROPERTIES

Leaf paste : Deep cuts by iron tools
Ripen fruits : To increase blood content
Shoot : Haemorrhoids

378. *Mucuna utilis* Wall. ex Wight

Family : Papilionaceae
Common names : S: Atmagupta H: Kivach E: Cowhage
Description : Slender climbing annual herb. Branches striate, downy-pubescent. Leaves trifoliate, leaflets ovate-rhomboid, entire. Flowers dark purple with yellow shade on standard petal. Pods curved at ends, prominently S-shaped. Seeds dark brown.

USEFUL PARTS AND THEIR CURATIVE PROPERTIES

Pod : Anthelmintic
Root & fruit : Hypoglycaemic, spasmolytic, nervine tonic
Root : CNS active, attracting the opposite sex, to break illusions, aphrodisiac, filariasis, paralysis, fever, psychological disorders
Seed powder : Drug for Parkinsonism, weakness, headache, impotency, laxative, irregular menstruation, fractures, aphrodisiac, depression, snake bite, scorpion sting
Fruit hairs : Intestinal worms
Leaf juice : Rotten teeth, paralysis, scorpion sting

379. *Mukia maderaspatana* (L.) Roem.

Family : Cucurbitaceae
Common names : S: Trikosaki H: Agumaki E: Gwala kakri

Description : Climbing herb. Tendril simple. Leaves suborbicular, 5-angled, irregularly dentate, cordate, apex acuminate. Corolla yellow. Fruits sessile.

USEFUL PARTS AND THEIR CURATIVE PROPERTIES

Leaf / fruit paste : Back ache
Leaf juice : Bile, diabetes
Seed : Diabetes

380. *Murraya koenigii* (L.) Spreng

Family : Rutaceae
Common names : S: Kaidaryah H: Kari patha E: Curry leaf tree
Description : Shrub, bark grey, leaves pinnate, leaflets spiral, oblong to lanceolate, pale green. Flowers small, white in terminal corymbs. Berry subglobose, shining, pale yellow, purplish black when ripe. Pulp whitish. Seeds green, globose.

USEFUL PARTS AND THEIR CURATIVE PROPERTIES

Aerial part : Spasmolytic, antiprotozoal
Root : Antiprotozoal, CVS active, effect on nictitating membrane, dysentery
Leaf : Hypoglycaemic, indigestion, dandruff, dysentery, belching, hair tonic, stomachache, diarrhoea, high fever, jaundice, vomitings, cough
Stem bark paste : Cuts, wounds, skin eruptions, bites

381. *Murraya paniculata* (L.) Jack.

Family : Rutaceae
Common names : S: Ekangi E: Orange jassamine
Description : Small evergreen tree, leaves imparipinnate, leaflets 3-7, flowers solitary or corymbs. Berry oblong or ovoid. Seeds solitary.

USEFUL PARTS AND THEIR CURATIVE PROPERTIES

Mexolide from stem bark : Antibacterial
Coumarins from leaves : Antifungal, diarrhoea, dysentery, arthritis, inflammated joints, stomachache, bone fracture
Alkaloid yuahchukene : Antiimplantational
Root powder : Stomach ache
Stem : Rheumatic pains

382. *Musa paradisiaca* L.

Family : Musaceae
Common names : S: Kadali H: Kela E: Plantain
Description : A stoloniferous plant, leaves large, spikes drooping, fruits oblong, sweet.

USEFUL PARTS AND THEIR CURATIVE PROPERTIES

Root : Gonorrhoea, sterilization

Fruit : Boils, peptic ulcers, heart pains
Leaf : Diarrhoea
Pseudostem : Irregular menstrual cycle, diabetes
Inflorescence : Rheumatism, headache
Rhizome : Kidney and bladder stones, peptic ulcers
Sap : Diarrhoea

383. *Myristica fragrans* Houtt.

Family : Myristicaceae
Common names : S: Jatiphalah H: Jayphal E: Nutmeg tree
Description : Moderate sized, aromatic, evergreen tree. Leaves elliptic, shiny. Flowers creamy yellow, fragrant, umbellate cymes. Anthers 10-14. fruits yellow, globose.

USEFUL PARTS AND THEIR CURATIVE PROPERTIES

Oil : Antibacterial, herbicidal, antitumour, perfumes, soaps, dental paste, flavouring chewing gums, chewing tobacco
Fruit : Dental caries, pyorrhoea, boils
Rhizome : Kidney and bladder stones
Stem : Diabetes
Root : sterilization

384. *Naravelia zeylanica* DC.

Family : Ranunculaceae
Common names : S: Dhanavalli
Description : Climbing shrubs. Leaves 3-foliolate, flowers panicles, bisexual, sepals 4 - 5, petals 6 -12. stamens many. Achenes long.

USEFUL PARTS AND THEIR CURATIVE PROPERTIES

Leaves : Astringent, anthelmintic, depurative, anti-inflammatory, cold
Stem : Toothache, headache
Whole plant : Pyorrhoea, rheumatism, helminthiasis, wounds, ulcers, stomach pains, jaundice, toothache, skin diseases

385. *Nardostachys grandiflora* DC.

Family : Valerianaceae
Common names : S: Jatamamsi H: Jatamamsi E: Spikenard
Description : An erect perennial herb, rhizome highly aromatic. Leaves radical, spathulate, sessile, glabrous. Flowers rosy in dense cymes. Fruits covered with dense white hairs and crowned with calyx teeth.

USEFUL PARTS AND THEIR CURATIVE PROPERTIES

Rhizome : Astringent, emollient, antiseptic, anodyne, digestive, carminative, laxative, stomachic, liver stimulant, nervine tonic, diuretic, fever, emmenagogue, asthma, bronchitis, foul ulcers, grey hair, convulsions, dyspepsia, colic, flatulence, leprosy, epilepsy, general debility

386. *Naregamia alata* Wt. & Arn.

Family : Meliaceae
Common names : S: Amlavalli H: Tinparni E: Goanese ipecacaunha
Description : A small undershrub, pungent, aromatic roots. Leaves trifoliate, alternate, petioles winged. Flowers white, large. Fruits globose, ovoid capsules. Seeds curved.

USEFUL PARTS AND THEIR CURATIVE PROPERTIES

Whole plant : Cooling, aromatic, vulnerary, emetic, expectorant, antipyretic, cough, asthma, scabies, splenomegaly, catarrh, bronchitis, chronic and malarial fevers, dyspepsia, dysentery

387. *Naringi crenulata* (Roxb.) Nicolson

Family : Rutaceae
Common names : S: Bilvaparni
Description : A small tree. Leaves 3-5 foliate. Leaflets elliptic-ovate, oil dotted, glabrous. Flowers pale green in axillary subumbellate racemes. Fruits globose black.

USEFUL PARTS AND THEIR CURATIVE PROPERTIES

Stem : Antiamoebic, CVS active, spasmolytic, dysentery, puerperal fevers, piles
Leaf : Diabetes
Fruit : Deworming

388. *Nelumbo nucifera* Gaertn.

Family : Nymphaeaceae
Common names : S: Padma H: Kanwal E: Sacred lotus
Description : Large perennial herb with milky juice and long creeping subterranean rhizomes. Leaves about a meter high above water, orbicular. Flowers white or rose coloured, fragrant, solitary, anthers yellow in white flowered and orange in rose coloured forms. Seeds with spongy coats.

USEFUL PARTS AND THEIR CURATIVE PROPERTIES

Rhizome : CNS depressant, diuretic, diarrhoea
Nuciferine : Neuroleptic
Flower paste : Blood purification
Perianth : Conjunctivitis
Seed : Diuretic, refrigerant, tonic

389. *Neolamarckia cadamba* (Roxb.) Bosser

Family : Rubiaceae
Common names : S: Kadambah H: Kadamb E: Kadam
Description : A medium sized deciduous tree. Leaves elliptic to oblong. Flowers yellow or orange in globose heads. Fruits globose pseudocarps, yellow when ripe.

USEFUL PARTS AND THEIR CURATIVE PROPERTIES

Bark : Astringent, anodyne, digestive, carminative, galactagogue, diuretic, febrifuge, expectorant, constipating, antiemetic, tonic, fever, cough

Leaves : Ulcers, wounds, metrorrhoea

Fruits : Gastric irritability and fever

390. *Neptunia oleracea* Lour.

Family : Mimosaceae

Common names : S: Alambusa H: Lajjalu E: Sensitive water plant

Description : A floating annual herb. Leaves bipinnate, leaflets 8-15 pairs, small. Flowers minute, yellow, axillary heads. Fruits stalked, deflexed. Seeds 6-9 compressed.

USEFUL PARTS AND THEIR CURATIVE PROPERTIES

Whole plant : Astringent, refrigerant, diuretic, anthelmintic, anodyne, otalgia, cephalalgia, syphilis, dypsia, diarrhoea, strangury

391. *Nervilia aragoana* Gaud.

Family : Orchidaceae

Common names : S: Padmakarini H: Sthalakamal

Description : Small tuberous herb. Tubers globose. Leaf appears after flowering, solitary, long petioled. Lamina broadly ovate, cordate at base, glabrous. Flowers pale green, with yellow near base.

USEFUL PARTS AND THEIR CURATIVE PROPERTIES

Tubers : General debility, wounds

Whole plant : Cooling, galactagogue, diuretic, tonic, epilepsy, diarrhoea, asthma, cough, vomiting, haemoptysis

392. *Nigella sativa* L.

Family : Apiaceae

Common names : S: Karavi H: Kalomji E: Kalonji

Description : Small herb, leaves compound, flowers pale blue, solitary, long peduncles, Seeds trigonous, black, rugulose - tubercular.

USEFUL PARTS AND THEIR CURATIVE PROPERTIES

Uses : Seeds contain aromatic oil, laxative, carminative, anthelmintic, regulates menstruation, lactation, contraction of uterus, headache, indigestion, boils, scorpion sting, cough, bronchitis, skin care, cosmetics

393. *Nyctanthes arbor-tristis* L.

Family : Oleaceae

Common names : S: Sephalika H: Parja E: Coral jasmine

Description : A bushy shrub or small tree. Leaves opposite, coarse, flowers yellow or white, sessile, axillary on long peduncles, capsule obcordate.

USEFUL PARTS AND THEIR CURATIVE PROPERTIES

Leaves : Blood purifier, skin diseases, malarial fever

Fruit : Cold, cough, bronchitis
Seed : Dandruff, lice eradication
Bark : Mouth ulcers, gum bleeding, throat pains, epilepsy

394. *Nymphaea nouchali* Burm. f.

Family : Nymphaeaceae
Common names : S: Kumuda H: Chhota-sundi E: Indian water lily
Description : Floating, aquatic, rhizomatous herb. Leaves long-petioled, peltate, orbicular, purple below, entire or wavy, cordate at base. Flower solitary, blue, white, rose or purple; anthers brown with creamy appendages. Berry green, spongy, ovoid. Seeds numerous.

USEFUL PARTS AND THEIR CURATIVE PROPERTIES

Flowers : Astringent, cardiotonic, retaining elasticity of muscles after delivery
Leaf paste : Eczema

395. *Ocimum basilicum* L.

Family : Lamiaceae
Common names : S: Arjakah H: Ban Tulsi E: Sweet basil
Description : Erect, aromatic, undershrub to 1 m, leaves elliptic ovate or lanceolate, entire to serrulate. Flowers simple or much branched thyrsoid racemes. Calyx lobes hairy within. Corolla white. Fruiting pedicel recurved with enlarged calyx.

USEFUL PARTS AND THEIR CURATIVE PROPERTIES

Essential oil : Antibacterial, antifungal
Leaf : Blindness, earache, fever, headache, epilepsy, hemicrania
Seed : Dysentery, aphrodisiac, asthma, bronchitis, piles
Uses : Cosmetics, culinary purposes, drugs, flavouring, perfumery

396. *Ocimum canum* Sims

Family : Lamiaceae
Common names : S: Gramya E: Hoary basil
Description : Herbs or slightly woody undershrubs. Leaves opposite or whorled. Flowers small. Racemes elongate, calyx villous, stamens 4, ovary 4 partite.

USEFUL PARTS AND THEIR CURATIVE PROPERTIES

Plant extract : CNS effect
Leaf extract : Antibacterial
Essential oil : Antifungal

397. *Ocimum gratissimum* L.

Family : Lamiaceae
Common names : S: Ramatulasi H: Ram tulsi E: Shrubby basil

Description : Aromatic, profusely branched subshrub to 1 m, branches quadrangular, glabrescent. Leaves obovate, acute, deeply serrate, apex acute to shortly acuminate. Flowers pale greenish yellow in close whorls. Calyx lobes hirsute without. Nutlets 4 or one aborts. Calyx enlarged in fruit.

USEFUL PARTS AND THEIR CURATIVE PROPERTIES

Essential oil : Antibacterial, antifungal
Plant : Spasmolytic, diuretic, CNS active, scurvy, skin allergies
Seed : Burning micturition, leucorrhoea, diarrhoea, urinary troubles
Leaf : Eczema, fever, rheumatism, paralysis, refrigerant, scorpion poison
Uses : Cosmetics, drugs, flavouring, perfumery

398. *Ocimum kilimandscharicum* Guerke

Family : Lamiaceae
Common names : S: Karpuratulasi H: Kapurtulsi E: Camphor basil
Description : An aromatic undershrub. Leaves simple, opposite, serrate, acute. Flowers in racemes, corolla 2-3 times the length of calyx, fruits nutlets.

USEFUL PARTS AND THEIR CURATIVE PROPERTIES

Oil : Perfumes, insecticide, tooth paste, explosives, toilet articles
Leaves : Thermogenic, antibacterial, appetizer, cough, bronchitis, catarrh, foul ulcers and wounds, anorexia

399. *Ocimum tenuiflorum* L.

Family : Lamiaceae
Common names : S: Tulasi H: Kala-tulsi E: Sacred basil
Description : Aromatic, subshrub to 1 m; branchlets hispid, terete. Leaves elliptic-oblanceolate, truncate, serrate-undulate, apex apiculate. Flowers in terminal racemes. Calyx purplish green, glabrous within. Corolla white, purplish within; Calyx not much enlarged in fruit. Pedicel spreading, longer than calyx.

USEFUL PARTS AND THEIR CURATIVE PROPERTIES

Leaf : Hypoglycaemic, spasmolytic, bronchitis, cough, fever with shivering, night blindness, cold, dandruff, malarial fever, rheumatism, gastric trouble, contraceptive, black patches, asthma, earache, eczema, fertility, foul breath, sterilization, respiratory troubles, jaundice, stomachache, wounds, toothache, boils, cuts, antiseptic, urinary troubles, tuberculosis (all types)
Root : Fever
Seed : Burning of feet, painful micturition.
Whole plant : Bronchitis, ringworm, rat bite
Inflorescence : Hypoglycaemic
Uses : Perfumery, flavouring

400. *Opuntia stricta* (Haw.) Haw.

Family : Cactaceae
Common names : S: Nagaphana H: Nag phana E: Prickly pear
Description : Shrub to 2 m; areoles raised,densely elongate-bristly, glochidiate;spines 5-7 per areole, yellow. Leaves deciduous. Flowers to 5 cm across. Perianth yellow. Berry obovoid, purple when ripe; seeds many.

USEFUL PARTS AND THEIR CURATIVE PROPERTIES

Fruit : CNS active, diuretic, excessive menstruation
Leaf pulp : Reduces excess of heat
Flowers : Tumours on body

401. *Oroxylum indicum* (L.) Benth. ex Kurz.

Family : Bignoniaceae
Common names : S: Syonakah H: Sonapatha E: Indian Trumpet tree
Description : A small tree, leaves long. Leaflets ovate-acuminate, flowers in terminal racemes. capsule flattened, seeds winged.

USEFUL PARTS AND THEIR CURATIVE PROPERTIES

Fruit : Spasmolytic
Bark : Diuretic
Root bark : Dysentery, rheumatism, wounds, fractures, dropsy, leucoderma, astringent, tonic, leprosy, antifertility
Stem bark : Flatulence, paralysis, jaundice, hepatic stimulant, diarrhoea, fever, muscular pain, general weakness, stomach pain, dysentery, bone fracture, ulcers, arthritis, piles
Root paste : Fertility, precaution for recurrence of abortion, diarrhoea
Seed : Snake bite, joint pain, scorpion sting
Leaves : Joint pains, gastroenteritis, bronchitis, lactation

402. *Ougeinia oojeinensis* (Roxb.) Hochr.

Family : Papilionaceae
Common names : S: Tinisah H: Sandan E: Sandan
Description : Medium sized deciduous tree. Leaves pinnately trifoliate, flowers numerous, white or pink, fascicled racemes, fruits linear, flat pods.

USEFUL PARTS AND THEIR CURATIVE PROPERTIES

Root : Tumour, menstrual disorder
Stem bark : Blood dysentery, diarrhoea, cataract, constipation, astringent, gonorrhoea, leprosy, leucoderma, haemorrhage, fever, anaemia

403. *Oxalis corniculata* L.

Family : Oxalidaceae
Common names : S: Kangeri H: Amrul E: Indian sorret
Description : Diffuse herb, rooting at lower nodes. Leaves digitately trifoliate; leaflets obcordate, pilose, cuneate, entire, apex emarginate. Flowers yellow in axillary umbels. Capsule oblong, 5-angled, tipped with persistent style.

USEFUL PARTS AND THEIR CURATIVE PROPERTIES

Leaf : Dysentery, indigestion, skin diseases, tonic for nursing mothers, chronic cough, headache, insomnia, prolapse of the rectum, diarrhoea, conjunctivitis, gastro-intestinal disorders

Whole plant : Stomach troubles, snake bite, dysentery, diarrhoea, fractures

404. *Pandanus fascicularis* Lamk.

Family : Pandanaceae

Common names : S: Ketaki H: Keura E: Screw pine

Description : Much branched shrub or small tree. Trunk with basal prop roots. Leaves linear, armed with white prickles on margins and dorsal midrib. Flowers yellow, fragrant. Female inflorescence solitary, terminal cephalium, pendulous fruit.

USEFUL PARTS AND THEIR CURATIVE PROPERTIES

Leaf paste : Body swellings

Root decoction : Fertility

Inflorescence : Skin diseases

Uses : Perfumery, flavouring for food and beverages

405. *Papaver somniferum* L.

Family : Papaveraceae

Common names : S: Aphukam H: Afin E: Opium poppy

Description : Annual or perennial herbs with milky juice. Leaves lobed or cut, flowers on long peduncles. Ovary 1-celled. Capsule short. Seeds small.

USEFUL PARTS AND THEIR CURATIVE PROPERTIES

Whole plant : Hypnotic drug in Materia Medica and used in relieving pain and also preventing pain after delivery. Poppy heads are used in diarrhoea, dysentery and all kinds of fluxes. The seeds are ground in cold water and is given in diarrhoea and dysentery. The roasted seeds are considered as tonic

406. *Passiflora foetida* L.

Family : Passifloraceae

Common names : S: Mukkopara E: Passion flower

Description : Climbing herb; tendrils simple. Leaves spiral, ovate, 3-lobed, cordate, glandular pubescent, subentire to ciliate, apex acute. Flowers axillary, often solitary. Berry subglobose; orange when ripe.

USEFUL PARTS AND THEIR CURATIVE PROPERTIES

Aerial part : CVS active, anticancer, diuretic, galactagogue

Fruit : Anti-narcotic effect, dandruff

Leaf : Asthma, headache, skin diseases

Root : Abortion

407. *Pavonia zeylanica* (L.) Cav.

Family : Malvaceae

Description : Woody viscid herb. Leaves ovate, deeply 3-lobed, 3-5 nerved from base, margin crenate-dentate. Epicalyx lobes 8-12, linear. Corolla white to pink. Mericarps smooth, glabrous.

USEFUL PARTS AND THEIR CURATIVE PROPERTIES

Root decoction : Dysentery

Whole plant paste : Tumours on the body

408. *Pedalium murex* L.

Family : Pedaliaceae

Common names : S: Gokshura H: Bada gokhru

Description : Erect, much branched herb. Leaves spiral to opposite, subsucculent, truncate, apex emarginate. Flowers solitary, axillary, emarginate, corolla yellow. Drupe indehiscent, apex conical, spiny along the angles.

USEFUL PARTS AND THEIR CURATIVE PROPERTIES

Plant : Diuretic, larvicidal, synergistic, gonorrhoea, joint pains, snake bite, nephroprotector

Fruit : Fertility, hydrocele, syphilis, diuretic, antiseptic, aphrodisiac

Root : Fever

Leaves : Dysmenorrhoea, menorrhagia, gonorrhoea

Seed : Joint pains

409. *Pedilanthus tithymaloides* (L.) Poit.

Family : Euphorbiaceae

Common names : S: Vilayatisij E: Slipper plant

Description : Erect or scandent subshrub to 1.5 m; branchlets zigzag subsucculent. Leaves spiral, distichous, elliptic to ovate, brittle, green to variegated, attenuate, apex acute, subsessile, deciduous, lateral obscure. Cyathia stalked, terminal, cymose, subtended by petaloid, lanceolate, caduceus bracts. Involucre scarlet red. Staminate floret ca.25 and pistillate floret single. Fruit not seen.

USEFUL PARTS AND THEIR CURATIVE PROPERTIES

Aerial part : CNS active, hypothermic

Latex : Cuts, joint pains, rheumatism, wounds, sprains

410. *Pelargonium graveolens* L. Herit

Family : Geraniaceae

Common names : H: Geranium E: Geranium

Description : Bushy, aromatic plant. Leaves alternate, stipulate, simple, highly aromatic. Inflorescence umbellate, pink. Stamens 10, ovary hairy, superior.

USEFUL PARTS AND THEIR CURATIVE PROPERTIES

Uses : Leaves yield geranium oil which is a substitute of Otto of roses in the manufacture of perfumes and soaps

411. *Pergularia daemia* (Forsk.) Chiov.

Family : Asclepiadaceae

Common names : S: Kurutakah H: Dudhi E: Whitlow plant

Description : Perennial, twining milky shrub with foetid smell. Stem clothed with spreading hairs. Leaves thin, broadly ovate to orbicular, cordate, apex acute. Raceme umbelliform, axillary; corolla greenish yellow. Follicles sticky, curved, covered with soft spines.

USEFUL PARTS AND THEIR CURATIVE PROPERTIES

Plant : Effect on respiration, CVS and CNS active, spasmolytic, hypothermic, antagonism to amphetamine hyperactivity, antibacterial, musclotropic, eczema

Leaves : Catarrhal affection, infantile diarrhoea, uterine, tonic, fractured bones, expectorant and emetic, incurring gynaecological conditions such as excessive bleeding and also cures rheumatic pains, scabies, inflammations, swellings, asthma, fever, epilepsy, abortion, easy delivery

Root : Stomach pain, rheumatic swellings, purgative, diabetes

Flower : Galactagogue

Fruits : Scabies

Stem : Fever, whooping cough

Latex : Boils, lymph gland swellings, migraine

412. *Phoenix sylvestris* (L.) Roxb.

Family : Areacaceae

Common names : S: Kharjura H:Khejur E: Wild date palm

Description : Tree; trunk to 15 m, leaves 2-4 m long, leaflets glaucous, rigid, base narrow, apex acuminate, spinous, lower leaflets spiny; spadices to 1m; spathes as long as spadices. Spikes in clusters. Drupe oblong ellipsoid.

USEFUL PARTS AND THEIR CURATIVE PROPERTIES

Leaf : Effect on respiration, CVS and CNS active, hypothermic, mouth ulcers, diarrhoea, dysentery

Toddy : Nervine tonic, digestive

413. *Phyla nodiflora* (L.) Green

Family : Verbenaceae

Common names : S: Jalapippali H: Jalpapli E: Purple lippia

Description : A creeping herb. Leaves obovate, flowers in long peduncled heads. Fruit capsule, minute.

USEFUL PARTS AND THEIR CURATIVE PROPERTIES

Whole plant : Cough, cold, gonorrhoea, toothache, fever, asthma, bronchitis, ulcers, dyspepsia, anorexia, flatulence, colic, diuretic, febrifuge, aphrodisiac, constipation, appetizer, cooling, stomachic

Leaf : Haematuria, stones in ureter, toothache

414. *Phyllanthus amarus* Schum. & Thonn.

Family : Euphorbiaceae

Common names : S: Bhumyaamlaki H: Jaramal E: Kirinelli

Description : Erect, annual glabrous, small herb. Flowers unisexual, minute, axillary. Seeds with longitudinal parallel ribs on the back.

USEFUL PARTS AND THEIR CURATIVE PROPERTIES

Leaf & root : Antibacterial, antihepatotoxic, antiulcer, molluscicidal, antiviral

Leaf : Hypoglycaemic, heart complaints, jaundice, antiseptic

Root : Jaundice, urinary diseases

Plant juice : Hiccups, diabetes, jaundice, corneal diseases, scorpion sting, hepatic stimulant, anaemia, constipation, dysmenorrhoea, fertility, migraine, diarrhoea, toothache, headache

415. *Phyllanthus emblica* L.

Family : Euphorbiaceae

Common names : S: Amalaki H: Amla E: Gooseberry

Description : Trees, leaves small, linear, oblong. Flowers monoecious, calyx 5-6, petals 0, glands in male flowers very small. Stamens 3, ovary 3-celled.

USEFUL PARTS AND THEIR CURATIVE PROPERTIES

Fruit : Antiviral, CVS active, mild cholinergic, antispasmodic, phyllemblin – CNS depressant, spasmolytic, antibacterial ,antifungal, antidiabetic, eye troubles, gonorrhoea, leucorrhoea, dandruff, stomach ulcers, asthma, cold, cough, scurvy, bleeding nose, ulcers and fissures in the mouth, urinary troubles, jaundice, dyspepsia

Bark and fruit decoction : Vomiting

Fruit powder and bark juice : Stomach trouble

Seed : Syphilis, leucorrhoea, stomach ulcers, asthma

Stem galls : Fractured bones

Leaf : Diarrhoea, skin diseases

416. *Phyllanthus maderaspatensis* L.

Family : Euphorbiaceae

Common names : S: Bhumyamalaki H: Ranavali

Description : Erect herb to 70 cm, leaves linear to obovate, glaucous below, cuneate, apex retuse or obtuse. Flowers axillary. Staminate flowers above and pistillate below. Capsule globose, trilobed; seed triquetrous, vertically muriculate.

USEFUL PARTS AND THEIR CURATIVE PROPERTIES

Leaf : Stomach ache, eczema, itching
Whole plant : Tumours on body.

417. *Phyllanthus reticulatus* Poir.

Family : Euphorbiaceae
Common names : S: Krishna kamboji H: Kala-maimuda E: Black honey shrub.
Description : Scandent or erect shrub upto 4 m, leaves oblong elliptic, acute at both ends. Staminate flowers 5-7 in axillary fascicles; pistillate flowers fewer. Berry globose, dark blue; seeds trigonous; testa crustaceous.

USEFUL PARTS AND THEIR CURATIVE PROPERTIES

Plant : Antiprotozoal, antiviral, spasmolytic, CVS active
Leaves : Bone fracture, piles, bleeding wounds
Root : Cough, asthma
Stem bark : Rotten teeth, swellings, anasarca, haemor-rhoids

418. *Phyllanthus simplex* Retz.

Family : Euphorbiaceae
Description : Erect herb to 75 cm, leaves oblong lanceolate, rounded, apex obtuse to acute, apiculate, subsessile. Flowers solitary in axils, staminate flowers few in lower axils; pistillate flowers many in upper axils. Capsule globose, 3 lobed; seeds trigonous, minutely tuberculate.

USEFUL PARTS AND THEIR CURATIVE PROPERTIES

Root : jaundice
Leaf decoction : Stomachache
Whole plant paste : Tumours on body

419. *Physalis angulata* L.

Family : Solanaceae
Common names : S: Tankari
Description : Erect, widely branched, annual herb. Stems angular-ribbed, glabrous. Leaves oblique, acuminate, glabrous. Flowers solitary, terminal, axillary. Corolla yellow, small, brown spots inside. Anthers violet or blue. Fruit greenish yellow.

USEFUL PARTS AND THEIR CURATIVE PROPERTIES

Fruit : Indigestion
Leaf extract : Malarial fever

420. *Physalis minima* L.

Family : Solanaceae
Common names : S: Tankari H: Tulatipati E: Country gooseberry
Description : Erect or prostrate, annual herb. Stems angular, ribbed, hairy. Leaves ovate, acute or acuminate, thinly pilose. Flowers solitary, pedicels hairy. Calyx hairy outside, corolla yellow. Anthers yellow.

USEFUL PARTS AND THEIR CURATIVE PROPERTIES

Aerial part : Diuretic
Physaline : X – abortifacient
Fruits : Indigestion
Leaf extract : Malarial fever, stomach swellings

421. *Pimenta dioica* (L.) Merr.

Family : Myrtaceae
Common names : E: Pimento
Description : Small evergreen tree. Flowers white, branch trichotomously in the axils of upper leaves, dioecious. Stamens numerous.

USEFUL PARTS AND THEIR CURATIVE PROPERTIES

Uses : Flavouring agent in culinary preparations like soups, sauces, ketchups, pickles, meat, curry powder, bakery items and in liquor industry

422. *Pimpinella anisum* L.

Family : Apiaceae
Common names : E: Anise

USEFUL PARTS AND THEIR CURATIVE PROPERTIES

Uses : Flavouring agents, cosmetics, perfumes, beverages

423. *Piper longum* L.

Family : Piperaceae
Common names : S: Pippali H: Pipli E: Indian long pepper
Description : A creeping aromatic herb, leaves ovate-oblong, long petioled, flowers unisexual. Fruit ovoid, 7-ribbed.

USEFUL PARTS AND THEIR CURATIVE PROPERTIES

Essential oil : Antibacterial, antimicrobial, anthelmintic
Fruit : Anti-inflammatory, severe headache, hypoglycaemic, cough, asthma, cold, fevers, rheumatism
Root powder : Antifertility activity, improving digestion, bronchitis, jaundice, paralysis, hair fall, asthma, throat infection, stomach pain, epilepsy, cough, fever, abortifacient, asthma, puerperal fever
Plant : Hypoglycaemic, spasmogenic
Piperine : Hypotensive, antipyretic, CNS stimulant, analgesic.
Seed : Asthma, cough, hair loss

424. *Piper nigrum* L.

Family : Piperaceae
Common names : S: Maricha H: Golki E: Black pepper
Description : A stout climbing shrub. Leaves ovate, flowers in spikes. Berries ovoid - globose, 5-9 ribbed.

USEFUL PARTS AND THEIR CURATIVE PROPERTIES

Fruit oil : Antibacterial, antifungal
Fruit : Taenicidal, larvicidal
Leaf : Hypertensive, cough and cold
Root : Dysentery, gumache, emetic

425. *Plantago ovata* Forsk.

Family : Plantaginaceae
Common names : S: Snigdhabijah H: Isabgol E: Isubgol
Description : Short stemmed, annual herb. Leaves simple, linear, flowers small. Fruits ellipsoid capsules, seeds smooth, yellowish brown, boat-shaped.

USEFUL PARTS AND THEIR CURATIVE PROPERTIES

Whole plant : Aphrodiasiac, cooling, demulcent, diuretic, expectorant, chronic diarrhoea, constipation, gastro-intestinal and genito-urinal tracts troubles, rheumatism and gout (paste applied).

426. *Plumbago indica* L.

Family : Plumbaginaceae
Common names : S: Davanah H: Raktacitra E: Fire plant
Description : Perennial shrub, leaves simple, alternate, flowers bright red, terminal spikes. Corolla tube slender, as long as calyx.

USEFUL PARTS AND THEIR CURATIVE PROPERTIES

Root : Rheumatism, ulcers, syphilis, piles, abortifa-cient, leprosy, bronchitis, piles, dyspepsia, cough, leucoderma, scabies, amenorrhoea, anaemia, digestive

427. *Plumbago zeylanica* L.

Family : Plumbaginaceae
Common names : S: Chitraca H: Chitta E: White leadwort
Description : Spreading undershrub, with ascending branches. Leaves elliptic-ovate, truncate to attenuate, apex apiculate. Corolla white. Capsule glandular-hairy, globose. Seed solitary, enclosed in calyx.

USEFUL PARTS AND THEIR CURATIVE PROPERTIES

Root : Uterine stimulant, leprosy, maggot infested sores, scabies, skin diseases, ring worm, sun paste, temporary birth control, aphthae, pyorrhoea, eczema, leprosy, piles, psoriasis, sterilization, bladder stones,hydrocele, liver enlargement, rheumatism, white spots, diarrhoea, dysentery, abdominal pain, stomach trouble, abscess, asthma, fever, conception, nephrocalcinosis, leucoderma, abortifacient, cancer, filariasis, tumours and ulcers in stomach and intestine
Root and fruits : Antiimplantation, blisters, jaundice, birth control Plumbagin induces antiimplantation, abortifacient, antiovulatory, antibacterial, antifungal, anticoagulant

Root and leaf decoction : Stomach trouble, rheumatism, dental caries, abortion
Root bark : Piles, snake bite, appetizer
Whole plant : Boils, skin diseases, contraction of uterus after child birth
Seed : Diarrhoea
Leaf : Leucorrhoea, headache, fever, jaundice, skin diseases, chest pain, muscle pain, sprains, wounds

428. *Plumeria alba* L.

Family : Apocynaceae
Common names : S: Kananaka ravira H: Safed Champa E: Pagoda tree
Description : Small tree. Leaves crowded in terminal branches. Flowers fragrant, white in lateral or terminal panicles.

USEFUL PARTS AND THEIR CURATIVE PROPERTIES

Root bark : Gonorrhoea, deworming, abortifacient, leprosy, stomach pain
Latex : Toothache, itch, boils

429. *Podophyllum hexandrum* Royle.

Family : Berberidaceae
Common names : H: Papra E: Podophyllum
Description : A succulent erect herb. Flower bearing branch is erect. Leaves 2, deeply lobed, toothed, purple spotted, cup-shaped, usually solitary. Fruit ovoid, scarlet.

USEFUL PARTS AND THEIR CURATIVE PROPERTIES

Whole plant : Blood purifier, cholagogue, hepatic stimulant, constipation, many skin diseases and tumorous growths, cancerous tissues, purgative

430. *Pogostemon cablin* L.

Family : Lamiaceae
Common names : E: Pacholi

USEFUL PARTS AND THEIR CURATIVE PROPERTIES

Uses : Oil - perfume industry, incense sticks, toilet articles

431. *Pogostemon perilloides* (L.) Mansf.

Family : Lamiaceae
Common names : E: Patchouly
Description : Erect branched, pubescent herb. Leaves ovate, coarse, simple, tomentose. Spikes terminal, axillary and panicled. Corolla pink. Filaments violet.

USEFUL PARTS AND THEIR CURATIVE PROPERTIES

Uses : Cosmetics, drugs, flavouring, insecticides and perfumery

432. *Polianthes tuberosa* L.

Family : Amaryllidaceae
Common names : H: Gulshaba E: Tuberose

Description : Tuberous root stock. Leaves long, narrow, pale green. Flowers pure, white, waxy-textured raceme of blooms. Tube long, funnel-shaped. Ovary 3-celled.

USEFUL PARTS AND THEIR CURATIVE PROPERTIES

Uses : Boutonnieres, cut flowers, flavouring, ornamental purposes, perfumery

433. *Polycarpaea corymbosa* (L.) Lam.

Family : Caryophyllaceae

Common names : S: Agnimantah

Description : Erect, annual herb; internodes glabrous or with scattered hairs. Leaves decussate or in false whorls, linear axillary to subulate, glabrescent, entire, acute, stipules scarious, much fimbriate. Cymes axillary or terminal, sepals lanceolate, not coloured. Capsules oblong, 3- valved.

USEFUL PARTS AND THEIR CURATIVE PROPERTIES

Shoot paste : Inflammatory body swellings

Plant decoction : Snake bite, febrifuge, jaundice, weakness after fever

434. *Pongamia pinnata* (L.) Pierre

Family : Papilionaceae

Common names : S: Karanjah H: Karanj E: Indian Beech

Description : Densely foliaceous tree. Leaves imparipinnate; leaflets 3-5 pairs, opposite, obovate, coriaceous, glossy above, entire, apex acuminate. Inflorescence panicles. Corolla blue. Pod obliquely oblong, woody, indehiscent.

USEFUL PARTS AND THEIR CURATIVE PROPERTIES

Seed oil : Leprosy, boils, blisters, skin diseases, scabies, sores, gonorrhoea

Root paste : Psoriasis, ulcers, dandruff, paralysis

Flower decoction : Diabetes, nephroprotector

Fruit : Whooping cough

Seed powder : Piles, corneal opacity, bronchitis, whooping cough, psoriasis

Root powder : Blood purification, arthritis, earache

Stem bark : Leucorrhoea, post patrum recovery, dental caries, fertility, bleeding piles, ulcers and dandruff, leprosy, rheumatism

435. *Prunus dulcis* (Mill.) D. A. Webb.

Family : Rosaceae

Common names : S: Vatadah H: Badam E: Almond

USEFUL PARTS AND THEIR CURATIVE PROPERTIES

Uses : Scented oils, soaps, perfumes, cosmetics

436. *Psoralea corylifolia* L.

Family : Papilionaceae

Common names : S: Bakuci H: Babchi E: Babchi

Description : Undershrub. Leaves simple, ovate, pubescent, base obtuse, dentate, apex acute. Racemes axillary. Flowers apically aggregated, purplish-violet. Pod ovoid or oblong, indehiscent; seed solitary, reniform.

USEFUL PARTS AND THEIR CURATIVE PROPERTIES

Seed paste : Skin diseases, blood purifier, laxative, anthelmintic, stomachic, stimulant, aphrodisiac, diuretic, diaphoretic, leucoderma, ulcers, scabies, leprosy, dermatitis

Tender shoot paste : toothache

437. *Pterocarpus marsupium* Roxb.

Family : Papilionaceae

Common names : S: Araktacandana H: Bijasal E: Indian kino tree

Description : Tree upto 15 m, leaves imparipinnate, leaflets 3 pairs, spiral, elliptic oblong, coriaceous, pubescent below, obtuse-truncate, entire, apex emarginate. Corolla golden yellow. Pods stipulate, wings broad.

USEFUL PARTS AND THEIR CURATIVE PROPERTIES

Root bark : Dysentery

Stem bark : Effect on respiration, nictitating membrane, CVS active, heart pains, blood pressure control, red and white leucorrhoea, diabetes, jaundice, piles, blood vomiting, fertility Gum is astringent used for diarrhoea and tooth aches

Wood : Diabetes

Latex : Burns and ulcers

Flowers : Nose bleeding, leprosy, blood motions, stomach pain, herpes, abscess, gonorrhoea, rheumatism

438. *Pterospermum acerifolium* Willd.

Family : Sterculiaceae

USEFUL PARTS AND THEIR CURATIVE PROPERTIES

Flowers : Indigestion, body dehydration, passing of blood with urine

439. *Pueraria tuberosa* (Willd.) DC.

Family : Papilionaceae

Common names : S: Vidari H: Sural E: Indian kanda

Description : Large tuberous climber. Leaves trifoliate, leaflets ovate; laterals oblique, silky-tomentose, coriaceous, obtuse, ciliate, apex acute, mucronate. Panicles dense, corolla pale violet.

USEFUL PARTS AND THEIR CURATIVE PROPERTIES

Tuber : Antiimplantational, hypoglycaemic, aphrodisiac, dyspepsia, peptic ulcers, tympanitis, rheumatism, skin diseases, prevents conception

440. *Punica granatum* L.

Family : Punicaceae
Common names : S: Dadimah H: Anar E: Pomegranate
Description : A glabrous, deciduous large shrub to small tree with thorny branches and dark grey bark. Leaves opposite or whorled, oblong, obovate, membranous. Flowers sessile, bright red, terminal, solitary or 3-flowered cymes; calyx greenish-red. Petals membranous. Fruit a globose, berry, seeds angled, aril filled with an acidic sweet juice.

USEFUL PARTS AND THEIR CURATIVE PROPERTIES

Pericarp : Antifertility effect, Rind, flowers, leaf and stem bark – antibacterial, diarrhoea
Leaf : Dysentery, nasal bleeding, diarrhoea
Aerial part : CNS depressant, diuretic, hypothermic.
Epicarp of fruit : Dysentery, diarrhoea, sexual vigour, toothache, anaemia, peptic ulcers
Seed : Vomiting, scabies
Root bark : Deworming
Flower : Nasal bleeding

441. *Rauvolfia serpentina* (L.) Benth. ex Kurz.

Family : Apocynaceae
Common names : S: Sarpagandha H: Chhotachand E: Serpentina
Description : Undershrub upto 1 m, leaves oblanceolate, attenuate, apex acute or shortly acuminate. Corymbs axillary, calyx lobes almost free. Corolla whitish red. Drupes connate except at top, ripe black.

USEFUL PARTS AND THEIR CURATIVE PROPERTIES

Reserpine : Hypotensive, tranquilizer, useful for mental disorders and certain forms of insanity
Ajmalicine : Hypotensive, tranquilizer
Rescinnamine : Hypotensive
Deserpidine : Hypotensive, sedative juice of leaves is instilled into eyes as a remedy for the opacities of the cornea. Decoction of roots is employed to increase uterine contraction, rheumatism, fever. The root is bitter tonic, narcotic, antidote to the bites of poisonous reptiles and stings of insects, febrifuge, minimises blood pressure, expels worms in children, relieve stomachache and also expel thread worms, fever, insanity, skin infection, epilepsy, eczema, chest pain, rabies

442. *Rhinacanthus nasutus* (L.) Kurz.

Family : Acanthaceae
Common names : S: Yuthikaparni H: Palakjuhi E: White-flowered justicia

Description : Erect herb to undershrub upto 1.5 m; young branches pubescent. Leaves elliptic-lanceolate, tapering, entire, apex acute, pubescent on both sides. panicles terminal or axillary, trichotomously branched. Corolla white; seeds tuberculate.

USEFUL PARTS AND THEIR CURATIVE PROPERTIES

Root paste : Eczema, snake bite, impotency in males, antiseptic, herpes

Leaf paste : Scorpion sting, cancer, aphrodisiac, prickly heat

443. *Rhus mysorensis* Heyne

Family : Anacardiaceae

Common names : H: Dansara

Description : Shrub or small tree upto 4 m; branches reddish, hirtellous. Leaves trifoliate, lateral leaflets obovate, terminal oblanceolate, coriaceous, cuneate, sinuate- toothed, puberulous. Flowers pale green in terminal and axillary panicles.

USEFUL PARTS AND THEIR CURATIVE PROPERTIES

Leaf : Piles and allergy

444. *Rhynchosia minima* (L.) DC.

Family : Papilionaceae

Description : Twining herb; branches slender, glabrescent; leaflets rhomboid, acute. Raceme 7-9 flowered. Corolla yellow. Pod oblong, slightly bent upwards, sparsely pubescent. Seeds 2, estrophiolate.

USEFUL PARTS AND THEIR CURATIVE PROPERTIES

Root decoction : Ephemeral fever

Leaf decoction : Termination of foetus

445. *Ricinus communis* L.

Family : Euphorbiaceae

Common names : S: Erandah H: Erandi E: Castor oil seed

Description : Evergreen shrub to 3 m, leaves spiral, palmatifid, 6-10 lobed; each 1-nerved with many lateral nerves, peltate. Racemes terminal; staminate flowers below and pistillate flowers below. Capsule 3-lobed, prickly; seeds oblong; testa smooth, marbled, shiny, carunculate.

USEFUL PARTS AND THEIR CURATIVE PROPERTIES

Root and stem : Antiprotozoal, anticancer, induces sterility in women, paralysis, abortifacient, toothache

Root, stem / leaf : Hypoglycaemic, rheumatism, irregular menstruation

Seed : Diuretic, purgative, gonorrhoea, laxative, abortion

Leaf paste : Termination of 2-3 months old foetus, rheumatism, body swellings, headache, jaundice, paralysis, stomachache, painful menstruation, boils, pimples, haemorrhoids, sores

Latex : Cures gums

446. *Robinia pseudoacacia* L.

Family : Papilionaceae
Common names : E: Acacia

USEFUL PARTS AND THEIR CURATIVE PROPERTIES

Uses : Perfumes, cosmetics

447. *Rosa damascena* Mill.

Family : Rosaceae
Common names : S: Shataputri H: Fasli gulab E: Otto of roses
Description : Perennial shrub. Stems moderately hooked. Leaf stipulate, compound, imparipinnate, stipules adnate. Flowers in terminal, axillary corymbs, sweet scented, pink. Fruit pseudobacate made of several hard achenes.

USEFUL PARTS AND THEIR CURATIVE PROPERTIES

Uses : Rose oil is most priced and most expensive of perfume oils, confectionery, drugs, food and beverages, liquor

448. *Rosmarinus officinalis* L.

Family : Lamiaceae
Common names : H: Rusmari E: Rosemary
Description : Hard, dense, evergreen herb. Leaves opposite, sessile, smooth, green. Flowers in clusters. Calyx 2-lipped. Fruit oval, 4-sectioned cremocarp.

USEFUL PARTS AND THEIR CURATIVE PROPERTIES

Uses : Cosmetics, culinary purposes, flavouring, perfumery

449. *Rubia cordifolia* L.

Family : Rubiaceae
Common names : Euphorbiaceae
Description : Climbing herb, branches prickly, leaves ovate, exstipulate, flowers in cymes. Berries globose.

USEFUL PARTS AND THEIR CURATIVE PROPERTIES

Leaves : Mouth ulcers, blood purifier, vermifuge, jaundice
Root : Ulcers, eczema, skin inflammation, stomach pain, giddiness, blood purifier, spleen disorders, dysentery, antiseptic, jaundice, anaemia, diabetes, vermifuge
Whole plant : Ringworm, leucoderma and other skin diseases

450. *Ruellia tuberosa* L.

Family : Acanthaceae
Common names : E: Menow-weed.
Description : Erect herb upto 50 cm; tender parts hispid, nodes often purplish. Leaves obovate to lanceolate, cuneate to attenuate, apex subacute. Flowers in axillary dichasial cymes. Corolla blue to violet. Seeds orbicular, hairy.

USEFUL PARTS AND THEIR CURATIVE PROPERTIES

Tuberous root paste : Body swellings, abortion
Tuberous root decoction : Gonorrhoea

451. *Rumex vesicarius* L.

Family : Polygonaceae
Common names : S: Chukra H: Chuka E: Bladder dock
Description : Erect succulent, stout herb; stem fleshy, stipules membranous. Leaves spiral, elliptic, cordate to hastate, apex obtuse to acute, succulent. Inflorescence in panicles. Flowers pink, arranged in clusters, polygamous. Seed ovoid, black.

USEFUL PARTS AND THEIR CURATIVE PROPERTIES

Leaf : Dysentery, snake bite, toothache
Seed powder : Scorpion sting

452. *Salvia officinalis* L.

Family : Lamiaceae
Common names : E: Sage

USEFUL PARTS AND THEIR CURATIVE PROPERTIES

Uses : Perfumes, cosmetics, flavouring agents

453. *Sansevieria roxburghiana* Schult. & Schult. f.

Family : Agavaceae
Common names : S: Muruva H: Murva E: Bow string hemp
Description : Stout, fleshy herb. Root stock rhizomatous. Leaves cylindric. Flowers greenish white, in clusters on a terminal scape. Fruits membranous, indehiscent.

USEFUL PARTS AND THEIR CURATIVE PROPERTIES

Leaf extract : Snake bite, trypanosomiasis, glandular enlargements
Root paste : Minimizes excess of heat, snake bite, haemorrhoids
Rhizome : Cooling effect

454. *Santalum album* L.

Family : Santalaceae
Common names : S: Candanah H: Chandan E: White sandal tree
Description : Small, evergreen tree with drooping branches. Leaves opposite, acute, entire, apex subacute. Inflorescence in paniculate cymes, shorter than leaves, terminal and axillary. Drupe globose, beaked with the basal part of style.

USEFUL PARTS AND THEIR CURATIVE PROPERTIES

Stem : CVS active
Sandalwood oil : Incense perfumery, soaps, fixative, blends Urs – 12 – en – 3B – yl palmitate – insect growth inhibitor. The oil obtained from the heartwood is used in the treatment of dysuria *i.e.,* to promote and facilitate

urination, cystitis (inflammation of bladder), gonorrhoea and cough, tuberculosis of gall bladder, contraceptive, headache, menorrhagia, wounds

Leaf : Leucorrhoea, jaundice, hyperacidity, liver disease, cardiac tonic, T.B Oil from the seed - skin diseases, gastero-enteritis, aphrodisiac. Stem bark paste - insect bite, tuberculosis, jaundice, leprosy, dysmenorrhoea

455. *Sapindus emarginatus* Vahl

Family : Sapindaceae

Common names : S: Arista H: Ritha E: Soapnut

Description : Medium sized tree. Leaves paripinnate, leaflets 3-4 pairs, elliptic-oblong, coriaceous, obtuse, emarginate, base cuneate, entire. Flowers brownish yellow in terminal panicles. Drupe ovoid-tomentose, 3-10 lobed. Seeds 1 in each locule, black.

USEFUL PARTS AND THEIR CURATIVE PROPERTIES

Fruit : Bath powder, scorpion sting, tonsils, lice, dandruff, pus and pain in the ear, sinusitis

Seeds : Night blindness, snake bite, dandruff

Leaf : Cooling

456. *Sarcostemma acidum* (Roxb.) Voigt.

Family : Asclepiadaceae

Common names : S: Chadra vallari H: Soma lata E: Moon creeper

Description : Leafless, climbing, succulent, jointed shrub with pendulous branches. Stem green, glabrous, joints 10-20 cm long. Flowers fragrant, creamy, sessile in terminal umbellate cymes.

USEFUL PARTS AND THEIR CURATIVE PROPERTIES

Stem : Bone fracture, maddog bite

Latex : Sprains

Root : Dog bite

Whole plant : Rheumatism

457. *Sarcostemma secamone* (L.) Bennet

Family : Asclepiadaceae

Common names : S: Dudhialata H: Dudhi E: Rosy milk weed

Description : Twining herb; branchlets purplish green. Leaves linear to oblong, sub-coriaceous, truncate, apex mucronate. Flowers white or rose; corolla marked with purple veins. Follicles ovate and lanceolate.

USEFUL PARTS AND THEIR CURATIVE PROPERTIES

Latex : Galactagogue and wounds

Leaves : Boils and wounds

458. *Sassafras albidum* Nees.

Family : Lauraceae

Common names : E: Sassafras

USEFUL PARTS AND THEIR CURATIVE PROPERTIES

Uses : Cosmetics, flavouring, perfumes

459. *Sauropus quadrangularis* (Willd.) Muell-Arg.

Family : Euphorbiaceae

Common names : S: Aruni E: Triplinerved lizard foot

Description : Undershrub upto 1 m, monoecious; branchlets quadrangular. Leaves elliptic - oblong, acute to obtuse at base, entire, apiculate. Flowers in axillary in cymes; staminate 2-3, pistillate solitary. Drupe depressed globose.

USEFUL PARTS AND THEIR CURATIVE PROPERTIES

Whole plant extract : Malaria

Leaf : Sores

460. *Schleichera oleosa* (Lour.) Oken.

Family : Sapindaceae

Common names : S: Kosamra H: Kussum E: Lac tree

Description : Tree, bark smooth grey. Leaves abruptly pinnate; leaflets 2 - 4 pairs, acute, entire, base acute. Flowers yellowish green, drooping racemes and crowded near the ends of branches. Fruit 1-celled, smooth.

USEFUL PARTS AND THEIR CURATIVE PROPERTIES

Stem bark : Swellings of arms and legs, rheumatic pains, tuberculosis, ulcerous wounds, chest pain, fractured bones

Seed oil : Skin diseases

Root bark : Snake bite

461. *Schleichera trijuga* Willd.

Family : Sapindaceae

Common names : H: Kosum E: Lac tree

Description : Trees. Leaves alternate, flowers polygamo-dioecious. Calyx 4-6, petals 0. stamens 5-8. ovary 3-celled.

USEFUL PARTS AND THEIR CURATIVE PROPERTIES

Uses : Macassar oil stimulates and cleanses scalp, hair growth, itches, aches, skin diseases, rheumatism, headache backaches and joint pains

462. *Schrebera swietenioides* Roxb.

Family : Oleaceae

Common names : S: Ksarasresthah H: Ban-palas E: Weaver's bean tree

Description : Medium sized tree. Leaves imparipinnate; leaflets opposite, elliptic-ovate, coriaceous, oblique to attenuate, apex acute. Cymes trichotomous. Flowers bisexual; corolla white with brown center. Capsule obovoid, pustulate, loculicidal; seeds flat, winged, exalbuminous.

USEFUL PARTS AND THEIR CURATIVE PROPERTIES

Aerial parts : CNS active, hypothermic
Root bark : Leprosy
Leaf paste : Ulcers

463. *Scoparia dulcis* L.

Family : Scrophulariaceae
Description : Herb, leaves rhomboid or elliptic, flowers axillary, solitary or 2 on slender pedicles. Capsule globose.

USEFUL PARTS AND THEIR CURATIVE PROPERTIES

Whole plant : Dysentery, menstrual disorders, spermatorrhoea, kidney stones, fever, headache, jaundice
Leaf paste : Burning sensation during urination, eye sores, body pain
Root : Removal of placenta, dysentery, warts

464. *Securinega virosa* (Willd.) Baill.

Family : Euphorbiaceae
Common names : H: Dalme E: Small Indian snow berry
Description : Shrub to 5m; leaves pubescent, variable, elliptic to obovate, cuneate at base, entire, acute. Flowers in axillary clusters. Capsule 4 mm, globose.

USEFUL PARTS AND THEIR CURATIVE PROPERTIES

Aerial parts : Spasmolytic, antagonism of amphetamine hyperactivity
Stem bark decoction : Insect bite
Whole plant : Diarrhoea, dysentery

465. *Semecarpus anacardium* L. f.

Family : Anacardiaceae
Common names : S: Bhallatakah H: Bhilawa E: Marking nut tree
Description : Tree upto 15 m. Leaves simple, oblong-elliptic, thick, rusty-villous below, nerves 16 pairs, obtuse, subacute or cordate, entire, apex rotund, retuse. Panicles terminal. Flowers unisexual, sometimes bisexual, rarely polygamous. Drupes globose-ovoid, reniform; hypocarp, fleshy.

USEFUL PARTS AND THEIR CURATIVE PROPERTIES

Fruit : Anticancer, antirheumatic, hypoglycaemic, CVS active, anthelmintic, antimicrobial, antiamoebic, piles, abortion, vermifuge, expel maggots from sores, cuts, heel cracks, sprains, skin diseases, leprosy, liver tonic
Stem bark : Headache, wounds due to burns, debility, venereal infections, ulcers
Seed paste : Kibes, epilepsy, corns, leucoderma, abdominal swellings and pain
Leaves : Leprosy
Seed oil : Headache
Whole plant : Snake bite
Resin : Tumours, leucoderma, diabetes, warts

466. ***Sesamum orientale*** **L.**

Family : Pedaliaceae
Common names : S: Tilah H: Til E: Gingelly
Description : Euphorbiaceae

USEFUL PARTS AND THEIR CURATIVE PROPERTIES

Oil cake : Nematicidal, leprosy, abortion
Seeds : Antidiabetic
Flowers : Eye diseases

467. ***Sesbania grandiflora*** **(L.) Pers.**

Family : Papilionaceae
Common names : S: Agastyah H: Basna E: Sesban
Description : Tree upto 12 m, branchlets pubescent. Leaflets 18-28 pairs, oblong, pubescent, obtuse, entire, apex emarginate. Racemes 3-5 flowered. Pod pendulous, 45 cm, seeds pale brown.

USEFUL PARTS AND THEIR CURATIVE PROPERTIES

Flowers : Haemolytic activity, night blindness, cataract, conjunctivitis, kidney and bladder stones, alopecia
Aerial parts : Spasmolytic, CNS active, hypothermic, depressant, diuretic.
Seed paste : Cough
Stem bark decoction : Fever, small pox, chicken pox, tonic, infusion in small pox
Leaf : Kidney, bladder stones, jaundice

468. ***Sida acuta*** **Burm. f.**

Family : Malvaceae
Common names : S: Bala H: Kharenti E: Hornbean leaved sida
Description : Erect herb to undershrub. Leaves oblong-lanceolate to elliptic, 3-5 nerved at base, serrate, acute at apex. Stipules of each pair different. Flowers solitary or in clusters of 2-5. schizocarp ovoid, acute, wrinkled, with 6-9 mericarps.

USEFUL PARTS AND THEIR CURATIVE PROPERTIES

Cryptolepine : Hypotensive, antimicrobial
Plant : Antiarrhythmic, nervous disorders
Leaf paste : Rheumatism, fractures
Root decoction : Venereal diseases, cholic pain
Root paste : Waist pain, boils, cuts, wounds

469. ***Sida cordifolia*** **L.**

Family : Malvaceae
Common names : S: Bala H: Khareti E: Bala

Description : A velvety undershrub. Leaves ovate, 5-7 nerved, base rounded or cordate, serrate, apex obtuse or subacute. Flowers yellow, axillary, solitary, rarely 2-6 in clusters. Schizocarp exceeding the calyx, rugulose, mericarps 8-10, trigonous.

USEFUL PARTS AND THEIR CURATIVE PROPERTIES

Whole plant : Plant possesses antifertility activity, spasmolytic, antiprotozoal, CVS active, Plant also possesses acetyl choline like activity, cures gonorrhoea, diarrhoea

Seed oil : Headache, paralysis, aphrodisiac

Roots : Intermittent fever

Leaf : Scorpion sting, wounds, ulcers

Leaf and stem decoction : Gonorrhoea, concentration of semen, excessive menstruation

470. *Siegesbeckia orientalis* L.

Family : Asteraceae

Common names : S: Lickura

Description : Herbs, leaves opposite, heterogamous heads, corollas of female flowers 2-3 lobed, bisexual flowers 5 lobed. Anther-bases obtuse. Achenes glabrous.

USEFUL PARTS AND THEIR CURATIVE PROPERTIES

Whole plant : Plant antiviral, hypoglycaemic, CVS active, spasmolytic

Root : Urinary trouble

471. *Smilax zeylanica* L.

Family : Liliaceae

Common names : E: Sarsaparilla

Description : A shruby climber with tendrils, prickly, leaves ovate, stipules modified into tendrils. Flowers in pedunculate umbels. Fruit globose.

USEFUL PARTS AND THEIR CURATIVE PROPERTIES

Root decoction : Weakness, spermatorrhoea, anaemia, leucorrhoea, haematuria, paralysis, cooling, venereal diseases, skin diseases, sores, swellings, abscess, boils

Tuber : Fertility, paralysis, venereal diseases, throat ulcers

Stem : Toothbrush in toothache, spongy gum and worn out teeth

Leaf : Spermatorrhoea

472. *Solanum americanum* Mill.

Family : Solanaceae

Common names : S: Kakamari H: Kamuni E: Black night shade

Description : Annual erect herb. Leaves ovate, with cuneate base, glabrous. Flowers nodding, in umbelliform, extra axillary inflorescence, corolla white or blue. Berry globose, glabrous. Seeds many, ovate-reniform.

USEFUL PARTS AND THEIR CURATIVE PROPERTIES

Plant : CVS active, spasmolytic, hypothermic
Leaf juice : Cough with blood
Ripe fruits : Fever

473. *Solanum anguivi* Lam.

Family : Solanaceae
Common names : S: Brhati H: Barhanta E: Indian night shade
Description : Perennial undershrub with sharp yellowish spines. Stem stout, purplish, covered with stellate hairs. Leaves ovate, oblong,subcordate, apex subacute or obtuse. Flowers in lateral, cymose corymbs. Corolla blue. Fruit orange-yellow.

USEFUL PARTS AND THEIR CURATIVE PROPERTIES

Plant : CVS active, anticancer, asthma, antidote for snake bite, jaundice
Fruit : Hair growth, asthma, cough, dropsy, rheumatism, sore throat, fever

474. *Solanum surattense* Burm. f.

Family : Solanaceae
Common names : S: Kanta kari H: Kateli E: Dwarf lid brinjal
Description : Perennial, very prickly, diffuse herb. Leaves pinnatifid, attenuate, entire, apex acute, stellately pubescent, prickles yellow. Flowers bluish purple, in 2-6 flowered cymes. Fruit yellow.

USEFUL PARTS AND THEIR CURATIVE PROPERTIES

Root : Asthma, sore throat, cough, malaria
Fruit : Paralysis, asthma, cough, intestinal worms, toothache, digestion
Seeds : Toothache
Whole plant : Toothache, chest ailments
Flower : Diarrhoea

475. *Solanum virginianum* L.

Family : Solanaceae
Common names : S: Kantakari H: Kateli E: Yellow berried night shade

USEFUL PARTS AND THEIR CURATIVE PROPERTIES

Plant : Antiviral, spermicidal, syphilis, cough, dysuria, asthma
Plant & fruit : Anticancer
Fruit : CVS active, spasmolytic, antiarrhythmic
Root : Fertility, whooping cough
Seed : Toothache

476. *Solena amplexicaulis* (Lam.) Gandhi

Family : Cucurbitaceae
Common names : S: Sukakamdah

Description : Vine. Leaves polymorphic, cordate, denticulate, apex obtuse-retuse, tendrils simple. Flowers dioecious, white. Staminate flowers in umbels, pistillate flowers solitary. Fruit oblong-ovoid, apically beaked, turgid, smooth.

USEFUL PARTS AND THEIR CURATIVE PROPERTIES

Aerial part : CNS active, hypothermic, diuretic
Root decoction : Burning micturition
Leaf paste : Skin eruptions

477. *Sophora glauca* Lesch. ex DC.

Family : Papilionaceae
Description : EuphorbiaceaeClimbing shrub. Leaflets 25-31, elliptic, oblong, subacute. Calyx distinctly 5-toothed, corolla pink or violet. Pod velvety, 5-seeded.

USEFUL PARTS AND THEIR CURATIVE PROPERTIES

Leaf paste : Dysentery, headache

478. *Soymida febrifuga* (Roxb.) A. Juss.

Family : Meliaceae
Common names : S: Patranga H: Rohan E: Indian red wood
Description : Tree upto 15 m, leaves spiral, paripinnate. Leaflets 5-6 pairs, opposite, oblong, coriaceous, glabrous, entire, apex obtuse. Flowers white in panicles. Fruit woody, 5-celled capsule; seeds oblong, winged.

USEFUL PARTS AND THEIR CURATIVE PROPERTIES

Stem bark : Acute pain in stomach, piles, trypanosomiasis, fever and cough, diarrhoea, indigestion, gout, urinary problems, bone fracture, dysentery, weakness
Leaf : Lactation
Flower : Earache, headache

479. *Spermacoce articularis* L. f.

Family : Rubiaceae
Common names : S: Madanaghanti
Description : An erect or diffuse annual herb . Leaves ovate, flowers pale pink. Capsule oblong-ellipsoid.

USEFUL PARTS AND THEIR CURATIVE PROPERTIES

Plant : Diuretic, CNS active
Root : Bone fracture, toothache, gum troubles, snake bite
Leaf : Diarrhoea

480. *Sphaeranthus indicus* L.

Family : Asteraceae
Common names : S: Mundi H: Gorakh mundi E: East Indian gole-thistle
Description : Prostrate aromatic herb. Stem cylindric with toothed wings more or less glandular hairy. Leaves sessile, flowers pink to purple, heterogamous globose heads. Fruit achene, angled, smooth, glabrous.

USEFUL PARTS AND THEIR CURATIVE PROPERTIES

Essential oil	:	Antifungal, antibacterial
Plant	:	Hypoglycaemic, abnormal labour pains, jaundice, headache, health tonic, mumps, ante-partum treatment, leucoderma, nephrocalcinosis, ureteral stones, easy delivery
Leaf	:	Diarrhoea, filariasis, ringworm
Flowers	:	Eye diseases and inflammed eyes, malaria
Garland from fruits	:	Chicken-pox and mumps, stomach worms, filariasis
Root juice	:	Epilepsy, impotency, cures bleeding, diarrhoea
Fruit	:	Chicken pox, jaundice

481. *Spondias pinnata* (L. f.) Kurz.

Family	:	Anacardiaceae
Common names	:	S: Amratakah H: Amra E: Wild mango

USEFUL PARTS AND THEIR CURATIVE PROPERTIES

Stem bark	:	CVS and CNS active, hypothermic, diuretic, dysentery, refrigerant, diarrhoea, rheumatism, fever, gonorrhoea, arthritis, antiseptic, scorpion sting
Leaves	:	Tetanus, eczema

482. *Stachytarpheta urticaefolia* (Salisb.) Sims.

Family	:	Verbenaceae
Common names	:	S: Chirchiti E: Aarows rod
Description	:	A woody herb. Leaves elliptic, flowers blue, spikes. Fruit oblong, ribbed.

USEFUL PARTS AND THEIR CURATIVE PROPERTIES

Plant	:	CNS active, hypothermic, snake bite
Leaves	:	Cuts, wounds
Bark	:	Diarrhoea

483. *Stephania japonica* Miers

Family	:	Menispermaceae
Description	:	Climbing shrubs. Leaves peltate, heads of flowers in stalked umbels, male flower sepals 6-10, petals 3-5, anthers 6. female flower sepals 3-5. Drupe glabrous. Seeds almost annular.

USEFUL PARTS AND THEIR CURATIVE PROPERTIES

Root	:	Stomachaches, diabetes, indigestion, deworming, arthritis, urinary troubles

484. *Sterculia urens* Roxb.

Family	:	Sterculiaceae
Common names	:	S: Arjuna H: Gulu E: Sterculia

Description : Deciduous, soft wooded tree. Leaves simple, 3-5 lobed, coriaceous, velvety below, cordate, entire. Panicles viscid terminal. Flowers foetid, greenish yellow. Follicles 4-5 lobed, oblong with ferruginous stiff hairs. Seeds oblong, dark.

USEFUL PARTS AND THEIR CURATIVE PROPERTIES

Gum : Improving stamina, suppress the phenol content in the body, dysentery, cooling effect, constipation, diarrhoea

Stem bark : Minimises pains during delivery, rheumatism, peptic ulcers, spermatorrhoea, leucorrhoea

485. *Streblus asper* Lour.

Family : Moraceae

Common names : S: Sakhotah H: Khorus E: Siamese rough bush

Description : Small tree to 6m, leaves obovate to rhomboid, cuneate, apex acute. Staminate flowers in clusters. Drupe enclosed by enlarged perianth.

USEFUL PARTS AND THEIR CURATIVE PROPERTIES

Aerial part : Anticancer, insecticidal, antiviral

Leaf : Anti-smoking, increase potency, eye infection

Latex : Dysentery, cuts, measles, dental caries

Roots/tender shoots : Toothache

Stem bark : Leucorrhoea, chest pain, rib muscle pain, epilepsy, fever, dysentery, diarrhoea, abdominal pain

Gum : Constipation

486. *Strychnos nux-vomica* L.

Family : Loganiaceae

Common names : S: Karaskarah H: Bailewa E: Strychnine tree

Description : Tree upto 12 m; bark smooth and grey. Leaves orbicular, shining, 3-nerved, obtuse, acuminate, entire. Flowers greenish-yellow in terminal racemes. Berries globose, orange when ripe; seeds many.

USEFUL PARTS AND THEIR CURATIVE PROPERTIES

Leaf and fruit : Spasmolytic, skin diseases, paralysis, wounds, itching, epilepsy

Root bark : Muscle relaxant, snake bite, cholera

Seed : Scorpion sting, snake bite, bitter stomachic, tonic, stimulate respiratory and cardio-vascular systems, rat bites, venomous reptile bites, ulcers, rheumatism, alcoholism, corns, menorrhagia, regain the lost hair, fevers, dysentery, menstrual disorders, dyspepsia, blood pressure, diabetes, psoriasis

Stem bark : Acute diarrhoea, leprosy, snake bite, diabetes, nervous disorders, asthma, dysentery, dyspepsia, fevers, gastritis

Stem : Inflammations, swellings

487. *Strychnos potatorum* L. f.

Family	:	Loganiaceae
Common names	:	S: Katakah H: Nirmali E: Clearing nut tree
Description	:	Small tree upto 8 m; bark black, cracked and scaly; trunk often irregularly fluted. Leaves ovate-elliptic, glabrous, shining, 5-nerved, truncate, apex acuminate. Flowers white in axillary, sessile cymes. Berries globose, black when ripe.

USEFUL PARTS AND THEIR CURATIVE PROPERTIES

Total alkaloids	:	Convulsant, hypotensive
Alkaloid diaboline	:	Hypotensive
Aerial parts	:	CNS depressant
Seeds	:	Cleaning of water, impotency, diarrhoea, snake and dog bites, jaundice, cataract, conjunctivitis, gonorrhoea, diabetes, scorpion sting, whooping cough, fever, bronchitis
Fruit powder	:	Tape worms in children
Stem bark	:	Puerperal fever

488. *Syzygium aromaticum* (L.) Merr. & Perry

Family	:	Myrtaceae
Common names	:	E: Clove
Description	:	Tree, leaves opposite, entire, glabrous, flowers small, in terminal axillary or lateral cymes. Petals 4-5, ovary 2-celled, fruit berry, globose.

USEFUL PARTS AND THEIR CURATIVE PROPERTIES

Uses	:	Medicines, perfumes, soaps, foods and in histological and microscopic work

489. *Syzygium cuminii* (L.) Skeels

Family	:	Myrtaceae
Common names	:	S: Jambuh H: Jamun E: Black plum
Description	:	Tree to 20 m, bark grey. Leaves coriaceous, elliptic, shortly acuminate, shining, base cuneate. Flowers tetramerous, subsessile in trichotomous lateral panicles from scars of fallen leaves. Petals united into a calyptra and falling off in one piece. Berries ovoid or oblong, juicy, 1-seeded.

USEFUL PARTS AND THEIR CURATIVE PROPERTIES

Leaf	:	Antibacterial, diabetes, dysentery, antiseptic, ulcers
Aerial part	:	CVS active
Seed	:	Hypoglycaemic, diabetes, leucorrhoea, earache, soft clear voice, controls frequent urination, small pox, dysentery, asthma, blood purifier
Fruits	:	Diabetes, kidney stones, urinary troubles, sore throat, gastro - enteritis
Wood	:	Diabetes
Stem bark paste	:	Body pain, leucorrhoea, cough, dysentery, dyspepsia, diabetes, diarrhoea, venereal diseases, wounds, burns

490. *Tabernaemontana divaricata* (L.)R. Br.ex Roem.&Schult.

Family : Apocynaceae

Description : A perennial shrub. Leaves simple, opposite, lanceolate, entire, acute. Flowers terminal, in corymbs. Corolla white 5, hypocrateriform. Fruit drupe.

USEFUL PARTS AND THEIR CURATIVE PROPERTIES

Leaf paste : Headache and fever, wounds, inflammation

Whole plant : Antihelmintic

Flowers : Burning sensation in eyes, sore eyes

Root : Dental caries and pyorrhoea, corneal diseases

491. *Tacca leontopetaloides* (L.) O. Kuntze

Family : Taccaceae

Common names : H: Diva E: Indian Arrow root

Description : Erect herb, about 1 m; root stocks tuberous. Leaves about 80 cm across, 3 partite, each irregularly pinnatifid, glabrous; flowers gree 1 cm across, drooping, in umbels. Perianth green, segments oblong. Berries ovoid with persistent perianth; seeds numerous, striate.

USEFUL PARTS AND THEIR CURATIVE PROPERTIES

Root stock : Dysentery, piles

Tuber : Mental depression

Whole plant : Kidney troubles

492. *Tamarindus indica* L.

Family : Caesalpiniaceae

Common names : S: Amlika H: Imli E: Tamarind

Description : Tree, about 15 m, branches glabrous, bark fissured. Leaves even pinnate, oblong, glabrous or puberulous, base and apex obtuse, entire. Flowers yellow with pink striations in terminal, few- flowered racemes.

USEFUL PARTS AND THEIR CURATIVE PROPERTIES

Leaves : Swelling due to wounds, burning micturition, diarrhoea, eye diseases

Epidermis of stem bark : Scorpion sting, diarrhoea, anorexia, stomach pain

Fruit : Menorrhagia, backache, anaemia, weakness, sprains, dysentery

Flower : Jaundice, blood dysentery, eye diseases, gonorrhoea, diarrhoea

Seed : Scorpion sting, fistula

493. *Tephrosia purpurea* (L.) Pers.

Family : Papilionaceae

Common names : S: Banah H: Sarpanka E: Wild indigo

Description : Erect perennial, undershrub. Leaves compound imparipinnate. Flowers bluish pink to purple, in terminal racemes. Calyx teeth triangular. Pod glabrescent.

USEFUL PARTS AND THEIR CURATIVE PROPERTIES

Plant	:	CNS active, antiprotozoal, antihepatotoxic, eczema, gonorrhoea, headache, indigestion
Root bark	:	Pulmonary diseases
Root	:	Conjunctivitis, diabetes in children, giddiness, earache, fertility, post partum treatment, stomach pain, aphthae, paralysis, snake bite, arthritis, rheumatism, fever, indigestion, colic pain, impotency, hydrocele, conception, spermatorrhoea, scorpion sting
Stem	:	Pyorrhoea
Leaves	:	Cough, headache, cooling effect, bodyache, joint pains, skin diseases, jaundice

494. *Teramnus labialis* Spreng

Family	:	Papilionanceae
Common names	:	S: Meshaparni
Description	:	Slender twining herbs. Leaflets ovate, acute, racemes very slender, calyx tube campanulate, corolla little exserted, stamens monadelphous, ovary many ovuled. Pod glabrous, seeds slightly oblong.

USEFUL PARTS AND THEIR CURATIVE PROPERTIES

Seed oil	:	Hypoglycaemic, anticancer
Leaf	:	Vertigo (hot sensation in the head)
Fruit	:	Astringent, antipyretic, stomachic, nervine tonic

495. *Terminalia alata* Heyne ex Roth

Family	:	Combretaceae
Common names	:	S: Asana H: Saj E: Black murdah
Description	:	Densely foliaceous tree upto 25 m, leaves spiral to opposite, oblong or elliptic, coriaceous, nerves 13-15 pairs, parallel ,glabrous above, tomentose below, base and apex obtuse; glands on the midnerve. Spikes axillary, in dense panicles. Drupe ovoid, glabrous, 5-winged.

USEFUL PARTS AND THEIR CURATIVE PROPERTIES

Stem bark	:	Earache, fever
Upper epider-mis of stem	:	Snake bite
Gum	:	Black spots

496. *Terminalia arjuna* (Roxb. ex DC) Wt. & Arn.

Family	:	Combretaceae
Common names	:	S: Arjunah H: Arjun saadadaa E: Arjun
Description	:	Large tree upto 20 m, leaves spiral to subopposite, oblong or obovate, nerves 14-17 pairs, obtuse-subcordate, crenate-serrate, apex obtuse, spikes axillary in panicles. Drupes 5-angled, 5-winged, wings oblique, apex notched.

USEFUL PARTS AND THEIR CURATIVE PROPERTIES

Stem bark : CVS and CNS active, antagonism of amphetamine hyperactivity, diuretic, abortifacient, abdominal pain, vomiting, diarrhoea, excessive menstruation, high blood pressure, increase potency, scorpion sting, ulcers, heart disorders, leucorrhoea, epilepsy, styptic, tonic, febrifuge, cirrhosis of liver, cough, dysentery, respiratory problems, emetic

Leaf juice : Earache, blood pressure

Aerial part : CNS depressant, semen coagulant, cardiac diseases

Stem paste : Vomiting and loose motions

497. *Terminalia bellirica* (Gaertn.) Roxb.

Family : Combretaceae

Common names : S: Bibhitakah H: Badami E: Belleric myrobalan

Description : Deciduous tree with large crown; branchlets with persistent leaf-scars. Leaves broadly ovate or elliptic, coriaceous, glabrous, cuneate-attenuate or obtuse, oblique, leaves densely clustered at the ends of branches. Petiole eglandular. Spikes axillary, solitary or clustered. Drupe subglobose, obscurely 5-ridged, horned.

USEFUL PARTS AND THEIR CURATIVE PROPERTIES

Fruit : Alcoholic extract of the fruit possesses bile stimulating activity, Anticancer, cough, sores in mouth, diarrhoea, fever, contraceptive, loose bowels, headache, strength, vigour, vitality, astringent, laxative, tonic, asthma, bronchitis, eye diseases, peptic ulcers, haemorrhoids, diabetes, leucorrhoea, indigestion

Flower : Apermicidal The dried fruits constitute the drug bahera which are useful in stomach disorders such as indigestion, diarrhoea, as a brain tonic, eye lotion, treatment of piles, leprosy, dropsy and fever

Gum : Urinary disorders

Seeds : Anti-alcoholism, hair tonic, strength, vigour, vitality, purgative

Stem bark paste : Jaundice, gastritis

498. *Terminalia chebula* Retz.

Family : Combretaceae

Common names : S: Haritaki H: Harara E: Chebulic myrobalan

Description : Deciduous tree upto 20 m, leaves spiral or opposite, ovate or elliptic-obovate, coriaceous, nerves 7-9 pairs, woolly below, rounded, entire, apex sub-acute. Spikes axillary, simple or branched. Drupe obovoid, glossy, horned, faintly angled.

USEFUL PARTS AND THEIR CURATIVE PROPERTIES

Chebulin : Antispasmodic

Flowers : Antiviral

Stem bark and fruit : Semen coagulant, hypoglycaemic, conjunctivitis, dysentery, piles

Stem bark : CVS active, cough, gastric troubles, disinfectant, diurectic, cardiotonic
Leaf and fruit : Antiviral, diabetes, muscle and rheumatic pains, wounds
Wood of stem : Oxytocic. hypothermic The dried fruits constitute the drug chebulic myrobalan or harra. This can be applied externally on ulcers, wounds and scalps or used as a gargle in inflammation of mucous membrane of mouth. Myrobalans are used as laxative, they have also been found to have some effect on blood pressure as cardiac tonics, diabetes, diarrhoea, bleeding, brain tonic, constipation, cough, fevers, jaundice, ulcers, stomachache, asthma, antifungal
Seed : Strength, vitality, purgative, vigour
Galls : Asthma

499. *Thespesia lampas* (Cav.) Dalz. ex Dalz. & Gibs.

Family : Malvaceae
Common names : S: Karpasi H: Ran-bendy
Description : Shrub to 1.5 m, stems woody. Leaves generally trilobed, cordate at base, pubescent-tomentose beneath, glandular on midrib at base adaxillary. Flowers yellow with maroon center, epicalyx segments 5, small, linear. Capsules ovoid, faintly stellate puberulous; seeds many, black, sparsely pubescent.

USEFUL PARTS AND THEIR CURATIVE PROPERTIES

Root extract : Heart stroke, malaria, typhoid
Leaf paste : Insect bite, loose bowels
Stem bark : Skin diseases
Dried roots and fruits : Bronchitis
Seed : Spermatorrhoea, tuberculosis, diabetes

500. *Thespesia populnea* Cav.

Family : Malvaceae
Common names : S: Parisha H: Paras papal E: Portia
Description : Trees, leaves entire, flowers solitary, axillary, bracteoles 5, calyx truncate, petals 5, staminal tube toothed at the top. Ovary 5-celled.

USEFUL PARTS AND THEIR CURATIVE PROPERTIES

Fruit : Antiviral, spasmolytic, anticancer, antifertility, antimalarial and antitumour effects due to gossypol and decreased sperm counts in men, eczema
Stem bark : Arthritis, dandruff
Leaf : Swellings

501. *Thymus vulgaris* L.

Family : Lamiaceae
Common names : H: Banajwain E: Thyme linalool

Description	:	Evergreen, perennial undershrub. Leaves lanceolate, sessile. Flowers purplish to white, bilabiate, tubular. Fruit nutlet, brown, smooth, 4-sectioned.

USEFUL PARTS AND THEIR CURATIVE PROPERTIES

Uses	:	Soap perfumery, mouth washes, dentrifices, anthelmintic, insecticides

502. *Tinospora cordifolia* (Willd.) Miers ex Hook. f.

Family	:	Menispermaceas
Common names	:	S: Guduci H: Gulancha E: Guluncha
Description	:	Woody climber. Bark corky and papery; petiole twisted at base. Leaves ovate, cordate, glabrous, membranous. Flowers yellow, fleshy, clasping the stamens in male. Drupelets turning red with age.

USEFUL PARTS AND THEIR CURATIVE PROPERTIES

Stem	:	Antiviral, hypoglycaemic, anticancer, cough, cold, fever, diabetes, flatulence, hair tonic, jaundice, eye diseases, rheumatic fever, malaria, paralysis, brain tonic, cuts, wounds, obesity, vaginal infection
Plant & stem	:	Spasmolytic, spermatorrhoea, antidote for snake bite, gonorrhoea
Root	:	Cold, cough, headache, hiccough, heart stroke, piles, skin diseases and whooping cough, high blood pressure, chronic fevers, tonic, snake bite
Tuber and aerial root	:	Leucoderma, snake bite, scorpion sting, stomach ulcers
Leaf	:	Fever, leucorrhoea, hepatic problems, diabetes, snake bite, scorpion sting
Whole plant	:	Aphrodisiac, stomachache, syphilis, jaundice, antipyretic, snake bite, arthritis, vomiting

503. *Toddalia asiatica* (L.) Lam.

Family	:	Rutaceae
Common names	:	S: Tiksnaksah H: Kanj E: Forest pepper
Description	:	Armed straggler, terminal prickles recurved, leaves trifoliate, sessile. Staminate or pistillate flowers in axillary or terminal panicles. Fruits ripen in black, globose, 5-lobed, fleshy.

USEFUL PARTS AND THEIR CURATIVE PROPERTIES

Aerial part	:	Hypoglycaemic, spasmolytic, anticancer, diuretic
Stem bark decoction	:	Indigestion, menorrhagia
Leaf	:	Bowel pains, bone fractures
Root bark	:	Gonorrhoea, diaphoretic, ulcers in the mouth, aromatic, pungent, stomachic, fever, diarrhoea, gonorrhoea, cough, influenza

504. *Trachyspermum ammi* (L.) Sprague

Family	:	Apiaceae
Common names	:	H: Ajuan E: Bishop's weed

Description : Slender herb to 50 cm. Leaves spiral, 2-3 pinnate, ultimate segments filiform; petioles sheathing at base. Flowers white. Fruits ovoid, ribbed, muricate.

USEFUL PARTS AND THEIR CURATIVE PROPERTIES

Leaf : Cold, cough, wounds, indigestion, sore throat
Seed : Irregular menstruation
Fruit : Asthma

505. *Tragia involucrata* L.

Family : Euphorbiaceae
Common names : S: Dusparsa H: Barhanta E: Indian nettle
Description : Climbing herb, stems with stinging hairs. Leaves elliptic, hispidly hairy, flowers in axillary racemes. Capsules long, seeds glabrous.

USEFUL PARTS AND THEIR CURATIVE PROPERTIES

Aerial part : Hypothermic, diuretic
Root : Gout, rheumatic pains, skin diseases, urination, bowel movement
Leaves : Tumours on thighs, sterility
Whole plant : Severe headache, fever, hypoglycaemic, vomiting

506. *Trema orientalis* (L.) Blume

Family : Ulmaceae
Common names : S: Jivanthi H: Jiban E: Indian nettle
Description : Evergreen tree, tender parts appressed pubescent. Leaves obovate to broadly lanceolate, obliquely cordate, serrulate, apex acuminate. Cymes axillary, in clusters. Flowers pentamerous, unisexual. Drupe globose, tipped by the style.

USEFUL PARTS AND THEIR CURATIVE PROPERTIES

Stem bark : Epilepsy
Root decoction : Haematuria
Root bark : Epilepsy

507. *Trianthema portulacastrum* L.

Family : Aizoaceae
Common names : S: Punarnava H: Santhi E: Horse-purslane
Description : Prostrate fleshy, much branched herb. Branchlets glandular-tomentose or sub- glabrous. Leaves broadly ovate, glabrous, petiole expanded into sheath at base. Flowers sessile, standing simply inside the sheath of petiole. Calyx white or pinkish.

USEFUL PARTS AND THEIR CURATIVE PROPERTIES

Whole plant : CVS active, spasmolytic, antagonism of amphetamine hyperactivity
Leaf : Bone fracture, bronchitis, wounds, vaginal discharges
Root : Eye diseases

508. *Tribulus terrestris* L.

Family : Zygophyllaceae

Common names : S: Gosksura H: Chologokhuru E: Land caltrops

Description : Prostrate herb, leaves opposite or spiral, paripinnate, leaflets 4-7 pairs, oblong, villous, oblique, entire, tip mucronate. Flowers yellow, axillary or leaf opposed, solitary. Fruit globose, spiny of 5 cocci, each coccus hairy, each with 2 long, hard, sharp divaricate spines.

USEFUL PARTS AND THEIR CURATIVE PROPERTIES

Whole plant : Burning micturition, excessive menstruation, urinary infections, jaundice, cystitis, stomachache, health tonic

Root : Recheck sterility in males, gonorrhoea

Fruit decoction : Urinary disorder, impotency, hiccups, nephroprotector, jaundice

509. *Trichosanthes anguina* L.

Family : Cucurbitaceae

Common names : S: Chichinda H: Chachinga E: Snake gourd

Description : Climbing shrub, tendrils branched. Leaves orbicular, shallowly 3-9 lobed, distantly denticulate, deeply cordate. Flowers white, staminate flowers in racemes; pistillate flowers solitary, axillary. Berries linear, cylindric, glaucous.

USEFUL PARTS AND THEIR CURATIVE PROPERTIES

Root : Dysentery, syphilis

510. *Tridax procumbens* L.

Family : Asteraceae

Common names : S: Jayanti E: Mexican daisy

Description : Annual decumbent herb to 30 cm. Leaves ovate, opposite, strigose on both sides, acute, coarsely serrate, apex acute. Heads solitary, terminal, yellow, heterogamous. Achenes obconical, ribbed.

USEFUL PARTS AND THEIR CURATIVE PROPERTIES

Plant : Homeostatic, styptic, antiseptic, astringent, jaundice, cuts, wounds, diarrhoea, decayed fingers

Leaf : Ulcers in stomach, uncontrolled bleeding wounds, eye diseases, carious teeth, cuts, bruises, aphrodisiac in males, piles

Root and leaf paste : Headache, stomach pain

Flower : Toothache

511. *Trigonella foenum-graecum* L.

Family : Apiaceae

Common names : E: Fenugreek

Description : Annual herb, leaves light green, pinnately trifoliate, flowers papilionaceous. Fruits legume, long, narrow, small deeply furrowed seeds.

USEFUL PARTS AND THEIR CURATIVE PROPERTIES

Whole plant : Constipation, indigestion, stimulates spleen and liver, appetizer and diuretic

512. *Triumfetta rotundifolia* Lam.

Family : Tiliaceae
Common names : S: Gippita H: Mendurli
Description : Erect undershrub. Branchlets stellate tomentose. Leaves rhomboid, orbicular, coriaceous, velvety below, base cuneate, crenate or serrate. Flowers yellow, in terminal racemes. Capsule ovoid or globose. Seeds ovoid, beaked.

USEFUL PARTS AND THEIR CURATIVE PROPERTIES

Leaf paste : Eczema, scabies, tumours on body

513. *Tylophora indica* (Burm. f.) Merr.

Family : Asclepiadaceae
Common names : S: Latakshiri H: Antamul E: Indian ipecacuanha
Description : Climber; leaves cordiform, oblong to lanceolate, subcoriaceous, truncate to cordate, apex acute, umbels compound; umbellules 2-4. Flowers greenish yellow outside, purple inside, in cymes. Follicle cylindric, acute at ends.

USEFUL PARTS AND THEIR CURATIVE PROPERTIES

Leaf : Antiallergic, asthma, cough, epilepsy in children, jaundice, snake bite, body pains
Leaf and stem decoction : Anticancer, backache
Tylophorine : Anti-inflammatory
Desmethyltylophorine : Antileukaemic
Root paste : Whooping cough, jaundice

514. *Uraria picta* (Jacq.) Desv.

Family : Papilionaceae
Common names : S: Prishniparni
Description : Erect herb. Leaves 5-7 foliate; leaflets linear-oblong, acute, glabrous above, minutely pubescent beneath. Raceme cylindric. Corolla purple. Joints of pod 3-6, glabrous.

USEFUL PARTS AND THEIR CURATIVE PROPERTIES

Root : Malaria, to increase potency, antidote for snake bite

515. *Urena lobata* L.

Family : Malvaceae
Common names : S: Atibala H: Kunjuya
Description : Shrub. Leaves deeply lobed, truncate, crenate-dentate. 2-serrate, apex acute. Flowers axillary, solitary, 2 or 3 in a cluster. Epicalyx segments 4. petals pinkish. Schizocarp globose; mericarps 5, trigonous.

USEFUL PARTS AND THEIR CURATIVE PROPERTIES

Whole plant : Rheumatism
Leaf paste : Wounds, cuts, dandruff, premature fall of hair
Root : Fever, syphilis, urinary trouble, anthelmintic

516. *Valeriana jatamansi* Jones.

Family : Valerianaceae
Common names : H: Tagar E: Indian valerian
Description :

USEFUL PARTS AND THEIR CURATIVE PROPERTIES

Whole Plant : Aphrodisiac, antiseptic, cardiac, stimulant, carminative, diuretic, emmenagogue, expectorant, febrifuge, nervine tonic, ophthalmic, sedative, suppurative and tonic. Useful in excitability of nervous system, insomnia, cardiovascular neurosis, gastrointestinal spasms. Indicated in abscess, colic, epilepsy, eye troubles, fever, headache, hysteria, liver trouble, neurosis, rheumatism, shell-shock and swoon.
Leaf : Diarrhoea

517. *Vernonia cinerea* (L.) Less.

Family : Asteraceae
Common names : S: Sahadevi H: Sahadevi E: Ash coloured fleabane
Description : Annual erect herb to 75 cm. Leaves ovate, broadly elliptic or lanceolate, cuneate-attenuate, entire, apex acute. Heads in terminal corymbose panicles, homogamous, pink. Achenes oblong, villous.

USEFUL PARTS AND THEIR CURATIVE PROPERTIES

Plant : Antiviral, spasmolytic, anticancer, piles, malaria, boils, blisters, abdominal pain
Leaf paste : Conjunctivitis, anthelmintic, amoebiasis, ringworm, eczema, extraction of guinea worms
Root : Malaria, filariasis, helminthiasis, stomach pain
Seed : Leucoderma

518. *Vetiveria zizanioides* Nash.

Family : Poaceae
Common names : S: Sevyah H: Khas-khas E: Vetiver, khus khus root
Description : Perennial herbs with stout rhizome, root stock with spongy, aromatic roots. Culms tufted, stout. Leaves distichous, panicle, sessile spikelets, upper lemma entire. Lodicules 2. stamens 3, styles 2, grain oblong.

USEFUL PARTS AND THEIR CURATIVE PROPERTIES

Uses : Root – mats for air cooling, diuretic, perfumery
Oil – aromatic, cool drinks, soaps, skin care creams, Ayurvedic medicines

519. *Viscum album* L.

Family : Loranthaceae
Common names : H: Banda

USEFUL PARTS AND THEIR CURATIVE PROPERTIES

Whole plant : Whole plant is used in medicine as a resolvent and laxative. It has been used in epilepsy, asthma, frost bite. In homoeopathy, it is used in a variety of disorders like epilepsy, sterility, vertigo, depression, hypertension, menstrual disorders and it is antispasmodic. The use of this plant for curing cancer was first declared by Rudolf Steiner in 1904. Recently, the Germans extracted a medicine from this plant called ISCADOR and claimed that it can cure cancer in early stages when applied in the form of homoeopathic injections.

520. *Vitex altissima* L. f.

Family : Verbenaceae
Description : Lofty deciduous tree. Leaves trifoliate, leaflets sessile or subsessile, glabrous above, thinly pubescent below, petiole angular. Flowers pale pink or purple in terminal panicles. Corolla very small. Drupes globose.

USEFUL PARTS AND THEIR CURATIVE PROPERTIES

Stem bark decoction : Fever, snake bite
Leaf paste : Skin eruptions
Root bark : Syphilis

521. *Vitex negundo* L.

Family : Verbenaceae
Common names : S: Nirgundi H: Nirgondi E: Five leaved chaste tree
Description : An aromatic shrub, tender parts grey pubescent. Leaves 3-5 foliate, leaflets oblanceolate. Panicles terminal. Corolla purple to violet. Drupe globose.

USEFUL PARTS AND THEIR CURATIVE PROPERTIES

Leaf : Anti-inflammatory, analgesic and CNS depressant activities, epilepsy in children, headache, joint pains, partial paralysis, conjunctivitis, eczema, rheumatism, asthma, fever, migraine, bodyache, insect repellant, cold, dermal diseases, body swellings, cooling, diabetes
Root : Joint pains and spermatorrhoea, rheumatism, piles, ringworm infection
Seed : Impotency
Flower : Cholera
Whole plant : Antifertility, vermifuge, fever, liver troubles, malaria, snake bite, rheumatism

522. *Wattakaka volubilis* (L.F.) Stapf

Family : Asclepiadaceae
Common names : S: Nakchikni H: Haran dodi E: Cotton milk plant
Description : Extensive, perennial woody, twiner with watery sap. Leaves broad, ovate to cordiform, rounded, apex shortly acuminate, glandular near lamina. Umbel axillary, corolla greenish.

USEFUL PARTS AND THEIR CURATIVE PROPERTIES

Leaves : Antiseptic, anticancer activity, CNS depressant, snake bite
Bark paste : Sischarge of blood with urine, urinary troubles, bone fracture
Root : Rheumatism, snake bite

523. *Withania somnifera* Dunal

Family : Solanaceae
Common names : S: Asvagandha H: Asgand E: Asvagandha
Description : Unarmed shrubs. Leaves alternate, flowers polygamo-dioecious, calyx 5 - 6, corolla 3 - 6, stamens 5, ovary 2 - celled. Fruit berry.

USEFUL PARTS AND THEIR CURATIVE PROPERTIES

Leaf : CNS active, anti-inflammatory, antihepatotoxic, antibacterial
Root : Anti-inflammatory, urinary troubles
Plant : Antitumour, hypotensive, brabycardic, antispasmodic, hypnotic, antibacterial, antiarthritic, adaptogenic, rejuvenate, respiratory stimulant activities, cataract
Bark : Rectal disease, itches, white patches, tuberculosis
Seed/fruit : Arthritis, asthma, eczema

524. *Woodfordia fruticosa* (L.) Kurz.

Family : Lythraceae
Common names : S: Dhataki H: Dhai E: Fire flame bush
Description : Large shrub, with spreading branches; bark reddish. Leaves ovate-lanceolate, rounded, entire, apex acuminate. Flowers in axillary clusters on slender pedicels, calyx bright red, petals white. Capsule enclosed by persistent calyx tube.

USEFUL PARTS AND THEIR CURATIVE PROPERTIES

Shoot : Antibiotic activity
Flower : Abortifacient, astringent and tonic, foul ulcers and wounds, stimulant, astringent, given in dysentery to check haemorrhages and leucorrhoea. Disorders of mucous membranes, haemorrhoids, derangements of liver. Safe stimulants in pregnancy, refrigerant, demulscent and aphrodisiac, diarrhoea Plant in small doses stimulant, which in large doses depresses the CNS, boils, swelling of the body
Stem bark : Bone fracture , snake bite, jaundice, cold
Root paste : Rheumatism, emmenagogue, stops bleeding from mouth and nose
Leaves : Wounds, ulcers, rheumatism, boils, blisters, burns, bruises, bodyache

525. *Wrightia tinctoria* (Roxb.) R. Br.

Family	:	Apocynaceae
Common names	:	S: Sveta kutajah H: Mitha indarjou E: Pala indigo plant
Description	:	Deciduous tree upto 10 m, leaves attenuate, apex acuminate. Flowers terminal, corymbose, dichotomous cymes. Corolla white. Fruit of 2 distinct deep green follicles cohering at the apex only.

USEFUL PARTS AND THEIR CURATIVE PROPERTIES

Leaf oil	:	Analgesic, anti-inflammatory, antipyretic
Leaf	:	Asthma, sore throat and cough, toothache
Tender shoot paste	:	Gonorrhoea
Root	:	Epilepsy, expel threadworms, snake bite, scorpion sting
Latex	:	Toothache, cuts, wounds, asthma, bronchitis, rheumatism, easy digestion
Stem bark	:	Stomach pain, dysentery, snake bite, skin diseases, ringworm, leprosy, cholera, piles, epilepsy
Seed	:	Carminative, laxative, helminthiasis

526. *Xanthium strumarium* L.

Family	:	Asteraceae
Common names	:	S: Kakubha E: Cockle-bur burweed
Description	:	A coarse annual herb. Leaves triangular-cordate. Heads in terminal or axillary racemes. Achenes 2 horned, densely covered hooked spines, pappus absent.

USEFUL PARTS AND THEIR CURATIVE PROPERTIES

Root	:	Antitumour; B-sitosterol glucoside – anti-inflammatory
Plant extract	:	Antimicrobial activity, leucorrhoea, gleet, menorrhagia, malarial fever
Leaf	:	Scrofula, herpes, cuts, wounds, menorrhoea, leucorrhoea

527. *Ximenia americana* L.

Family	:	Olacaceae
Common names	:	S: Kadaranji E: False sandal wood
Description	:	Bushy straggler. Spines axillary. Leaves ovate, coriaceous, ends obtuse, entire. Racemes umbellate. Flowers white. Drupe globose, ripening yellowish. Seed solitary.

USEFUL PARTS AND THEIR CURATIVE PROPERTIES

Root Bark	:	Astringent, diarrhoea
Fruit	:	Antidiabetic, blood purification, increase potency, diuretic, demulscent
Leaf	:	Maggot infested sores, skin diseases, ulcers
Seed	:	Lactation

528. *Zaleya decandra* (L.) Burm.f.

Family	:	Aizoaceae
Common names	:	S: Punarnavi H: Yadabani

Description : Prostrate herb. Leaves elliptic-oblong, cuneate, entire, obtuse. Flowers in dense umbel-like clusters in the axils of leaves, inner side of calyx white. Stamens 10. Capsule 4-seeded, not enclosed in the calyx tube.

USEFUL PARTS AND THEIR CURATIVE PROPERTIES

Leaves : Jaundice
Root : Malaria

529. *Zea mays* L.

Family : Poaceae
Common names : S: Makayah E: Maize
Description : Tall, stout, annual herbs. Leaves large, inflorescence monoecious, glumes membranous, lemmas similar, hyaline, lodicules 2, stamens 3, female spikelets lodicules 0, styles 2-fid, grain sub-globose.

USEFUL PARTS AND THEIR CURATIVE PROPERTIES

Plant : Diuretic, antilithic
Leaf : Cough, headache
Hairs of spike : Nephroprotector

530. *Zingiber officinale* Rosc.

Family : Zingiberaceae
Common names : S: Sunthi H: Soth E: Ginger
Description : Herb, leaves linear-lanceolate, sessile. Flowers in spikes, calyx shortly 3 lobed. Ovary 3-celled, fruit capsule, seeds globose, arillate.

USEFUL PARTS AND THEIR CURATIVE PROPERTIES

Rhizome : Antioxidant and antidiabetic, relieve labour pain and to facilitate child birth, migraine, dyspepsia, anorexia, cough, eye diseases, hypoglycaemic, diarrhoea, bone fractures, sprains, expectorant, stimulant, carminative, tonic, flatulent, colic, jaundice

531. *Ziziphus mauritiana* Lam.

Family : Rhamnaceae
Common names : S: Badarah E: Indian jujuba
Description : Thorny tree. Leaves suborbicular or ovate-elliptic. Flowers in axillary cymes. Drupe globose, yellow or red when ripe.

USEFUL PARTS AND THEIR CURATIVE PROPERTIES

Leaves : Anticholonergic activity, dysuria, hypoglycaemic
Fruit : Diarrhoea, blood dysentery, cooling
Buds : Measles
Root : Asthma, malaria
Bark powder : Dysentery and typhoid fever, fractures, diarhoea, burns

532. *Ziziphus oenoplia* (L.) Miller

Family : Rhamnaceae

Common names : S: Srigalakoli H: Makai E: Jackal jujuba
Description : Straggling shrub; thorns recurved. Leaves ovate-lanceolate, glabrescent above, subacute, denticulate, apex acuminate. Cymes axillary in umbellate clusters. Petals greenish, obovate. Drupe globose, rugose, woody. Seed 1, ovoid.

USEFUL PARTS AND THEIR CURATIVE PROPERTIES

Aerial part : Effect on respiration, nictitating membrane, hypotensive, diuretic
Fruit : Dysentery, indigestion
Root paste : Wounds, abdominal pain, loose motions
Stem bark : Dysentery, eczema, abscess, wounds, cuts
Leaves : Bone fractures

533. *Ziziphus rugosa* Lam.

Family : Rhamnaceae
Common names : H: Bhand ber
Description : Straggler, thorns stout, recurved. Leaves orbicular rotund, cordate, apex rotund, mucronate. Cymes in panicles, axillary or terminal. Peduncle with recurved spines. Drupe globose or pyriform, seed obovoid, turgid.

USEFUL PARTS AND THEIR CURATIVE PROPERTIES

Stem bark : Epilepsy, gastric troubles, menstrual disorders, stomach pains, diarrhoea, rheumatism

534. *Ziziphus xylopyrus* (Retz.) Willd.

Family : Rhamnaceae
Common names : S: Ghonta H: Kat-ber
Description : Small armed tree, thorns paired or solitary. Leaves ovate-oblong, glabrous above, tomentose below, base subcordate or obtuse, apex rounded. Cymes axillary divaricate. Petals greenish spathulate. Drupe globose, white tomentose; seeds oblong.

USEFUL PARTS AND THEIR CURATIVE PROPERTIES

Bark extract : CNS depressant activity, antinociceptive activity
Root : Anthrax, rheumatism, diarrhoea, dysentery
Stem bark paste : Snake bite, fever, cold, cholera
Seed : Piles
Leaf : Conception
Fruit : Anodyne, astringent, cooling, styptic, tonic

DIABETES MELLITUS
ETIOLOGY, COMPLICATIONS AND TREATMENT

SYED IBRAHIM RIZVI AND NEETI SRIVASTAVA

DEPARTMENT OF BIOCHEMISTRY, UNIVERSITY OF ALLAHABAD, ALLAHABAD, U.P.-INDIA

Chapter Outline

IN: HERBAL MEDICINE FOR HUMAN DISEASES: VOLUME-III, PAGES: 178-215

(EDITORS : IRFAN ALI KHAN AND ATIYA KHANUM), UKAAZ PUBLICATIONS - HYDERABAD (A.P)-INDIA

1. INTRODUCTION

Diabetes mellitus is recognized as one of the oldest known disease. Historical accounts reveal that as early as 700-200 B.C. Diabetes mellitus was a well-recognized disease in India, (Oubre *et al.*, 1997). Sushrut used the term "Madhumeha" for diabetes mellitus in 6th century. He described it as a disease of the rich, produced by over consumption of rice, flour and the sugar.

By definition, the term diabetes mellitus describes the metabolic disorder of multiple etiology characterized by chronic hyperglycemia with the disturbance in carbohydrate, protein and fat metabolism resulting from defects in insulin secretion, action or both. Diabetes mellitus is characterized by chronic elevation of circulating glucose (hyperglycemia), which is followed by development of micro and macro vascular complications.

The past two decades have seen an explosive increase in the number of people diagnosed with diabetes worldwide (Amos *et al.*, 1997; King, 1998). Pronounced changes in the human environment and in human behavior coupled with sedentary lifestyle that have accompanied globalization, have resulted in escalating rates of both obesity and diabetes. The combination of diabetes and obesity has resulted in the recent adoption of the term **'diabesity'** (Astrup *et al.*, 2000), which was first suggested by Shafrir some years ago (Shafrir *et al.*, 1997).

The long term effects of diabetes mellitus include progressive development of specific complications such as retinopathy, which effects eyes and lead to blindness; nephropathy in which the renal functions are altered or disturbed, and neuropathy which is associated with the risk of amputations, foot ulcers, and features of autonomic disturbances including sexual dysfunctions *etc*. People with diabetes are at increased risk of cardiovascular, peripheral vascular and cerebrovascular disease. All these complications substantially increase the rates of morbidity and mortality associated with the disease and reduces the quality of life of the diabetic individual.

It is, therefore, imperative that healthy individuals should adopt effective strategies to prevent the development of diabetes and for individuals with the disease, to seek the beneficial ways to help treatment in order to avoid complications.

There are various therapeutic approaches employed in the treatment of diabetes with a range of agents fighting hyperglycemia but the efficacy of these agents is compromised in various ways. This may be the reason that even after the much advancement in understanding of diabetes and designing of therapeutics, the disease profile of diabetes is still progressing. Present day drugs have prominent side effects like causing hyperglycemia at higher doses, liver problems, diarrhea *etc*. It is important that efforts are made to develop more efficacious agents with lesser side effects.

The role of medicinal plants in ameliorating the problem of diabetes is noteworthy because of their low cost, quick positive response and being safe on the body without apparent side effects. Therefore, investigations of these herbal agents for anti-diabetic activity is an important area of research.

In view of the importance of various herbal and medicinal plants, the present chapter has been compiled to create awareness about the disease, its causes and complications and most importantly role of selective Indian medicinal plants with pharmacologically established hypoglycemic potential in ameliorating the complications of diabetes.

2. DEVELOPMENT OF DIABETES

Carbohydrate from various dietary sources is the primary exogenous source of glucose, which is the main fuel providing energy to the body. A continuous supply of glucose is essential for the proper functioning and also survival of all organs. Mammals have evolved sophisticated system to maintain blood glucose level within narrow limits. Despite significant fluctuations in food intake the body maintains the level of glucose always towards normalcy, thus, protecting the body against hypoglycemic situations during periods of fasting and also against high levels following ingestion of carbohydrate rich diet.

These goals are chiefly met by hormonal modulations of production of glucose by liver, and peripheral uptake of glucose by skeletal, heart muscles and adipose tissue. When mammals fast, glucose homeostasis is achieved by triggering expression of gluconeogenic genes in response to glucagon and when rich carbohydrate diet is taken the action is taken over by insulin for its uptake and peripheral utilization. Thus, any impairment in glucose metabolism can lead to physiological imbalance with the onset of hyperglycemia and subsequently diabetes mellitus.

There are two main categories of this diabetes. Type 1 diabetes mellitus also called insulin-dependent diabetes mellitus (IDDM) and Type 2, the non-insulin dependent diabetes mellitus (NIDDM). IDDM represents a heterogeneous and polygenic disorder, with a number of non-HLA loci (about 20) contributing to the disease susceptibility (Tiwari and Rao, 2002). Though this form of diabetes accounts for 5 to 10% of all cases, the incidence is rapidly increasing in specific regions. It is estimated that incidence of Type 1 diabetes will be about 40% higher in the year 2010 than in 1997 (Tiwari and Rao, 2002) and yet there is no identified agent substantially capable of preventing this type of disease. NIDDM is far more common and results from a combination of defects in insulin secretion and action. This type of disease accounts for 90 to 95% of all diabetic patients. Treatment of Type 2 diabetes is complicated by several factors inherent to the disease process, typically insulin resistance, hyperinsulinemia, impaired insulin secretion, reduced insulin-mediated glucose uptake and utilization (Tiwari and Rao, 2002).

ROLE OF INSULIN

The hormone insulin exerts its short-term metabolic actions and its long-term growth-promoting action by binding to the insulin receptor on cell surfaces. In doing so it stimulates the uptake of simple sugars (monosaccharides) into cells and promotes the synthesis and storage of carbohydrates, fats and proteins while at the same time inhibiting enzymatic breakdown and release of these substances into the blood circulation. Insulin stimulates the cell stimulating lipogenesis, glycogen and protein synthesis and simultaneously inhibiting lipolysis, glycogenolysis, and breakdown of protein. Insulin increases the transport of glucose into fat and muscle cells by promoting movement of the glucose transporter GLUT4 from the interior of the cell to the cell membrane (Saltiel *et al. 2001)* Insulin is synthesized at blood glucose concentrations as low as 2–4 mmol/l, but released only at blood glucose concentrations above 4–6 mmol/l. This hormone, the only one that reduces blood glucose level, is rapidly cleared from the blood circulation and inactivated by specific insulin-metabolizing enzymes in the cells of the liver and other tissues.

3. PREVALENCE

The disease profile of the world is rapidly evolving of which diabetes is considered to be a major health problem and is one of the top five leading causes of death in most developed countries. Evidences suggest that it could reach epidemic proportion particularly in developing and newly industrialized countries (King *et al.*,1998).

By the year 2025, an estimated 300 million adults will be affected with diabetes and a major contribution to this number will be from India and China. The top ten countries in terms of diabetic patients are : India, China, USA, Indonesia, Japan, Pakistan, Russia, Brazil, Italy and Bangladesh. The increase in diabetic incidence in developing countries has been attributed to unhealthy diets, obesity and sedentary lifestyles.

The WHO estimate for the number of people with diabetes in 2000 is 171 million and this is likely to increase to at least 366 million by 2030. Around 3.2 million deaths every year are attributed to complications of diabetes, the sixth death every minute.

While talking about prevalence in India, WHO has estimated 19.4 million individuals affected with diabetes in 1995 and these numbers are expected to increase to 57.2 million by the year 2025.

Recent epidemiological studies have shown that migrant Asian Indian living in different part of the world show a much higher prevalence of diabetes than the host population of those countries (Pradeepa *et al.*, 2002a ; Pradeepa *et al.*, 2002b ; Zimmet *et al.*, 1983). This has been attributed to changes in environmental factors, such as increased affluence, which unmask an increased genetic or ethnic propensity of diabetes.

Direct health cost of diabetes ranges from 2.5 to 15 % of total healthcare budgets, depending on local diabetes prevalence and sophistication of treatment available.

ESTIMATED INCREASE IN DIABETES WORLD WIDE

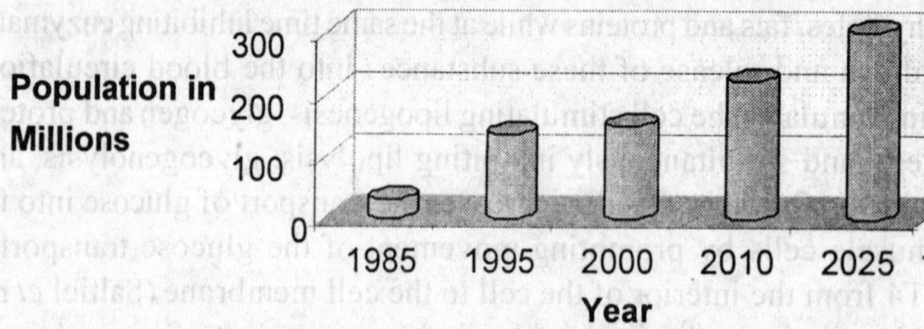

(Source : King *et al.,* 1998)

4. FACTORS RESPONSIBLE FOR SUCCEPTIBILITY TOWARDS DIABETES

The important factors contributing to risk for high prevalence of diabetes includes the following:

- Genetic predisposition
- Insulin resistance
- Obesity
- Rabid urbanization
- Ageing population

4.1 GENETIC FACTORS

Researchers while studying identical twins and the family tree of patients with diabetes have found that hereditary is an important factor contributing to the development of type 2 diabetes. A positive family history confers 2-4 fold increase risk of type 2 diabetes. Scientists have also identified several genes which seem to be involved. It may be possible to test family members to determine their risk of developing the condition. Genes responsible for several rare forms of autosomal dominant early onset of type 2 diabetes also known as Maturity Onset Diabetes of Young (MODY) have been identified. It has been estimated that 2-5 % patients with type 2 diabetes may have MODY forms of diabetes. Studies have indicated that insulin resistance is more pronounced in MODY compared to classical adult onset Indian type 2 diabetic subjects (Mohan et al.1985a ; Mohan et al., 1985b).

4.2 INSULIN RESISTANCE

Insulin resistance is an important clinical issue in patients with diabetes particularly in type 2 diabetes. However, its presence may be less evident in patients who are not obese. In a study carried by Mohan(2004) evidences of high prevalance rate of type 2 diabetes was found in Asian Indians which was attributed to the higher degree of insulin resistance compared to the caucasians (Chandalia *et al.,* 1999 ; Misra *et al.,* 2002). It was further demonstrated that Asian Indians have higher insulin levels to a glucose load compared to Europeans. Various studies have demonstrated that low birth weight is the predisposing factor for insulin resistance in Indian population. Patients with Insulin Resistance Syndrome have a group of related clinical findings : glucose intolerence , central obesity , dyslipidemia , hypertension , and altered fibrinolysis.

Insulin resistance occurs because of defective insulin mediated glucose uptake and utilisation, which reflects the inhibition of glucose transport . Insulin resistance is the major factor that contributes to hyperglycemia.

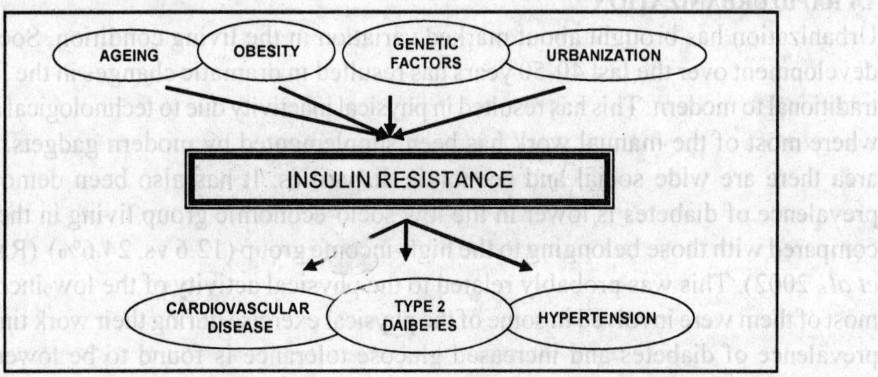

4.3 OBESITY

Insulin resistance is strongly associated with obesity and physical inactivity, and several mechanisms mediating this interaction have been identified. A number of circulating hormones, cytokines, and metabolic fuels, such as non-esterified (free) fatty acids (NEFA) originate in the adipose tissue and modulate insulin action. An increased mass of stored triglyceride, especially in visceral or deep subcutaneous adipose depots, leads to large adiposities that are themselves resistant to the ability of insulin to suppress lipolysis. This results in increased release and circulating levels of NEFA and glycerol, both of which aggravate insulin resistance in skeletal muscle and liver.

The role of obesity in pathogenesis of diabetes is complex and confounded by many heterogeneous factors. Indeed the relationship between diabetes and obesity has given the term diabesity to characterize the close association between these two disorders. Chan et al., 1994 have demonstrated that the relative risk of type 2 diabetes increases as body mass index (BMI) increases in the US population. Another study by Singh *et al.* 1998. showed that overweight / obesity and the central obesity were significantly associated with diabetes. Obesity has been on the increase in children, which might play a causative role in the escalating prevalence of diabetes in the young (Ehtisham *et al.,* 2004; Bloomgarden.2002). This increased occurrence of overweight in childhood may be the first sign of insulin resistance and future metabolic syndrome.

CENTRAL OBESITY

The android pattern of body fat typified by more upper body adiposity measured as waist hip ratio (WHR) has been found to be a greater risk factor for type 2 diabetes than the general obesity (Ramachandran *et al.* 2002).Studies have shown that central obesity is common in Indians despite low rates of obesity. The adverse effect of central obesity is manifested in increasing tertiles of BMI both in men and women. The effect being more evident in the women. This is probably one of the reasons for higher prevalence of diabetes in women in urban area.

4.4 RAPID URBANIZATION

Urbanization has brought about marked variation in the living condition. Socio-economic development over the last 40-50 years has resulted in dramatic changes in the lifestyle from traditional to modern. This has resulted in physical inactivity due to technological advancement where most of the manual work has been supplemented by modern gadgets. In the urban area there are wide social and economic disparities. It has also been demonstrated that prevalence of diabetes is lower in the low socio-economic group living in the urban areas compared with those belonging to the high-income group (12.6 vs. 24.6%) (Ramachandran *et al.*, 2002). This was probably related to the physical activity of the low-income group as most of them were involved in some of the physical exercise during their work time. Therefore prevalence of diabetes and increased glucose tolerance is found to be lower in the low-income group significantly. This indicates that the sedentary life style among the high-income group accompanies diabetes. In addition to sedentary life style, dietary pattern and high level of mental stress also effect insulin sensitivity, fuelling obesity leading to diabetes.

4.5 AGEING POPULATION

One of the most predictable and universal biochemical changes that occurs as we grow old is a progressive loss of glucose tolerance, characterized by prolonged post-meal elevations of glucose and insulin. As glucose tolerance continues to worsen, it increases our risk for obesity, hypertension, coronary artery disease and diabetes.

5. HYPERGLYCEMIA AND DIABETIC COMPLICATIONS

Diabetic complications are the major cause of morbidity and mortality in diabetic patients. Chronic hyperglycemia is the major initiator of diabetic micro vascular complications (*e.g.* retinopathy, neuropathy and nephropathy). Glucose processing uses variety of diverse metabolic pathway; chronic hyperglycemia can induce multiple cellular changes leading to complications. Two landmark studies conducted by The Diabetes Control and Complication Trial (DCCT),1993 and the United Kingdom Prospective Diabetes Study (UKPDS),1998 showed that intensive control of hyperglycemia can reduce the occurrence or progression of retinopathy, neuropathy and nephropathy in persons with Type 2 diabetes. Several predominant well-researched theories have been proposed to explain how hyperglycemia can produce the neuronal and vascular derangements that are hallmarks of diabetes. These theories can be separated into those that emphasize the toxic effect of hyperglycemia and its pathophysiological derivatives (such as oxidants, hyperosmolarity and glycation products) on tissues directly and those that ascribe pathophysiological importance to the sustained alteration in cell signaling pathway, such as changes in phospholipids or kinases induced by products of glucose metabolism (Bursell *et al.,* 1996).

All the mechanisms which have been implicated in glucose mediated vascular damage seem to reflect that hyperglycemia induces processes leading to overproduction of superoxide by mitochondrial electron transport chain. This integrating paradigm provide a new conceptual framework for future research and drug discovery.

COMPLICATIONS	ORGAN AFFECTED
Coronary heart disease	Heart
Dermopathy	Skin
Microangiopathy	Small blood vessels
Macroangiopathy	Large blood vessels
Nephropathy	Kidney
Neuropathy	Nerves
Peripheral vascular disease	Blood vessels of legs and feets
Retinopathy	Eyes

6. COMPLICATIONS OF DIABETES MELLITUS

6.1 CHRONIC STATE

The chronic complications of diabetes mellitus affect many organ systems and is responsible for majority of morbidity and mortality.

6.1.1 DIABETIC RETINOPATHY EFFECTING EYES

Diabetic retinopathy is deterioration of small blood vessels that nourish retina. This involves narrowing, hardening, bulging, hemorrhaging of several of veins and capillaries of retina. This is a serious complication and may lead to loss of vision, contraction of the visual field, changes in size of the object or photophobia.

In the more advanced stage, termed 'proliferative retinopathy', hemorrhages, retinal detachment and other serious forms of deterioration are observed. When the disease progresses to this late stage total blindness may occur. It usually takes between 10-13 years for diabetic retinopathy to develop and it is present in some degree in most diabetics who have had the disease for more than 20 years. In only about half of the diabetics who develop retinopathy the vision is markedly impaired and total blindness occurs in only about 6%. Still, diabetes is the leading cause of blindness in adults and is estimated to cause from 12,000 to 24,000 new cases each year. Two other complications of diabetes, cataracts and glaucoma, can also lead to loss of vision.

The development of laser therapy has reduced the prevalence of diabetes-induced blindness, however, this therapy is not without occasional side effects (hemorrhage, retinal detachment and loss of visual field) and is therefore indicated only for the more serious conditions.

Cataracts are clouding of the normally clear lens. A cataract develops over years and causes blurred vision when a large part of the lens becomes cloudy. Causes of cataracts include aging, eye injuries, disease, heredity, and birth defects. Cataracts can be treated by surgical removal of the lens. Eyeglasses, contact lenses, or intraocular lens implants restore vision following surgery.

6.1.2 DIABETIC NEPHROPATHY EFFECTING KIDNEYS

It is a complication of long-term diabetes. Nephropathy is less frequent than retinopathy and develops with long standing diabetes. Diabetes is the major cause of end stage renal disease in the U.S. Nephropathy results from damage to the bundle of capillaries which are involved in the formation of kidney filtering system. During diabetic nephropathy the kidney filtering becomes less efficient, and certain proteins leak out. Protein in the urine may be the first sign of nephropathy. Other signs include high blood pressure, weight gain from fluid retention, fatigue, and just feeling ill. Kidney function tests help determine the degree of kidney damage. Treatments for kidney failure include hemodialysis, peritoneal dialysis and kidney transplants.

6.1.3 DIABETIC NEUROPATHY AFFECTING NERVES

Diabetic neuropathies are among the most frequent complication of long-term diabetes. It is estimated that 60% to 70% of diabetics have mild to severe forms of nervous system damage. Neuropathy occurs in people with Type II diabetes due to metabolic changes with diabetes. Constant high blood sugar destroys both nerve fiber (**axon**) and the fatty insulation that surrounds it (**myelin**). Damaged nerves do not transmit proper signals, resulting in a loss of sensation, hyper sensation, or pain.

Peripheral neuropathy is the most common form. Varying from mild to severe, it causes changes in sensation that begin in the toes move up to the feet and legs. One may experience numbness, tingling, burning, dull ache, or stabbing pain and cramping, which is worse at night. The skin can become so sensitive that pressure from clothes is painful. Severe neuropathy may cause weakness and unbalanced walking. The greatest danger is foot ulcers, which result when lack of sensation causes people to continue walking on injured feet. Many treatments are available for peripheral neuropathy, including medications and topical creams. Not all are effective for everyone. Better diabetic control helps some patients. A painful neuropathy may change to a numb feeling after a while. Neuropathies sometimes disappear on their own. Autonomic neuropathy involves the nerve supply to small blood vessels and sweat glands of the skin, the stomach, the bladder, the heart, and the nervous system *etc*. It is most often associated with long-term diabetes, poor control, and elevated blood sugar.

6.1.4 MACROVASCULAR COMPLICATIONS AFFECTING BLOOD VESSELS

Cardiovascular disease is the leading cause of mortality among diabetics. Macrovascular disease is a change in somewhat medium to large sized blood vessels.The blood vessel wall thickens, becomes hard and non elastic (called as Arteriosclerosis), blood vessels also become clogged with mounds of plague (known as Atherosclerosis). Eventually the flow of blood may be blocked. Three types of this disease are recognised:

PERIPHERAL VASCULAR DISEASE

Arises from abnormality in blood vessels that supply the blood to legs and feet. This can cause weakness and pain while walking in the initial stage and when the artery wall is completely blocked it causes severe pain and the legs becomes cold and pale. Treatment includes replacing the diseased artery surgically or opening the blood vessels against artery wall.

CORONARY ARTERY DISEASE

This disease deals with diseased heart arteries. Cramping and angina may occur when the flow of blood is decreased and complete blockage results in myocardial infarction leading to heart attack. Treatments include coronary bypass surgery.

CEREBRAL VASCULAR DISEASE

The disease refers to diseased arteries in the brain. Temporal reduction in the supply of blood may cause partial blockage while a complete loss of blood supply to the area of brain due to clogging result in cerebro vascular stroke.

In addition to the above complications ulcers of the legs and feet occur in people with diabetes due to the combination of neuropathy and peripheral vascular disease. Neuropathy causes a loss of sensation; so that foot injuries may go untreated and become infected. Decreased circulation to the feet and legs slows healing. Proper nourishment does not reach damaged tissue, and infected material is not destroyed. Even a small injury may progress to an ulcer.

An increase in cavities and infectious periodontal disease has been found in people with poor diabetes control. Diabetic subjects also have a higher risk of some infections, including, lower extremity infections, re-activation tuberculosis, infections in surgical wounds and group B streptococcal infection. Population based data suggest a probable higher mortality from influenza and pneumonia.

7. MECHANISM OF HYPERGLYCEMIA INDUCED DIABETIC COMPLICTIONS

Many hypothesis about how hyperglycemia causes diabetic complications have generated large amount of data as well as several clinical trials based on specific inhibitors of these mechanisms. The mechanisms underlying the development of diabetic late complications have been reviewed by Brownlee *et al.*, 2001. The major theories are as follows: Aldose Reductase theory, Advanced Glycation End Product (AGE) Theory, Activation of Protein Kinase C (PKC) Isoform Theory, and Increase in Hexosammine Pathway Flux. In addition Reactive Oxygen Intermediate Theory has also been found to be responsible for diabetes complications.

7.1 ALDOSE REDUCTASE

It is the first enzyme in the polyol pathway. It is a cytosolic, monomeric oxidoreductase that catalyses the NADPH dependent reduction of glucose. Increased intracellular glucose in hyperglycemic environment results in its increased enzymatic conversion to the alcohol sorbitol, with concomitant decrease in NADPH. In the polyol pathway, sorbitol is oxidized to fructose by the enzyme sorbitol dehydrogenase, with NAD^+ being reduced to NADH. Cataract formation in diabetes and galactosemia results from accumulation in the lens of excessive sorbitol synthesized by the action of aldose reductase on glucose or galactose.

POLYOL PATHWAY

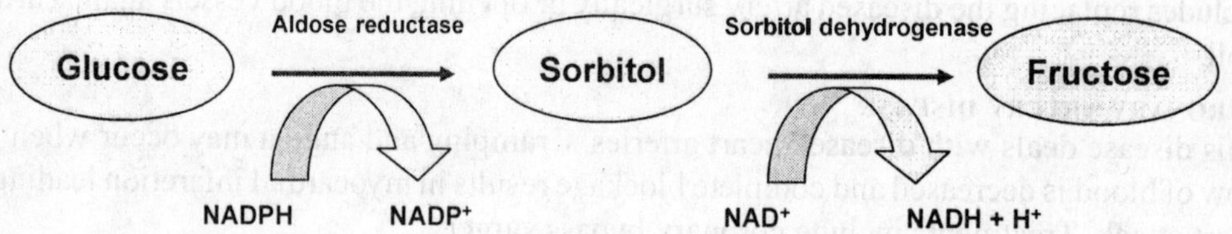

A number of mechanisms have been proposed to explain the potential detrimental effects of hyperglycemia induced increase in polyol pathway flux. These include sorbitol induced osmotic stress, decreased (Na^+, K^+) ATPase activity, an increase in cytosolic $NADH/NAD^+$ and a decrease in cytosolic NADPH. Hyperglycemia induced activation of PKC increases cytosolic phospholipase A_2 activity, which increases the production of two inhibitors of $Na^+ K^+$ ATPase, arachidonate and PGE2. It has also been proposed that reduction of glucose to sorbitol consumes NADPH. Since NADPH is required for regenerating reduced glutathione (GSH) this could induce or exacerbate intracellular oxidative stress.

7.2 ADVANCED GLYCATION END PRODUCTS

(AGEs) are found in increased amount in diabetic retinal vessels (Stitt *et al.*,1997) and renal glomeruli (Horie *et al.*,1997). AGE inhibitors partially inhibit various structural and functional manifestations of diabetic micro vascular diseases in retina, kidney and nerve (Saulis-Liporota *et al.*, 1991; Nakamura *et al.*, 1997; Hammes *et al.*, 1991). The AGE inhibitor amino guanidine lowered total urinary protein and slowed progression of neuropathy. Production of intracellular AGE precursors damages target cells by three general mechanisms; intracellular protein modified by AGEs have altered functions; extra cellular matrix components modified by AGE precursors interact abnormally with other matrix components and with the receptors from matrix proteins (integrins) on cells; and plasma proteins modified by AGE precursor bind to the receptors of AGE (RAGE) on endothelial cells, mesangial cells and macrophages inducing receptor mediated production of reactive oxygen species. The AGE receptor ligation activates pleiotropic transcription factors causing pathological changes in gene expression along with other cellular signaling events such as activation of mitogen activated protein (MAP) kinase or PKC which can lead to cellular dysfunction.

7.3 DIACYLGLYCEROL (DAG) AND PROTEIN KINASE

These are critical intracellular signaling molecules that can regulate many vascular functions including permeability, vasodilator release, endothelial activation and growth factor signaling. The PKC family comprises at least eleven isoforms, nine of which are activated by lipid second messenger DAG. Intracellular hyperglycemia increases the amount of DAG in cultured micro vascular cells and in the retina and renal glomeruli of diabetic animals (Koy and King,1998). Increased *de novo* synthesis of DAG leads to activation of beta isoforms of PKC, which have been shown to mediate the retinal and renal blood flow abnormalities (Ishii *et al.,* 1996). Activation of PKC by raised glucose also induces expression of permeability enhancing factor VEGF in smooth muscles cells (Williams *et al.*, 1997). Treatment with an inhibitor specific for PKC significantly reduced PKC activity in the retina and renal glomeruli of diabetic animal. Concomitantly, treatment significantly reduces diabetes induced increase in retinal mean circulation time, normalizes increase in glomerular filtration rate and partially corrected urinary albumin excretion.

7.4 HEXOSAMINE PATHWAY

The excessive flux of glucose or FFAs into a variety of cell types results in the activation of the hexosamine biosynthetic pathway (Marshall *et al.*, 1991; Boden *et al.*, 1994), which in turn leads to insulin resistance and the development of late complications of diabetes (Marshall *et al.*, 1991; Boden *et al.*, 1994; Schleicher *et al.*2000). Researches have implicated a hyperglycemia-induced increase in ROS formation in the activation of the hexosamine pathway (Brownlee *et al.,* 2001).

7.5 REACTIVE OXYGEN INTERMEDIATE THEORY

Hyperglycemia can increase oxidative stress through both enzymatic and non-enzymatic processes as mentioned earlier. Glucose metabolism through glycolytic pathway and TCA cycle produces reducing equivalents used to drive the synthesis of ATP via oxidative phosphorylation in mitochondria. By-products of mitochondrial oxidation include free radicals like superoxide anions whose generation increases with increase in glucose levels. Glucose oxidation also produces free radicals that damage cellular proteins as well as mitochondrial DNA. Increased oxidative stress reduces nitric oxide levels, damage cellular proteins and promote leukocyte adhesion to the endothelium while inhibiting the barrier function. Levels of antioxidants such as GSH, Vitamin C and Vitamin E have been reported to get decreased in diabetes.

There can be two approaches for designing treatment for prevention of hyperglycemia induced complications: First the neutralization of specific glucotoxins such as reactive oxygen species or AGE's and second, identifying and normalizing the activity of a common signaling pathway used by glucose and glucotoxins to exert their effects. Clinical trials are in progress using both these approaches. Reactive oxygen intermediate theory may be defined as one of the main culprits in causal of various diseases like diabetes.

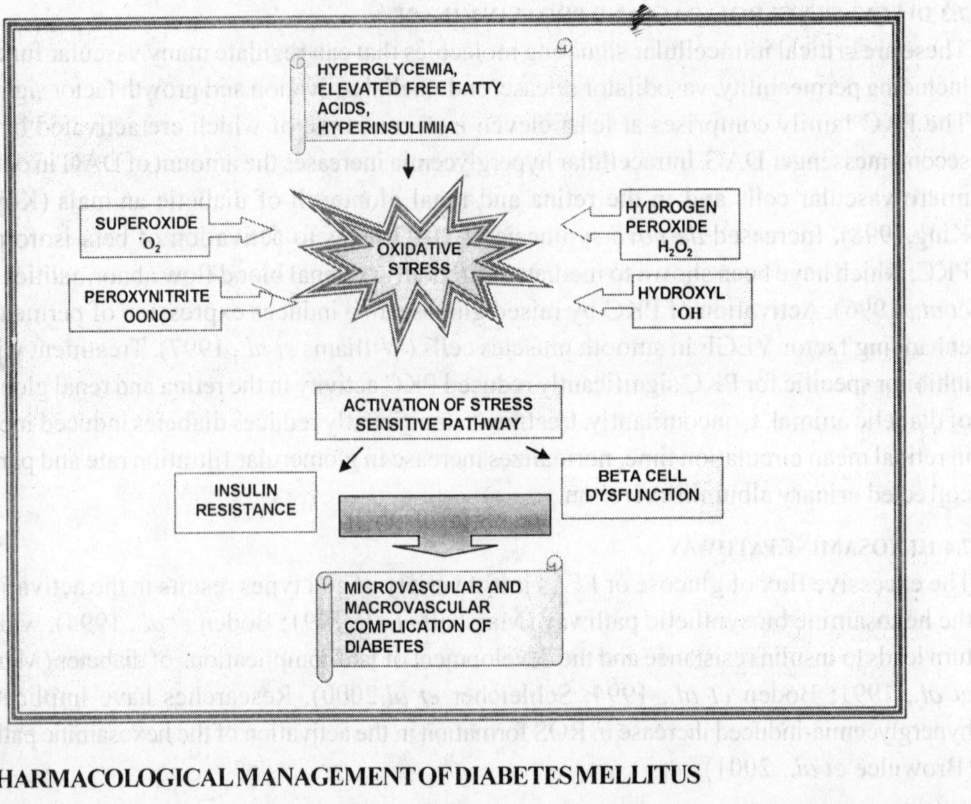

8. PHARMACOLOGICAL MANAGEMENT OF DIABETES MELLITUS

Hyperglycemia in patients with diabetes mellitus is always the result of mismatch between the quantity of insulin necessary to regulate the person's metabolic processes and the amount of insulin being secreted by the beta cells. Patients with insulin resistance start with relative insulin deficiency and with passing years frequently progress as to an absolute insulin deficiency. Oral antihyperglycemic agents such as Thiazolidinediones or Metformin decrease insulin resistance, alpha glucosidase inhibitors decrease postprandial insulin needs, insulin secretagogues improve and increase endogenous insulin secretion, and insulin and its analogues replace endogenous insulin secretion by exogenous secretion. Drug therapy for diabetes especially for type 2 diabetes is considered when diet, patient's education and increased physical activity have failed to achieve individual treatment goals.

9. CHEMOTHERAPEUTIC APPROACH IN THE TREATMENT OF DIABETES

It is now clear that aggressive control of hyperglycemia in patients with type 2 diabetes can attenuate the development of chronic complications such as retinopathy and nephropathy. Presently therapy for type 2 diabetes mellitus relies mainly on several approaches intended to reduce hyperglycemia. Given below are the description of some of commonly used antidiabetic chemotherapeutics along with their mechanism of action and associated side-effects.

9.1 THIAZOLIDINEDIONES

Two important agents belonging to Thiazolidinediones are Rosiglitazone and Proglitazone (Lebovitz *et al.,* 2002.) These agents bind to peroxisome proliferator activator receptor-gamma nuclear receptors affecting gene regulation in target cells. Interestingly, this alteration of gene transcription takes place in adiposities and the genes concerned primarily regulate fatty acid metabolism, the net result of which is to decrease serum FFA by approximately 20% to 40% (Phillips *et al.,* 2001; Fonseca *et al.* 2000; Yamasaki *et al.,* 1997). This reduction in FFA, in turn, improves insulin action in muscle tissue, thus, implicating elevated FFA as a major contributor to insulin resistance. Furthermore, this reduction in FFA improves β-cell function by decreasing lipotoxicity, a process whereby increased FFA eventually leads to β-cell death (Bell *et al.,* 2001). In various trials the TZDs have increased β-cell function significantly. However, the problem of weight gain and edema is also seen in some patients.

9.2 SULPHONYLUREAS

They are widely considered as first line drug treatment in NIDDM patients who are not obese. Sulphonylureas are the short acting insulin releaser and act directly on islet beta cells to close ATP sensitive potassium channels which leads to membrane depolarization and influx of calcium through voltage dependent channels this subsequently increases the secretion of insulin (Zimmerman, 1997).

The efficacy of these agents depends on the presence of enough beta cells with sufficient functional reserve. However, the endogenous insulin response to glucose is usually diminished in advance stage of type 2 diabetes mellitus.

The major acute problem associated with sulphonylureas is hypoglycemia, the risk of it varies somewhat among agents. It is generally accepted that Glyburide has twice the risk of hypoglycemia as compared to other second-generation sulphonylureas (Shorr *et al.,* 1996 ; McCall., 2001). This is due to the increase in duration of binding to suphonylurea receptor leading to hyperinsulemia with Glyburide, which is not seen in other Sulphonylurea.

In addition glyburide leads to suppression of several counter regulatory hormones. Weight gain is also one of the negative aspects with sulphonylurea agents. It also reduces the potential for decreasing myocardial protective mechanism (Langtry and Balfour,1998).

Various sulphonylurea agents and their metabolites are excreted by various degrees via kidneys and therefore caution has to be taken while using it for elderly peoples and peoples with renal insufficiency (Horrower, 1996).

9.3 NON-SULPHONYLUREA SECRETAGOGUES

Repaglinide and Nateglinide, these agents belong to different classes, as Repaglinide belongs to Meglitinide family while Nateglinide is a derivative of Phenylalanine.

The main difference between these agents and sulphonylurea is rapidity and duration of action exhibiting the secretion of insulin. Much has been said about efficacy of these agents to control post-prandial glucose because of their fast action. Despite the methods in which these newer insulin secretagogues have been marketed, there is little published evidence they control PPG better than the sulphonylureas.

9.4 BIGUINIDES

Metformin is the only established drug that deals with insulin resistance. The glucose lowering effect is mainly the consequence of reduced hepatic glucose output (gluconeogenesis and glycogenolysis) and increased insulin stimulated glucose uptake and glycogenesis in the skeletal muscles thus improving fasting hyperglycemia. (Hundal *et al.,* 2000). There is increased peripheral effect of increased insulin action in the muscles tissue, which may be related to the ability of Metformin to lower free fatty acids (Del Prato *et al.,*1995 ; Abbasi *et al.,* 1998). By increasing the insulin sensitivity, it also improves the variety of other factors related to increased cardiovascular risk (Palumbo.1998). Metformin induces weight loss through its appetite suppressing action. The main side effect associated with Metformin is gastrointestinal intolerance, which occurs approximately in 30% of patients. (Garber *et al.,* 1997) Metformin should also be avoided in patients with liver disease or the habits that expose them towards the risk (alcoholism) and other condition, which may predispose to acidosis.

9.5 ALPHA-GLUCOSIDASE INHIBITORS

The agents in this class are Acarbose and Miglitol. These agents delay the intraluminal production of monosaccaride, particularly glucose. Acarbose competitively inhibits alpha glycosidase that are associated with the brush border membrane of the small intestine and are responsible for the digestion of complex polysaccharide and sucrose. This slows carbohydrate digestion and lowers postprandial hyperglycemia. These drugs do not cause hypoglycemia or weight gain. However, because they affect only postprandial glucose level, the potency of this agent is less than most of the other agents. There is significant troublesome side effects of flatulence, abdominal pain and diarrhea.

Despite great improvements in modern medicine and research that goes in the development of drugs, these therapies have limited efficacies, limited tolerability and exhibit significant mechanism based side effects. Of particular concern is the tendency for most of these treatments to increase body weight. Several current approaches are associated with generation of hypoglycemia, and few of the available therapies adequately address underlying defects such as obesity and/or insulin resistance. Furthermore the multifactoral pathogenicity of diabetes demands multimode therapeutic approach. On account of all these drawbacks there is renewed interest in complimentary and alternative herbal medicines derived from medicinal plants. These traditional medicines contain a variety of herbal ingredients that incorporate synergistic, potentiative and antagonistic pharmacological agents and hence act on variety of targets by various modes of action.

DRUG CATEGORY	CHEMICAL CLASS	MODE OF ACTION	PROBLEMS ASSOCIATED
Insulin Sensitizers	Thiazolidineiones (Glitazones),(eg.pioglitazone Troglitazone, rosiglitazone)	Helps in reduction of peripheral Insulin resistance which has been the major culprit in most cases of type 2 diabetes by reduction of free fatty acids in the blood and consequent stimulation of glucose metabolism and reduction of endogenous glucose production in the liver (gluconeogenesis and the reduction of blood glucose levels)	Increases weight of the body
Substance that help to stimulate the secretion of Insulin	Sulphonylureas **First Generation Drugs-** Chlorpropamide, Tolbutamide Tolazamide, acetohexamide. **Second Generation** Drugs – Glyburide, glipizide. **Third generation drugs** – glimiperide	These reagents reduce glucose by increasing the insulin secretion from the pancreatic beta cells in patients with residual beta cell function half-life	Risk of hypoglycemia with over dosage, exhaustion of beta cell by over stimulation
Biguanides	Metformin	Increases sensitivity of Insulin by hepatic gluconeogenesis and increased effectiveness of AMP Kinase, which promote glucose uptake into the muscles and inhibits the synthesis of cholesterol. lipid and triglyceride in the liver.	Gastrointestinal symptoms and very rarely lactic acidosis
Inhibitors of carbohydrate absorption	Acarbose, miglitol	Inhibition of beta glucosidase which releases glucose from Starch, delayed release of glucose from dietary carbohydrates, reduction of postprandial hyperglycemia	Digestive Disturbance. Flatulence
Non-Susecretagogues	Repaglinide and Nateglinide	These agents are short acting insulin secretogoques. They act on ATP-dependent potassium channels in pancreatic beta cells allowing opening of Ca2+channels and increasing insulin release.	There is also evidence that increased PPG levels may translate into a greater risk of CVD.

10. THE HERBALAPPROACH COMBATING DIABETES

Healthy healing is an incredible resource for every patient. Fossil record date human use of plants as medicines at least to the middle Paleolithic age some 60,000 years ago (Solecki and Shanidar IV, 1975) The Indian medicinal system *viz* Ayurveda, Sidda and Unani system predominantly use plant based raw materials in most of their preparations and formulations. The interest in medicinal plants has increased due to failure of modern medicines to provide effective treatment of the chronic disease.

According to The World Health Organization estimates 80% population of the developing world rely on traditional medicines derived from medicinal plants. The plant-based raw materials are safe, preventive, curative and are particularly useful in achieving the goal of "Health to All" in a cost effective manner. Thus demand of medicinal plant is increasing in both developed and developing countries. (Government of India, Planning Commision March, 2000)

With the onset of scientific research in herbals it is becoming clearer that medicinal plants have a potential in today's synthetic era. With the progress of new technologies, new avenues have been opened in purifying active components from the plants and establishing their chemical structure or even to synthesize and modify them chemically. So the ancient knowledge coupled with scientific principles can come into the forefront and provide us with powerful remedies to treat different diseases.

India has about 45,000 plant species and among these several thousand have been claimed to possess medicinal properties. Research conducted in last few decades on plants, which have been traditionally used for medicinal purpose for diabetes, has shown that several plants and plant based products have strong anti diabetic property.

Interestingly in most cases the antidiabetic property has been attributed to phytochemicals derived from these medicinal plants, most of the phytochemicals are antioxidants e.g., epicatechin, a polyphenol flavonoid isolated from the bark of Indian tree *Pterocarpus marsupium* has significant antidiabetic effect.

The active principal present in medicinal plants have been observed to possess pancreatic beta cell regenerating property, insulin releasing, sparing or even ameliorating the problem of insulin resistance (Gymnema sylvestre, bitter melon and extract of Indian Kino tree).

Medicinal plants have been reported to affect various metabolic enzymes involved in diabetogenesis (Fenugreek, tinospora, Ivy guard and bitter melon) correcting the imbalanced glucose metabolic disturbances, improving the glucose uptake, inhibiting gluconeogenic enzymes and modulating glycolitic and lipolytic pathways in diabetic conditions.

In late complication of diabetes, it has been observed that medicinal plants (Bitter melon, tinospora, Bilberry *etc.*) attenuate renal hypertrophy, and ameliorate diabetic neuropathy and gastropathy.

Thus, medicinal plants play an important role in modifying the corrective factors which cause vitiation in normal/healthy homeostasis, biochemical and physiological process at cellular and tissue level.

Ethanobotanical information has reports of about 800 plants possessing antidiabetic potential. Many of them has been investigated for their beneficial use in different types of diabetes and reported in numerous scientific journals (Grover *et al.* 2002 ; reviewed by Mukherjee *et al.* 2006). Out of these, some of the selected Indian medicinal plants, which are anticipatory in context of diabetes, are mentioned herewith along with their important properties and mode of action.

1. *Allium cepa*

Family : Liliaceae
Common name : Onion
Part used : Seedling, Callus, Bulb *etc.*

It is an essential plant cultivated throughout India. Commonly known as **onion** and belongs to the family Liliaceae. Various parts such as seedling, callus cultures *etc.,* are known to possess antidiabetic activity. Several studies have indicated that it has hypoglycemic, hypolipedemic and antioxidant activity (Romon-Ramos *et al.,* 1995).

The relative potency of onion with respect to hypoglycemic and hypolipidemic effects on the diabetic condition and the association of these effects with potential against oxidative stress was studied in male Wistar rats. It was shown that the hypoglycemic and hypolipidemic actions of *Allium cepa* was associated with antioxidant activity since onion decreases superoxide dismutase activity (Campos *et al.,* 2003).

A study with seedling, seedling parts and callus cultures exhibited much higher hypoglycemic activity as compared to natural bulb of onion and the same can be used as an alternative source for the isolation of hypoglycemic compounds (Kelkar *et al.,* 2001)

Investigations reveal the presence of sulfur containing amino acid S-methyl cysteine sulphoxide (SMCS) in onion which when administered orally to alloxan-induced diabetic rats (200 mg/kg for 45 days) significantly controlled blood glucose and lipids in serum and tissues and normalized the activity of liver hexokinase, glucose-6-phosphatase and HMG-CoA reductase. The effect was in accordance with that of glibenclamide and insulin (Kumari *et al.,* 1995). Another compound S-allyl-cysteine sulphoxide was also found to be effective in reducing the blood glucose of alloxan induced diabetic rats. (Sheela *et al*., 1995)

Beneficial effect of fresh onion as a dietary aid has also been shown in a crossover designed clinical study. The onion diet decreased or maintained blood glucose level (Tjokroprawiro *et al.,* 1983). Onion is also an excellent source of Quercetin, a flavonoid that is an antioxidant. (Hollman *et al*., 1997)

2. *Allium sativum*

Family	:	Alliaceae
Common name	:	Garlic
Part used	:	Cloves of bulb

Another dietary component cultivated throughout India commonly known as garlic and it belongs to the family Alliaceae. The hypoglycemic activity of garlic has also been extensively studied and reported. Work carried by various researchers have proved the potent hypoglycemic activity of *Allium sativum* (Zacharias *et al*., 1980 ; Roman-Ramos *et al*., 1995; Kasuga *et al.* 1999).

Garlic contains S-allyl cysteine sulphoxide, a sulfur containing amino acid which has significant blood glucose lowering activity in experimental diabetic animals. (Sheela and Augusti,1992). Its administration decreased the concentration of serum lipids, blood glucose and activities of serum enzymes as alkaline phosphatase, acid phosphatase, lactate dehydrogenase, and liver glucose-6-phosphatase. It also increased the activity of HMG-CoA reductase and liver hexokinase (Sheela and Augusti,1992)

Garlic is also known to exhibit synergistic antioxidant property (Shobana and Naidu, 2000) Allicin, which is an antioxidant compound has also been shown to possess hypoglycemic activity when given orally to mildly diabetic rabbits (150mg/kg, IV.) (Jain and Vyas.1975). The hypoglycemic effect was comparable to tolbutamide, while its effect was negligible in severe diabetic animals (Mathew and Augusti,1973).

Aqueous extract of garlic increased hepatic glycogen, and free amino acid content when given orally to sucrose fed rabbits (10ml/kg/day). Garlic is known to decrease fasting blood sugar, triglyceride level in serum, liver and aorta and protein levels when compared with sucrose controls (Zacharias *et al.,* 1980)

Pretreatment with aged garlic extract in stress induced hyperglycemia model of mice significantly prevented adrenal hypertrophy, hyperglycemia, elevation of cortisone without altering serum insulin levels. The efficiency of treatment was same as that of diazepam (5mg/kg. Po) thus garlic extract may prevent stress induce risk of diabetes mellitus and its progression (Kasuga *et al.,* 1999). Garlic has also been reported to prevent cardiovascular complications (Patumraj *et al.,* 2000) Hypolipidemic effects of Allium sativum has also been described (Augusti and Mathew, 1973).

3. *Aloe barbadensis*

Family	:	Liliaceae
Common name	:	Aloe vera
Part used	:	Leaves

Commonly called as *Aloe vera* is a medicinal herb cultivated throughout India. Aloe has been used widely all over the world on account of its various beneficial effects. Leaf gel, leaf pulp and dried sap are known to possess antidiabetic and antioxidant activity.

The potential antioxidative activity of ethanolic extract of *Aloe vera* leaf extract in plasma and pancreas in streptozotocin induced diabetic rats was studied by Rajasekaran *et al.,* 2005. Oral administration of ethanolic extract at a concentration of 300 mg /Kg body weight for 21 days, proved more effective in controlling oxidative stress found in diabetes. (Rajasekaran *et al.,* 2005).

The extract of Aloe gum is effective in enhancement of glucose tolerance in normal as well as diabetic rats (Al-Awadi and Gumaa,1987). Hypoglycemic activity of Aloe and its bitter principle is thought to be mediated through stimulation of synthesis and/or release of insulin from the beta cells of islet of langerhans (Ajabnoor ,1990). *Aloe vera* is well regarded as the "Healing Herb" in various parts of the world; both Aloe vera and Aloe gibberellins (over a dose range 2 –100 mg/kg) inhibit inflammation in a dose responsive manner and improved wound healing in STZ diabetic mice (Davis and Maro,1989 ; Chithra *et al.,* 1998).

Also the dry sap of the plant has been found to reduce the blood glucose levels as well as HbA1c. *Aloe vera* maintains glucose homeostasis by controlling the carbohydrate metabolizing enzymes (Rajasekaran *et al*. 2004)

4. *Azadirachta indica*

Family : Meliaceae
Common name : Neem
Part used : Seeds

Large sized tree cultivated throughout India. The extract of plant is widely used as remedy for diabetes. It showed antidiabetic activity which has been observed in normal and glucose fed diabetic rats. The antidiabetic activity of seeds of *Azadirachta indica* was studied and it has been found that *Azadirachta indica* has significant hypoglycemic activity in type 2 diabetes. The antioxidative effect of kernel and husk of neem seeds have been studied by Gupta *et al.,* 2004 in diabetic wistar rats. They found that kernel and husk of neem seeds prevent oxidative stress caused by streptozotocin in heart and erythrocytes. Neem seeds have been reported to increase the glucose uptake and glycogen deposition (Chattopadhyay *et al*., 1987).

5. *Areca catechu*

Family : Arecaceae
Common name : betel nut
Part used : Nut

It is commonly known as betel nut, It is reported to contain large quantity of tannin, garlic acid, fixed oil gums, volatile oil, lignin and alkaloids like arecoline, guracine *etc*. Arecoline is reported to have hypoglycemic activity seen in animal model of diabetes upon subcutaneous administration (Chempakan., 1993)

6. *Beta vulgaris*

Family : Chenopodiaceae
Common name : Common beet
Part used : Roots

Commonly known as garden beet and its traditionally used in various parts of India for management of diabetes. Various glycosides such as beta vulgarosides 1-1V,isolated from roots of this plant were investigated for blood glucose lowering activity. This plant was found to be effective in inhibition of non-enzymatic glycosylation of skin proteins in streptozotocin induced diabetic rats (Tunali *et al.,* 1998).

7. *Caesalpinia bonducella*

Family : Caesalpiniaceae
Common name : Cinnamon
Part used : Generally seeds are used

It is a small shrub distributed in coastal regions of India. Different parts of the plant contribute to its antidiabetic activity. The antihyperglycemic activity in seed extract has been reported. The aqueous extract and ethanolic extract exhibit hypoglycemic activity in type 2 diabetic models with initiating the release of insulin from isolated islets (Chakrabarti *et al*., 2005).

8. *Cajanus cajan*

Family : Fabaceae
Common name : Pigeon pea
Part used : leaves, Seeds *etc.*

Cultivated throughout India and is used as folk medicine for treatment of diabetes. The effect of the roasted and unroasted seeds was examined on serum glucose levels of normal and alloxan induced diabetic mice by Amalraj and Ignacimuthu,1998. Aqueous fractions of the leaves and stem were also studied for glucose reducing tolerability. Hypolipidemic activity was also reported earlier (Prema and Kurup,1973 a,b). Significant hypoglycemic effect has been found in human volunteers on eating cooked diet of *Cajanus cajan* (Panlasigui *et al.* 1995).

9. *Coccinia indica*

Family : Cucurbitaceae
Common name : Ivy Guard
Part used : Leaves, Fruit

It is a creeper widely grown in many parts of the sub- continent. It is used in ayurveda and unani system of medicine for the treatment of diabetes (Chopra *et al.,* 1956). It also exhibits antioxidant activity.

Water-soluble alkaloid fraction of alcohol extract of leaves as well as the pectin showed significant hypoglycemic action (Mukhergee *et al.,* 1972) this effect was due to the presence of beta sitosterol. The leaf extracts also exhibit antioxidant activity, which has been proved by an experiment by Vankateshwaran *et al.*(2003) showing the antioxidant effect of ethanolic extract of *Coccinia indica* leaves in streptozotocin diabetic rats.

A single oral dose of plant extract have shown beneficial hypoglycemic effect in experimental animal and human diabetic subjects possibly through its insulin secreting effect or through the influence of enzymes which are involved in glucose metabolism (Platel and Srinivasan. 1997).

Study conducted by (Hossain *et al.,* 1992) suggested that hypoglycemic activity attributed to Coccinia indica was partially mediated through suppression of gluconeogenic enzyme: glucose-6-phosphatase. Overall it has an insulin secretagogue effect (Khan *et al.,* 1979 ; Platel and Srinivasan.1997).

10. *Camellia sinensis*

Family : Theaceae
Common name : Tea
Part used : Tea leaves

Commonly known as tea . It is small evergreen tree . Tea has been planted in tropical and sub-tropical areas.

The blood glucose lowering activity has been extensively investigated. Anti hyperglycemic activity of hot water extract of green tea in STZ induced diabetic rats was studied by Gomes *et al.,* 1995, these findings have been supported by Anderson and Polansky, 2002.

Tea polyphenols apart from their much cited anti-oxidant capacity, have also been reported to inhibit á-amylase. Furthermore these polyphenolics also inhibit glucose transport across the intestine by inhibiting sodium – glucose co-transporter (S-GLUT-1) (Tiwari and Rao, 2002) The compound epigallocatechin gallate present in the tea increases the activity of insulin and also prevents oxidative damage found to be responsible for hyperglycemic activity. This has also been proved by further experiments that green tea provides complete antioxidative mechanism and ameliorates oxidative stress in aorta and heart of diabetic rats. This suggests that green tea may provide useful therapeutic option in reversal of oxidative stress induced cardiac dysfunction in diabetes mellitus.

11. *Eucalyptus globulus*

Family : Myrtaceae
Common name : Eucalyptus
Part used : Leaves

It is an ornamental tree found in subtropical Indian regions. Eucalyptus belongs to the family Myrtaceae. *Eucalyptus globulus* represents an effective antihyperglycemic dietary adjunct for the treatment of diabetes. It has been reported that aqueous extract (0.5 gm/l) of eucalyptus increases peripheral uptake of glucose in mouse abdominal muscles and also stepwise enhancement of insulin secretion from clonal pancreatic beta cell line (Gray and Flatt,1998).

The insulin releasing effect attributed to the aqueous extract is found to be responsible for antihyperglycemic activity.

12. *Ficus bengalensis*

Family : Moraceae
Common name : Banyan tree
Part used : Bark

It is a very large tree distributed throughout India. Various components isolated from the plant including dimethoxy derivative of leucocyandin 3-O beta D galactosyl celloboiside, dimethoxy derivative of prelargonidin (*in vitro* secretion of insulin), rhamnoside, glycoside of leucopelargonidin (hypoglycemic, hypolipidimic, serum insulin raising effect), leucodelphendin (antioxidant) have been known for their hypoglycemic activity (Deshmukh *et al.,* 1960 ; Brahmachari andAugusti,1964 ; Kumar and Augusti,1994)

Studies carried by Daniel *et al.,* 2003 reveals that on treatment of alloxan diabetic dogs with a glycoside *viz* leucopelargonin derivative isolated from the bark of *Ficus bengalensis* caused a decrease in fasting blood sugar and glycosylated hemoglobin by 34-28% respectively.

The antioxidant property of the compound leucodelphinidin (Daniel *et al.,* 1998) have shown hypoglycemic action equal to that of glibenclamide (2mg/kg) in normal and alloxan diabetic rats.

Overall the components (glycosides) stimulate secretion of insulin from beta cells and inhibit insulin degradative proteoses.

13. *Gymnema sylvestre*

Family : Asclepidaceae
Common name : Gurmar
Part used : Leaves

Native of tropical regions of India. The leaves of this plant has blood sugar lowering effect. This multipurpose plant has also been emphasized to possess significant antidiabetic potential in Indian traditional medicine for over 2000 years. Chewing the leaf decreases the sensitivity of taste buds to sweet tastes, gymnema has also been called gurmar, which means, "sugar destroyer." This effect is reported to last several hours. In people who have had extracts of gymnema applied to their tongue, have experienced decrease in sensitivity to sweets resulting in short-term decrease in food consumption.

Gurmar leaves raise insulin level, reduce glucose absorption from the intestine, improve uptake of glucose into the cells and prevent adrenal hormone from stimulating the liver to produce glucose, thereby reducing the blood glucose levels, glycosylated hemoglobin and glycosylated protein.

The antihyperglycemic activity of dried leaf powder of *Gymnema sylvestre* has been reported to cause a decrease in activity of gluconeogenic enzymes and removal of pathological changes in the liver initiated during hyperglycemic phase in alloxan-induced rabbits (Shanmugasundaram *et al.,* 1983). The chemical constituent gurmarin present in the leaves when chewed interfere with the ability to taste sweetness . The primary application was for adult onset diabetes mellitus where it has been found that beta cells regenerated or repaired alone in type 2 diabetes on supplementation of *Gymnema sylvestre* leaves.

Various hypoglycemic principles of gurmar isolated from the saponin fraction of the plant are referred to as: Gymnemosides and Gymnemic acids. (Murakami *et al.* 1996 ; Yoshikawa *et al.,* 1997). The triterpine glycosides isolated from the plant inhibited glucose utilization in muscles. (Shimizu *et al.,* 1996). However, triterpine glycosides exhibited little or no inhibitory activity against glucose absorption in OGTT conducted in rats. Gymnema fractions inhibit glucose uptake in the intestine, (Shimizu *et al.,* 1997).

In further studies it has been found that in case of insulin dependent diabetes mellitus (Type 1), prolonged administration of *Gymnema sylvestre* extract improved blood glucose homeostasis and reduced insulin requirement, better controlled hyperlipidemia and increased beta cell function (Shanmugasundaram *et al.,* 1990)

14. *Hibiscus rosa sinensis*

Family : Malvaceae
Common name : Hibiscus
Part used : Leaves

These are large shrub or small tree growing to 15 feet in frost-free climates and native to south Asia. It has been well mentioned in Ayurveda for its medicinal purposes.

It has been found that ethanol extract of *Rosa sinensis* showed mild but significant hypoglycemic activity carried out in glucose-loaded rats. The action was found to be similar to tolbutamide and possibly due to insulin release by stimulation of pancreatic beta cells and increase of glycogen deposition in liver. (Sachdeva and Khemani,1999)

15. *Momordica charantia*

Family : Cucurbitaceae
Common name : Karela
Part used : Fruit

It is a slender, climbing annual plant commonly known as Bitter Guard or Karela growing in India and other parts of tropical countries. Since Ayurvedic times bitter guard has been used as folk remedy for diabetes.

Several earlier and recent studies have indicated the hypoglycemic activity of various parts of this plant. Laboratory experiments and clinical trials using extract of dried fruit from the plant indicate that it lowers blood sugar levels (Leatherdale.*et al.*1981 ; Sarkar *et al.*, 1996) particularly in NIDDM (Raman and Lau ,1996).

Polypeptide isolated from fruits, seeds and tissues of *Momordica charantia* showed significant hypoglycemic activity which was observed in animal models such as gerbils, langurs as well as humans. (Khanna *et al.*, 1981).

The pulp juice and saponin free metholic extract exerted significant hypoglycemic effect in fasting and post prandial states of normal and NIDDM rats but not in IDDM.

A peptide **Charantin** isolated from *Memordica charantia* was found to be homologous to that of insulin and showed consistent hypoglycemic effect in patients with diabetes mellitus.

Experiments in rat model have shown that two important constituents of *Memordica charantia i.e.* oleonolic acid 3-o-glucoronidin and momordin, exert antihyperglycemic effect possibly by inhibiting glucose transport at brush boarder of small intestine.

Aqueous extract of unripe fruit partially stimulate insulin release from isolated beta cells of obese hyperglycemic mice which differed from other insulin secretagogues in the manner that it is not suppressed by L-epinephrine, even being potentiated by removal of Ca^{2+} suggesting that insulin releasing action is the result of perturbation of membrane function. (Welihinda and Karunanayake,1986). *Momordica charantia* is also reported to exhibit antioxidant activity (Dhar *et al.*1999)

16. *Murraya koeingii*

Family : Rutaceae
Common name : Curry leaf
Part used : Leaves

Curry leaf tree is native of India and Sri Lanka and is a small tree with aromatic leaves. The leaves are used in traditional Indian healing. Its antidiabetic property is based upon inhibition of digestive enzymes (pancreatic amylase) which is involved in breakdown of dietary starch to glucose.

In one experimental study it has been found that oral administration of curry leaves for 60 days to normal rats showed hypoglycemic effect associated with increased glycogenesis and decreased glycogenolysis and gluconeogenesis (Khan *et al.*,1995).

The recent studies on curry leaves suggest their beneficial effect in improving the management of high cholesterol and type 2 diabetes (Xie *et al.*, 2006)

17. *Ocimum sanctum*

Family : Lamiaceae
Common name : Holy basil
Part used : Leaves

A tropical branched annual herb upto 18 inches tall; this unassuming little plant plays a central role in folk medicine commonly called as Tulsi in Sanskrit literature.

A controlled clinical trial showed a positive effect on post prandial and fasting glucose and experts predict that the herb could enhance function of beta cells and facilitate the insulin secretion process. The dried powder of leaves also mildly reduces cholesterol and triglyceride level that are integral to diabetes as well as other cardiovascular diseases. (Agrawal *et al.*, 1996).Crossover studies led to the conclusion that Holy basil may be valuable in mild to moderate diabetes.

18. *Pterocarpus marsupium*

Family : Fabaceae
Common name : Vijayasar
Part used : Bark

It is a well-known plant named as Vijayasar, found throughout India and most essentially advocated in treatment of diabetes. Different parts of the plant like bark, latex *etc.*, were investigated and shown to exhibit hypoglycemic activity.

Pterocarpus marsupium is a rich source of polyphenolic compounds. Various active components like (-) epicatechin, marsupin, pterosupin, and pterostillbine isolated from the bark and heartwood of the plant were found to possess blood sugar lowering activity (Manickam *et al.*, 1997). The flavonoid fraction of *P. marsupium* has been shown to cause pancreatic beta cell regranulation and may explain the antidiabetic mechanism of the plant. (Chakravarthy *et al.*, 1980)

19. *Syzigium cumini*

Family : Myrtaceae
Common name : Jamun
Part used : Seeds

Commonly known as Jamun, it is cultivated throughout India. It is also one of the most studied medicinal plant possesing antidiabetic property. Preliminary studies on *Syzigium cumini* seeds have also shown hypoglycemic effect. Fresh seeds are effective in diabetes; they reduce sugar in urine and allay the unquenchable thirst in diabetes.

Glucoside jamboline, one of the phenolic constituent found in Java Plum is said to have power of checking pathological conversion of starch to glucose in case of increased production of glucose.

Oral feeding of *Eugenia jambolana* (510 mg/rat for 15 days) caused 50% reduction in blood glucose of normal fasted rats while Chlorpropamide showed 52% reduction. In addition there was 2.4 - 6.8 fold increase in cathepsin B activity (Bansal *et al.,* 1981).

It has been found that oral administration of seed aqueous extract of *Syzygium cumini* (2.5 and 5.0 gm/kg for 6 weeks) showed hypoglycemic potential and it also exhibited antioxidant property.

20. *Trigonella foenumgraecum*

Family : Fabaceae
Common name : Methi
Part used : Seeds

It is generally used in seasoning of foods especially in Egypt, India and Middle East.

It is a well known hypoglycemic and hypolipidemic agent used in traditional Indian medicine and is beneficial in both types of diabetes. (Ribes *et al.,* 1984; Riyad *et al.,* 1988 ; Alarcon-Aquilara *et al.,* 1998)

Various extract of different parts of this plant: fibers, proteins and saponins isolated from seeds were studied and reported to exhibit hypoglycemia. The defatted seeds of the fenugreek plant contain ~50% fiber (similar to guar gum), along with a variety of bioactive saponins, alkaloids, coumarins, and 4-hydroxyisoleucine, the principle bioactive compound.

When these extract were given with meals for 21 days to alloxan induced diabetic rats there was significant hypoglycemic activity and anti glucosuric effect along with reduction in high plasma glucagons and somatostatin. (Ribes *et al.,*1984)

4-hydroxyisoleucine, a novel amino acid has been extracted and purified from fenugreek seeds found to increase glucose induced insulin release (ranging from 100 imol/l to 1mmol/l) through a direct effect on the isolated islets of langerhans in both rats and humans.

This pattern of insulin secretion was biphasic, glucose dependent, occurred in the absence of any change in pancreatic alpha and delta cells activity and without interaction with other agonist of insulin secretion (such as arginine, leucine, tolbutamide, glyceraldehydes) (Sauvaire *et al.,* 1998)

The antioxidant (Ravi Kumar and Anuradha,1999) and hypercholesterolimic activity is also described in literature. (Stark and Madar,1993)

21. *Tinospora cardiofolia*

Family : Menispermaceae
Common name : Guduchi
Part used : roots, leaves

It is a large climbing shrub found throughout India and used in various ailments as vitaliser and in diabetes mellitus and metabolic disorders.

Through various studies it has been found that plant has blood sugar lowering activity, which has been proved by experiment on normal and alloxan-induced diabetic rabbits. The hypoglycemic effect depends upon the functional status of pancreatic beta cells (Grover *et al.,* 2000).

Oral administration of water extract of *Tinospora cardiofolium* root is reported to show reduction in blood glucose, brain, lipid levels, hepatic glucose-6-phosphate, serum acid phosphatases, alkaline and lactate dehydrogenases and increase in body weight in alloxan induced diabetic rats. (Stanely *et al.* 2000). Antioxidant and hypoglycemic property was also highlighted by this plant (Prince and Menon, 1999).

22. *Vinca rosea*

Family : Apocyanaceae
Common name : Sadabahar
Part used : Leaves

Found throughout India. It has also shown dose-dependent reduction in blood glucose levels. Oral administration of water-soluble ethanol extract of *Vinca rosea* leaves show reduction in blood sugar levels (Chattopadhyay *et al*., 1991).

Aqueous extract of *Vinsa rosea* flowers along with *Piper nigrum* seeds were administered orally to alloxan induced diabetic rats showed significant blood sugar lowering effect and also reduction in serum lipid levels. The component may also be helpful in strengthing the antioxidant potential as they improved the activity of antioxidant enzymes (Kaleem *et al.,* 2005).

The antidiabetic activity of *Vinsa rosea* flowers may be attributed to beta cell rejuvenation, generation and stimulation (Ghosh *et al.,* 2001).

The hypoglycemic effect of *Vinsa rosea* leaves was comparable to that of tolbutamide (Chattopadhyay *et al.,* 1991).

23. *Zizipus jujuba*

Family : Zingeberaceae
Common name : Sweet Zinger, Zinger root
Part used : Leaves

It is a small spreading tree with drooping branches and is also reported to contain one of the hypoglycemic agents involved in ameliorating the syndrome of diabetes mellitus.

Antihyperglycemic and antihyperlipidemic activity of *Zizipus jujuba* was reported which was significant compared to Glibenclamide (Tiwari and Rao,2002)

The authors proposed that the alkaloid barberine present in the leaves of this plant is found to be responsible for hypoglycemic activity and also suggested that the chemical ingredient in *Zizipus* has the ability to release insulin from the pancreatic beta cells and protect the alloxan induced damage

11. PHYTOTHERAPEUTIC COMPOUNDS FROM MEDICINAL PLANTS

Various active components processing different chemical structure but same therapeutic activity have been isolated from different plant species. Some of the active principles originate from edible plants and are known to possess significant antidiabetic activities. Several of the active components present in plants include: flavonoids, alkaloids, glycosides, saponins, glycolipids, polypeptides and many more. They all have been reported to possess significant antidiabetic and antioxidant activity.

11.1 ANTIOXIDANT DEFENSE

Recent studies have shown that plasma antioxidants are depleted in diabetes and this depletion is the major cause of various diabetic complications and the onset of other disease conditions like atherosclerosis and coronary heart diseases. Antioxidant activity of variety of compounds isolated from plants has been studied and their benefit in oxidative stress and related disease conditions have been widely described. It appears that apart from acting on carbohydrate metabolism, compounds present in medicinal plants have a variety of beneficial activities and have the potential to impart beneficial effects in complicated disorders like diabetes and its complications. The properties of some of active components have been described below:

11.1.1 FLAVONOID

Flavonoids represent a group of naturally occurring compounds with hypoglycemic potentials. The flavonoids can be widely classified into different categories like flavonols, flavones, catechins, flavanones *etc*. Some flavonoids possess hypoglycemic properties because they improve altered glucose and oxidative metabolism of diabetic states. Quercetin is known to possess array of pharmacological activities. It also posseses significant antidiabetic activity probably by enhancing the release of insulin from pancreas islet of diabetic rats.

Flavonoids Hesperidin and Naringin both play important role in prevention and progression of hyperglycemia, partly by increasing hepatic glycolysis and glycogen concentration and by lowering hepatic gluconeogenesis (Jung *et al.*, 2004).

Proanthocyanins, the flavonoid with an oligomeric structure is found to improve the pathological oxidative state generated in diabetes.

Another flavonoid glycoside Kaempferitrin (Kaempferol-3,7-0-(alpha)-L-dirhamnoside)was found to have an acute lowering effect on blood glucose in diabetic rats and stimulate the glucose uptake as efficiently as insulin in muscles from normal rats *in vitro* suggesting that the blood glucose lowering activity of the compound is related to altered intrinsic activity of glucose transporter (Jorge *et al.*, 2004). Another important flavonoid epigallocatechin gallate found in green tea also exhibits glucose lowering effect. It does this by decreasing hepatic glucose production and increasing tyrosine phosphorylation of the insulin receptor. This along with some more findings suggests that this is an important hypoglycemic agent (Waltner-Law *et al.*, 2002)

Another flavonoid (-) Epicatechin that was isolated from Indian kino tree has been reported to possess insulin like activity. Epicatechin has been shown to mimic some of the effects of insulin on diabetic human erythrocytes (Rizvi *et al.* 1995 ; Rizvi and Zaid, 2001).

In addition to these flavonoids, various active components like saponins (charantin from Memordica charantia, beta sitosterol, gymnemic acid from Gymnema sylvestre) were found to possess significant hypoglycemic activity.

Various alkaloids like barberine from Trigonella cardifolia (Singh *et al.*,2003) and Catharanthine, Vindoline(XI), and Vindolinine(XII) (from *Catharathus roseous*) (Chattopadhyay *et al.*, 1999) have been found to possess blood sugar lowering activity.

12. CONCLUSION

Diabetes, which is a disorder of metabolism, is attributed to diminished production of insulin or mounting resistance to insulin. Diabetes is the root cause of various complications which if untreated becomes fatal for the body.

There are various therapeutic agents that are the mainstay in the treatment of diabetes and are effective in controlling hyperglycemia, but with the ongoing research it has been highlighted that these agents have prominent side effects and they fail to address the cause of diabetic complications.

As the knowledge of heterogeneity of this disease is increasing, there is need for agents which are more efficacious and have fewer side effects. The need of the hour is to come closer to herbal medicine. Studies on some traditional medicines have shown that these plants or their active compounds have potent antidiabetic effects. Moreover these plants have been used as therapeutic agents for a long time without any apparent side effects.

From the above reports of their potential effectiveness against diabetes it is assumed that these botanicals play a major role in management of diabetes which needs further exploration for the development of essential drugs and neutraceuticals from various herbal resources.

13. SELECTED INDIAN MEDICINAL PLANTS WITH ANTIDIABETIC POTENTIAL

S.No.	Botanical name	Common name	Family	Part used	Putative bioactive
1.	*Allium cepa*	Onion	Liliaceae	Seedling, Callus, Bulb etc.	S-methyl cysteine sulphoxide, S-allyl-cysteine sulphoxide
2.	*Allium sativum*	Garlic	Alliaceae	Cloves of bulb	S.allyl cysteine sulphoxide, Allicin,
3.	*Aloe barbadensis*	Aloe Vera	Liliaceae	Leaves	Fibre (glucomannon),aloin s,anthraquinones,bar baloin,polysaccharid es,salicylic acids
4.	*Azadirachta indica*	Neem	Meliaceae	Seeds	No authentic reports
5.	*Areca catechu*	Betel nut	Aracaceae	Nut	Alkaloids like arecoline, guracine etc.
6.	*Beta vulgaris*	Common beet	Chenopodiaceae	Roots	Beta vulgarosides I-1V
7.	*Caesalpinia bonducella*	Cinnamon	Caesalpiniaceae	Seeds	No authentic reports
8.	*Cajanus cajan*	Pigeon pea	Fabaceae	Leaves, Seed etc.	saponins
9.	*Coccinia indica*	Ivy Guard	Cucurbitaceae	Leaves, Fruit	Beta sitosterol
10.	*Camellia sinensis*	Tea	Theaceae	Tea leaves	Catechins especially Epigallocatechin gallate
11.	*Eucalyptus globulus*	Eucalyptus	Myrtaceae	Leaves	No authentic reports
12.	*Ficus bengalensis*	Banyan tree	Moraceae	Bark	Leucocyandin 3-o beta D galactosyl celloboiside, Dimethoxy derivative of prelargonidin leucopelargonidin, leucodelphendin
13.	*Gymnema sylvestre*	Gurmer	Asclepidaceae	Leaves	Gurmarin, Gymnemosides and Gymnemic acids, triterpine glycosides
14.	*Hibiscus rosa sinensis*	Hibiscus	Malvaceae	Leaves, flower	Flavonoids,glyc-osides etc.
15.	*Momordica charantia*	Karela	Cucurbitaceae	Fruit	Peptide Charantin, oleonolic acid 3-o-glucoronidin and momordin

16.	*Murraya koeingii*	Curry leaf	Rutaceae	Leaves	No authentic reports
17.	*Ocimum sanctum*	Holy basil	Lamiaceae	Leaves	No authentic reports
18.	*Pterocarpus marsupium*	Vijayasar	Fabaceae	Bark	(-) Epicatechin, marsupin, pterosupin, and pterostillbine
19.	*Syzigium cumini*	Jamun	Myrtaceae	Seeds	Jamboline
20.	*Trigonella foenum graecum.*	Methi	Fabaceae	Seeds	saponins, alkaloids, coumarins, and 4-hydroxyisoleucine
21	*Tinospora cardiofolia*	Guduchi	Menispermaceae	Roots ,Leaves	Barberine(Singh *et al.*2003)
22.	*Vinca rosea*	Sadabahar	Apocyanaceae	Leaves	Antioxidant compounds
23.	*Zizipus jujuba*	Sweet Zinger	Zingeberaceae	Leaves	Barberine

14. REFRENCES

Abbasi, F., Carantoni, M., Chen, Y.D.and Reaven, G.M. Further evidence for a central role of adipose tissue in the antihyperglycemic effect of metformin. Diabetes Care 21: 1301–1305 (1998).

Agrawal, P., Rai, V.,and Singh, R.B. Randomized placebo-controlled, single blind trial of holy basil leaves in patients with non-insulin dependent diabetes mellitus. Int.J.Pharmacol. Ther. 34: 406-409 (1996).

Ajabnoor, M.A.Effect of Aloes on blood glucose levels in normal and alloxan induced diabetic mice. J. Ethnopharmacol. 28: 215-220 (1990).

Alarcon-Aguilaria, F.J., Roman-Ramos, R., Perez-Gutierrez, S., Aguilar-Contreras, A., Contreras-Weber, C.C. and Flores-Saenz, J.L. Study of antihyperglycemic effect of plants used as antidiabetics. J. Ethnopharmacol. 61(2): 101-110 (1998).

Al-Awadi, F.M .and Gumaa, K.A. Studies on the activity of individual plants of a hypoglycemic plant mixture. Acta Diabetol. Lat. 24:37–41 (1987).

Amalraj, T. and Ignacimuthu, S. Hypoglycemic activity of Cajanus cajan (seeds) in mice. Ind. J. of Exp. Biol. 36:1032-1033 (1998).

Amos, A., Mc Carty, D. and Zimmet, P. The rising global burden of diabetes and its complications: estimates the projections to the year 2010. Diabetic Med. 14: 51-585 (1997).

Anderson, R.A. and Polansky, M.M .Tea enhances insulin activity. J. Agric. Food Chem. 50: 7182-7186 (2002).

Astrup, A. and Finer, N. Redefining type 2 diabetes: diabesity"or obesity dependent diabetes mellitus? Obesity Rev.1:57-59 (2000).

Augusti, K. T. and Mathew, P.T. Effect of long term feeding of an aqueous extracts of Onion (Allium Cepa Linn.) and garlic (Allium Sativum Linn.) on normal rats. Indian J. Exp.Biol. 11:239-241 (1973).

Azad Khan, A.K., Akhtar, S. and Mahtab, H. Coccinia indica in the treatment of patients with diabetes mellitus. Bangladesh Med. Res. Council Bull. 5(2):60-66 (1979).

Bansal, R., Ahmad, N. and Kidwai, J.R. Effects of Oral administration of Eugenia Jambolana seeds and chloropropamide on blood glucose levels and pancreatic cathepsin B in rat. Indian J. Biochem. Biophys. 18(5): 377 (1981).

Bell, D.S. and Ovalle, F. Tissue triglyceride levels in type 2 diabetes and the role of thiazolidinediones in reversing the effects of tissue hypertriglyceridemia: review of the evidence in animals and humans. Endocr. Pract. 7:135-138 (2001).

Bloomgarden Z.T.: New insights in obesity. Diabetes Care 25: 789-795 (2002).

Boden. G., Chen, X., Ruiz, J., White, J.V. and Rossetti L. Mechanisms of fatty acid-induced inhibition of glucose uptake. *J Clin Invest* 93 :2438 –2446 (1994).

Brahmachari, H.D. and Augusti, K.T. Isolation of orally effective hypoglycemic compounds from Ficus bengalensis Linn. Indian J. Physiol. and Pharmacol. 13: 60–64 (1964).

Brownlee, M.Biochemistry and molecular cell biology of diabetic complications. Nature 414 :813-820 (2001).

Bursell, S.E., Clermont, A.C. and Kinsley, B.T. Retinal blood flow changes in patients with insulin-dependent diabetes mellitus and no diabetic retinopathy. Invest. Ophthalmol. Vis. Sci. 37: 886-897 (1996).

Campos, K.E., Diniz, Y.S., Cataneo A.C., Faine, L.A., Alves, M.JQF. and Novel ECLB.Hypoglycaemic and antioxidant effects of onion,Allium cepa:Dietary onion addition,antioxidant activities and hypoglycaemic effects on diabetic rats. Int. J. Food Sci.Nutr. .54:241-246 (2003).

Chakrabarti,S., Biswas, T.K., Seal, T., Rokeya, B., Ali. L., Azad Khan A.k., Nahar, N., Mosihuzzaman, M.and Mukhergee, B.Hypoglycemic activity of Caecelpenia Bonducella in chronic type 2 diabetes model in long evans rats and evaluation of insulin secretatagogue property of its fractions in isolated islets. J. Ethanopharmacol.10. 97(1):117-22 (2005 Feb).

Chakravarthy, B.K., Gupta, S., Gambhir, S.S. and Gode, K.D. Pancreatic beta cell regeneration .A novel antidiabetic mechanism of Pterocarpus marsupium Roxb. Indian J. Pharmacol. 12:123-127 (1980).

Chandalia,M., Abate, N.,Garg, A.,Stray-Gundersen, J. and Grundy, S.M..Relationship between generalized and upper body obesity to insulin resistance in asian Indian men. J. Clin.Endocrinol. Metab.84:2329-35 (1999).

Chan ,J.M., Rimm, E.B., Colditz, G.A., Stampfer, M.J. and Willet ,W.C. Obesity, fat distribution, and weight gain as the risk factor for clinical diabetes in men. Diabetes Care 17: 961-969 (1994)

Chattopadhyay, R.R., Chattopadhyay, R.N., Nandy, AK.,Poddar,G. and Maitra,S.K. The effect of fresh leaves of Azadirachta indica on glucose uptake and glycogen content in the isolated rat hemi diaphragm. Bull. Calcutta School Trop. Med. 35:8-12 (1987).

Chattopadhyay, R.R., Sarkar, S.K., Ganguly, S., Banerjee, R.N. and Basu, T.K.Hypoglycemic and antihyperglycemic effect of leaves of Vinca rosea Linn. Indian J. Physiol. and Pharmacol. 35: 145–151 (1991)

Chattopadhyay,R.R.A comparative evaluation of some blood glucose lowering agents of plant origin. J. Ethanopharmacol. 67 (3): 367-372 (1999).

Chattopapadhyay, R.R., Sarkar, S.K.., Ganguly, S., Banergee, R.N. and T.K. Hypoglycemic and antihyperglycemic effect of leaves of Vinsa rosea Linn. Indian J. Physiol. Pharmacol. 35 (3): 145-151 (1991).

Chempakam, B. Hypoglycemic activity of arecoline of betel nut Areca catechu L. Indian J. Exp. Biol. 31 (5): 474-475 (1993).

Chithra, P., Sajithlal, G.B. Chandrakasan, G. Influence of Aloe Vera on the healing of dermal wounds in diabetic rats. J. Ethnopharmacol. 59:195-201, (1998).

Chopra, R.N., Nayar, S.L. and Chopra, I.C. Glossary of Indian Medicinal Plants. CSIR, New Delhi (1956)

Daniel, R.S., Devi, K.S., Augusti, K.T., Sudhakaran. And Nair, C.R. Mechanism of action of antiatherogenic and related effects of Ficus bengalensis Linn. Flavonoids in experimental animals. . Indian J Exp Biol. 41(4): 296-303 (2003).

Daniel, R.S., Mathew, B.C., Devi, K.S. and Augusti, K.T. Antioxidant effect of two flavonoids from the bark of Ficus bengalenesis Linn. in hyperlipidemic rats. Indian J. Exp. Biol. 36 (9):902-/906 (1998).

Davis, R.H. and Maro, N.P. Aloe Vera and gibberellin . Antiinflammatory activity in diabetes. J. Am. Pediat. Med. Assn. 79:24-26 (1989)

Del Prato, S., Marchetto, S., Pipitone, A., Zanon, M., Vigili de Kreutzenberg, S. And Tiengo A. Metformin and free fatty acid metabolism. Diabetes Metab Rev. 11: S33–S41 (1995).

Deshmukh, V.K., Shrotri, D.S. and Aiman, R. Isolation of a hypoglycemic principle from the bark of *Ficus bengalensis* Linn. A preliminary note. Indian J. Physiol. Pharmacol. 4: 182–185 (1960).

Dhar, P., Ghosh, S. and Bhattacharya, D.K. Dietary effects of conjugated octadecatrienoic fatty acid (9 cis, 11 trans, 13 trans) levels on blood lipids and nonenzymatic in vitro lipid peroxidation in rats. Lipids 34 (2):109-114 (1999).

Diabetes Control and Complications Trial Research Group. The effect of intensive treatment of diabetes on the development and progression of long-term complications in insulin-dependent diabetes mellitus. N Engl J Med. 329:977-986 (1993).

Ehtisham, S. and Barrett, T.G. The emergence of type 2 diabetes in childhood. Ann Clin Biochem .41:10-6 (2004)

Fonseca, V., Rosenstock, J., Patwardhan, R. and Salzman, A. Effect of metformin and rosiglitazone combination therapy in patients with type 2 diabetes mellitus: a randomized controlled trial. JAMA. 283:1695–1702 (2000).

Garber, A.J., Duncan, T.G., Goodman, A.M., Mills, D.J. and Rohlf, J.L. Efficacy of metformin in type II diabetes: results of a double blind, placebo-controlled, dose-response trial. Am J Med. 103: 491–497 (1997).

Ghosh, S. and Suryavanshi, S.A. effect of Vinca rosea extract in treatment of alloxan diabetes in male albino rats. Indian J. Exp. Biol. 39(8):748-59 (2001).

Gomes, A., Vedasiromani J.R., Das, M., Sharma, R.M. and Ganguly, D.K. Anti-hyperglycaemic effect of black tea (Camellia sinensis) in rat. J. Ethnopharmacol .45:223-226 (1995).

Gray, A.M. and Flatt, P.R. Antihyperglycemic actions of Eucalyptus globulus (Eucalyptus) are associated with pancreatic and extra pancreatic effects in mice. J. Nutr. 128 (12): 2319 -/2323 (1998).

Grover, J.K., Yadav, S., and Vats, V. Medicinal plants in India with Antidiabetic potential. J. Ethnopharmacol. 81: 81-100 (2002).

Grover, J.K., Vats, V. and Rathi, S.S. Anti-hyperglycemic effect of Eugenia jambolana and Tinospora cordifolia in experimental diabetes and their effects on key metabolic enzymes involved in carbohydrate metabolism. J. Ethnopharmacol. 73 (3): 461-470 (2000).

Gupta, S., Kataria, M., Gupta, P.K.,Murganandan, S. and Yashroy, R.C. Protective role of extracts of neem seeds in diabetes caused by streptozotocin in rats. J. Ethnopharmacol. 90(2-3): 185-9 (2004).

Hammes, H.P., Martin, S., Federlin, K., Geisen, K. and brownlee, M . Aminoguanidine treatment inhibits the development of experimental diabetic retinopathy. *Proc. Natl Acad. Sci. USA* 88: 11555–11559, (1991).

Harrower, A.D. Pharmacokinetics of oral antihyperglycaemic agents in patients with renal insufficiency. Clin Pharmacokinet.31: 111–119 (1996).

Hollman, P.C., van Trijp, J.M. and Mengelers, M.J. Bioavailability of the dietary antioxidant flavonol quercetin in man. ancer Lett. Mar 19;114(1-2):139-40 (1997).

Horie, K., Miyata, T., Maeda, K, Miyata, S., Sugiyama, S., Sakai, H., van Y prsole de strihou C., Monnier, V.M.,Witztum, J.L. and Kurokawa, K. Immunohistochemical colocalization of glycoxidation products and lipid peroxidation products in diabetic renal glomerular lesions. Implication for glycoxidative stress in the pathogenesis of diabetic nephropathy. J. Clin. Invest. 100: 2995–2999 (1997).

Hossain .M.Z.,Shibib,B.A. and Rahman,R.Hypoglycaemic effect of Coccinia indica: inhibition of key gluconeogenic enzyme ,glucose-6-phosphatase. Indian J. Exp. Biol. 30(5):418-420 (1992).

Hundal, R.S., Krssak, M., Dufour, S., Laurent, D., Lebon, V., Chandramouli, V., Inzucchi, S.E., Schumann, W.C., Petersen, K.F., Landau, B.R. and Shulman ,G.I. Mechanism by which metformin reduces glucose production in type 2 diabetes. Diabetes 49:2063–2069 (2000).

Ishii, H., Jirousek, M.R.,Koya, D.,Takagi,C., Xia, P., Clermont, A., bursell, S.E., Kern, T.S.,Ballas, L.m.,Heath, W.F.,Stramm, L.E.,Feener, E.P. and King, G.L. Amelioration of vascular dysfunctions in diabetic rats by an oral PKC beta inhibitor. Science 272: 728–731; (1996).

Jain, R.C. and Vyas, C.R. Garlic in alloxan-induced diabetic rabbits. Am. J. Clin. Nutr. 28: 684-685 (1975).

Jorge, A.P., Horst, H., de Sousa, E., Pizzolatti, M.G. and Silva, F.R. Insulin mimetic Effects of kaempferitrin on glycaemia and on 14C-glucose uptake in rat soleus muscle. Chem. Biol. Interact.149: 89–96 (2004).

Jung, U.J., Lee, M.K., Jeong, K.S. and Choi, M.S. The hypoglycemic effects of hesperidin and naringin are partly mediated by hepatic glucose regulating enzymes in C57BL/KsJ-db/db mice. J. Nutr. 134:2499–2503 (2004).

Kaleem, M., Sheema, Sarmad H. and Bano, B.protective effect of Piper Nigrum and Vinca rosea in alloxan induced diabetic rats. Indian J. Physiol. Pharmacol. 49(1): 65-71 (2005).

Kasuga, S., Ushijima, M., Morihara, N., Itakura, Y. and Nakata, Y. Effect of agedgarlic extract(AGE)on hyperglycemia induced by immobilization stress in mice. Nippon Yakurigaku Zasshi. 114:191-197 (1999).

Kelkar, S.M., Kaklij, G.S. and Bapat, V.A. Determination of hypoglycemic activity in Allium cepa (onion) tissue cultures. Indian J. Biochem. Biophys. 38: 277–279 (2001).

Khan, B.A., Abraham, A. And Leelamma, S. Hypoglycemic action of Murraya koeingii (curry leaf) and Brassica juncea (mustard): mechanism of action. Indian J. Biochem. Biophys. 32 (2): 106-/108 (1995).

Khanna, P., Jain, S.C., Panagariya, A. and Dixit, V.P. Hypoglycemic activity of polypeptide-p from a plant source. J. Nat. Prod. 44 (6):648-655 (1981).

King H, Aubert R.E. and Herman, W.H., Global burden of diabetes, 1995-2025: prevalence, numerical estimates, and projections. Diabetes Care 21: 1414-1431 (1998).

Koy, D. and King, G. L. Protein kinase C activation and the development of diabetic complications. Diabetes 47: 859–866 (1998).

Kumar, R.V. and Augusti, K.T.Insulin sparing action of a leucocyanidin derivative isolated from Ficus bengalenesis Linn. Indian J. Biochem. Biophys. 31 (1): 73-/76 (1994).

Kumari, K., Mathew, B.C. and Augusti, K.T. Antidiabetic and hypolipidemic effects of S-methyl cysteine sulfoxide isolated from Allium cepa Linn. Indian J. Biochem. Biophys 32 (1): 49-/54 (1995).

Langtry, H.D. and Balfour, J.A. Glimepiride. A review of its use in the management of type 2 diabetes mellitus. Drugs 55:563–584 (1998).

Leatherdale, B.A.,Panesar,R.K.,Singh, G.,Atkins, T.W.,Bailey, C.J. and Bignall A.H. Improvement in glucose tolerance due to Momordica Charantia. Br. Med. J. ,282:1823-1824,(1981).

Lebovitz, H.E., Kreider ,M. and Freed, M.I. Evaluation of liver function in type 2 diabetic patients during clinical trials: evidence that rosiglitazone does not cause hepatic dysfunction. Diabetes Care 25:815–821 (2002).

Manickam, M., Ramanathan, M., Jahromi, M.A., Chansouria, J.P. and Ray, A.B. Antihyperglycemic activity of phenolics from Pterocarpus marsupium. J. Nat. Prod. 60 (6): 609-/610 (1997).

Marshall, S., Garvey, W.T. and Traxinger, R.R. New insights into the metabolic regulation of insulin action and insulin resistance: role of glucose and amino acids. *FASEB J* 5 :3031 –3036 (1991).

Mathew, P.T. and Augusti, K.T. 1973. Studies on the effect of allicin (diallyl disulphide-oxide) on alloxan diabetes. Hypoglycemic action and enhancement of serum insulin effect and glycogen synthesis. Indian J. Biochem. Biophys 10:209-212 (1973).

McCall, A.L. Clinical review of glimepiride. Expert Opin Pharmaco Ther. 2:699–713 (2001).

Micchael T. and Sheehan MD. Current Therapeutic options in type 2 diabetes: A practical approach. Clin Med Res.1(3) :189-200 (2003).

Misra, A. and Vikram, N.K. Insulin resistance syndrome (Metabolic syndrome) and asian Indians.Current Sci. 83: 1483-96 (2002).

Mohan, V. Why are Indians more prone to diabetes? JAPI.52:468-472 (2004).

Mohan,V., Ramachandran,A., Snehalatha.C., Mohan,R., Bharani,G., and Visvanathan,M. High prevalence of maturity onset diabetes of the young (MODY) among Indians. Diabetes Care 8:374-374 (1985a).

Mohan,V.,Snehalatha,C.,Ramachandran,A.,Jayashree,R. and Vishvanathan,M. C peptide responses to glucose load in maturity onset diabetes of the young (MODY), Diabetes Care 1:69-71 (1985b).

Mukherjee Pulok K., Maitik Kuntal., Mukherjee Kalkali and Houghton Peter J. Leads from Indian medicinal plants with hypoglycemic potential .J. Ethnopharmacol. 106:1-28 (2006).

Mukherjee, K., Ghosh, N.C. and Datta, T. Coccinia indica Linn. As potential hypoglycemic agent. Indian J. Exp. Biol. 10 (5): 347-349 (1972).

Murakami, N., Murakami, T., Kadoya, M., Matsuda, H., Yamahara, J. and Yoshikawa, M. New hypoglycemic constituents in gymnemic acid from Gymnema sylvestre. Chem. Pharma. Bull. (Tokyo) 44 (2): 469-471 (1996).

Nakamura, S.,Makita ,Z., Ishikawa, S.,Yasumura, K.,Fujii, W.,Yanagisawa, K., kawata, T. and Koite, T. Progression of nephropathy in spontaneous diabetic rats is prevented by OPB-9195, a novel inhibitor of advanced glycation. Diabetes 46: 895–899 (1997).

Oubre, A.Y., Carlson, T.J. King, S.S. and Reaven, G.M. From plant to patient; an ethanomedical approach in identification of new drugs for treatmant of NIDDM. Diabetologia 40(5):614-617 (1997).

Palumbo, P.J. Metformin: effects on cardiovascular risk factors in patients with non-insulin-dependent diabetes mellitus. J Diabetes Complications.12: 110–119 (1998).

Panlasigui, L.N., Panlilio, L.M. and Madrid, J.C. Glycemic response in normal subjects to five different legumes commonly used in the Philippines. Int. J. Food Sci.Nutr. 46 (2): 155-160 (1995).

Patumraj, S., Tewit, S., Amatyakul, S., Jaryiapongskul, A., Maneesri, S., Kasantikul, V. and Shepro, D. Comparative effects of garlic and aspirin on diabetic cardiovascular complications. Drug Delivery 7:91-96 (2000).

Phillips, L.S., Grunberger, G., Miller, E., Patwardhan, R., Rappaport, E.B. and Salzman. A. The Rosiglitazone Clinical Trials Study Group, author. Once- and twice-daily dosing with rosiglitazone improves glycemic control in patients with type 2 diabetes. Diabetes Care 24:308–315 (2001).

Platel, K. and Srinivasan, K. Plant foods in the management of diabetes mellitus: vegetables as potential hypoglycemic agents. Die Nahrung 41 (2): 68-/74 (1997).

Pradeepa R, Deepa R and Mohan V.epidemiology of diabetes in India-current prospective and future projections .JIMA 100: 144-148 (2002a).

Pradeepa, R. and Mohan, V.The changing scenario of the diabetes epidemic: implications for Indian J Med Res. 116:121-132 (2002b).

Prema, L. And Kurup, P.A. Hypolipidemic activity of the protein isolated from Cajanus Cajan in high fat-cholesterol diet fed rats. Indian J. Biochem. Biophys 10: 293-/296 (1973a).

Prema, L. and Kurup, P.A. Effect of protein fractions from Cajanus cajan (redgram) and Dolichos biflorus (horsegram) on the serum, liver and aortic lipid levels in rats fed a high-fat cholesterol diet. Atherosclerosis 18:369-377 (1973b).

Prince, P.S. and Menon, V.P. Antioxidant activity of Tinospora cordifolia roots in experimental diabetes. J. Ethnopharmacol. 65 (3): 277-/281 (1999).

Rajasekaran, S., Sivagnanam, K., Ravi, K. and Subramaniam, S. Hypoglycemic effect of Aloe Vera gel on streptozotocin induced diabetes in experimental rats .J Med Food. 7(1): 61-6 (2004 spring).

Rajasekarans, Sivagnanam, K. and Subramaniam, S . Modulatory effects of Aloe Vera leaf gel extract on oxidative stress in rats treated with streptozotocin. J Pharm Pharmacol. 57(2): 241-6 (2005Feb).

Ramachandran, A.,.Snehalatha, C,.and Viswanathan Vijay.Burdern of type 2 diabetes and its complications-The Indian Scenario. Curr Sci. 84,.12.Dec (2002).

Raman A and Lau C. Antidiabetic property and phytochemistry of Momordica Charantia L.(Cucurbitaceae). Phytomedicine .2(4):349-362 (1996).

Ravikumar, P. And Anuradha, C.V. Effect of fenugreek seeds on blood lipid peroxidation and antioxidants in diabetic rats. Phytotherapy Res. 13 (3): 197-201 (1999).

Ribes, G., Sauvaire, Y., Baccou, J.C., Valette, G., Chenon, D., Trimble, E.R. and Loubatieres-Mariani, M.M. Effects of fenugreek seeds on endocrine pancreatic secretions in dogs. Ann. Nutr. Metab. 28 (1): 37-/43 (1984).

Riyad, M.A., Abfdul-Salam, S.A. and Mohammad, S.S. Effect of Fenugreek and lupine seeds on the development of experimental diabetes in rats. Planta Med. 54 (4): 286-290 (1988).

Rizvi, S.I., Abu Zaid, M. and Suhail, M. Insulin-mimetic effect of (-) epicatechin on osmotic fragility of human erythrocytes. Indian J. Exp. Biol. 33: 791–792 (1995)

Rizvi, S.I. and Zaid, M.A. Insulin-like effect of (-)-epicatechin on erythrocyte membrane acetyl cholinesterase activity in type 2 diabetes mellitus. Clin. Exp. Pharmacol. Physiol. 28: 776–778 (2001).

Roman-Ramos, R., Flores-Saenz, J.L., Alarcon-Aguilar, F.J. 1995. Anti-hyperglycemic effect of some edible plants. J. Ethnopharmacol. 48:25-32,(1995).

Sachdewa, A., Khemani, L.D. A preliminary investigation of the possible hypoglycemic activity of Hibiscus rosa-sinensis. Biomed. Environ. Sci. 12:222–226(1999).

Saltiel, A.R., Kann, C.R Insulin signaling and the regulation of glucose and lipid metabolism. Nature 414:799-806,(2001).

Sarkar, S.et al.Demonstration of the hypoglycemic action of Momordica Charantia in a validated animal model of diabetes. Pharmacol. Res. 33(1): 1-4,(1996).

Sauvaire, Y., Petit, P., Broca, C., Manteghetti, M., Baissac, Y., Fernandez-Alvarez, J., Gross, R., Roye, M., Leconte, A., Gomis, R., Ribes, G. 4-Hydroxyisoleucine: a novel amino acidpotentiator of insulin secretion. Diabetes 47 (2): 206-/210(1998).

Schleicher, E.D. and Weigert, C. Role of the hexosamine biosynthetic pathway in diabetic nephropathy. Kidney Int 58 (Suppl. 77) : 13 – 18 (2000).

Shafrir, E.Development and consequences of Insulin Resistance: lessons from animals with hyperinsulinaemia.Diabetes.Metab.22:131-148 (1997).

Shanmugasundaram, E.R., Rajeswari, G., Baskaran, K., Rajesh Kumar, B.R., Radha Shanmugasundaram, K., Kizar Ahmath, B. Use of Gymnema sylvestre leaf extract in the control of blood glucose in insulin-dependent diabetes mellitus. J. Ethnopharmacol. 30 (3): 281-/294 (1990).

Shanmugasundaram, K.R., Panneerselvam, C., Samudram, P., Shanmugasundaram, E.R. Enzyme changes and glucose utilization in diabetic rabbits: the effect of Gymnema sylvestre, R.Br. J. Ethnopharmacol. 7 (2): 205-/234 (1983).

Sheela, C.G., Augusti, K.T. Antidiabetic effects of S-allyl cysteine sulphoxide isolated from garlic Allium sativum Linn. Indian J. Exp. Biol. 30: 523-526 (1992)

Sheela, C.G., Kumud, K. and Augusti, K.T. Anti-diabetic effects of onion and garlic sulfoxide amino acids in rats. Planta Med. 61 (4): 356-357 (1995).

Shimizu, K., Abe, T., Nakajyo, S., Urakawa, N., Atsuchi, M. and Yamashita, C. Inhibitory effects of glucose utilization by gymnema acids in the guinea-pig ileal longitudinal muscle. J. Smooth Muscle Res. 32 (5): 219-228 (1996).

Shimizu, K., Iino, A., Nakajima, J., Tanaka, K., Nakajyo, S., Urakawa, N., Atsuchi, M., Wada, T. and Yamashita, C.Suppression of glucose absorption by some fractions extracted from Gymnema sylvestre leaves. J. Vet. Med. Sci. 59 (4): 245-/251 (1997).

Shobana, S. and Naidu, K.A. Antioxidant activity of selected Indian spices. Prostaglandins Leukot Essent Fatty Acids. 62(2): 107-10 (2000).

Shorr, R.I., Ray, W.A., Daugherty, J.R. and Griffin, MR. Individual sulfonylureas and serious hypoglycemia in older people. J Am Geriatr. Soc.44: 751–755 (1996).

Singh ,R. B,Bajaj, S.,Niaz M.A, ,Rastogi, S.S. and Moshiri, M.Prevalance of type 2 diabetes mellitus and risk of hypertension and coronary artery disease in rural and urban population with low rates of obesity. Int J Cardiol.66:65-72 (1998).

Singh, S.S., Pandey, S.C., Srivastava, S., Gupta, V.S., Patro, B. and Ghosh, A.C. Chemistry and medicinal properties of Tinospora cordifolia (Guduchi). Indian J. Pharmacol. 35:83–91 (2003).

Solecki, R. and Shanidar, IV. A Neanderthal flower burial in northern Iraq. Science 190: 880-881 (1975).

Soulis-Liparota T., Cooper, M., Papazoglou, D., Clarke, B. and Jerums, G. Retardation by aminoguanidine of development of albuminuria, mesangial expansion, and tissue fluorescence in streptozocin-induced diabetic rat. Diabetes 40: 1328–1334 (1991).

Stanely, P., Prince, M. and Menon, V.P. Hypoglycemic and other related actions of Tinospora cordifolia roots in alloxan-induced diabetic rats. J. Ethnopharmacol. 70 (1): 9 -/15 (2000).

Stark, A. and Madar, Z. The effect of an ethanol extract derived from fenugreek (Trigonella foenum-graecum) on bile acid absorption and cholesterol levels in rats. Br. J. Nutr. 69(1): 277-287 (1993).

Stitt, A. W.,Li,Y.M., Gardiner,T.A.,Bucala,R., Archer, D.B. and Vlassara,H. Advanced glycation end products (AGEs) co-localize with AGE receptors in the retinal vasculature of diabetic and of AGE-infused rats. Am. J. Pathol. 150: 523–528 (1997).

Tiwari A.K. and Madhusudana Rao J.Diabetes Mellitus and multiple therapeutic approaches of phytochemicals: present status and future prospectives. Curr. Sci. 83.30-38 (2002 July).

Tjokroprawiro, A., Pikir, B.S., Budhiarta, A.A., Pranawa, Soewondo, H., Donosepoetro, M., Budhianto, F.X., Wibowo, J.A., Tanuwidjaja, S.J. and Pangemanan, M. Metabolic effects of onion and green beans on diabetic patients. Tohoku J. Exp. Med. 141 (Suppl.): 671-/676 (1983).

Tunali, T.,Yarat, A.,Yanardag, R.,Ozcelic, F.,Ozsoy, O.,Ergenekon, G. and Emekli, N. The effect of chard(beta vulgaris L. var. cicla) on the skin of streptozotocin induced diabetic rats . Die Pharmazie.53:638-640 (1998).

UK Prospective Diabetes Study (UKPDS) Group. Intensive blood-glucose control with sulphonylureas or insulin compared with conventional treatment and risk of complications in patients with type 2 diabetes (UKPDS 33). Lancet 352:837-853 (1998)

Venkateswaran, S. and Pari, L. Effect of Coccinia indica leaves on antioxidant status in streptozotocin induced diabetic rats. J. Ethnopharmacol. 84(2-3):163-168 (2003).

Waltner-Law, M.E., Wang, X.L., Law, B.K., Hall, R.K., Nawano, M. and Granner, D.K. Epigallocatechin gallate, a constituent of green tea, represses hepatic glucose production. J. Biol. Chem. 277:34933–34940 (2002).

Welihinda, J. and Karunanayake, E.H. Extra-pancreatic effects of Momordica charantia in rats. J. Ethnopharmacol. 17 (3): 247-/255 (1986).

Williams, B., Gallacher, B., Patel, H. and Orme, C. Glucose-induced protein kinase C activation regulates vascular permeability factor mRNA expression and peptide production by human vascular smooth muscle cells in vitro. Diabetes 46: 1497–1503 (1997).

Xie, J.T., Chang, W.T., Wang, C.Z., Mehendale, S.R., Li.J., Ambihaipahar, R., Ambihaipahar, U., Fong, H.H. and Yuan, C.S. Curry leaf (Murraya koenigii Spreng.) reduces blood cholesterol and glucose levels in ob/ob mice. Am. J. Clin. Med. 34(2): 279-84 (2006).

Yamasaki, Y., Kawamori, R., Wasada, T., Sato, A., Omori, Y., Eguchi, H., Tominaga, M., Sasaki, H., Ikeda, M., Kubota, M., Ishida,Y., Hozumi, T., Baba, S., Uehara, M., Shichiri, M. and Kaneko, T. Glucose Clamp Study Group, Japan, author. Pioglitazone (AD-4833) ameliorates insulin resistance in patients with NIDDM. AD-4833 Tohoku J Exp Med. 183:173–183 (1997).

Yoshikawa, M., Murakami, T. and Matsuda, H. Medicinal foodstuffs. X. Structures of new triterpene glycosides, gymnemosides-c, -d, -e, and -f, from the leaves of Gymnema sylvestre R.Br.: influence of gymnema glycosides on glucose uptake in rat small intestinal Fragments. Chem. Pharm. Bull. (Tokyo) 45(12): 2034-2038 (1997).

Zacharias, N.T., Sebastian, K.L., Philip, B. and Augusti, K.T. Hypoglycemic and hypolipidemic effects of garlic in sucrose fed rabbits. Indian J. Physiol. Pharmacol. 24: 151-154 (1980).

Zimmerman, B.R. Sulfonylureas. Endocrinol Metab Clin North Am.26:511–522 (1997).

Zimmet, P., Taylor,R. and Ram, P. Prevalance of diabetes and impaired glucose tolerance the biracial Melanesian and Indian population of Fiji.a rural urban comparison. Am J Epidemiol. 118:673-688 (1983).

DIABETES MELLITUS
INTRODUCTION, COMPLICATIONS AND HERBAL THERAPY

IRFAN ALI KHAN AND ATIYA KHANUM

P.G. DEPARTMENT OF BOTANY, NAWAB SHAH ALAM KHAN CENTRE FOR POST GRADUATE STUDIES AND RESEARCH, ANWARUL ULOOM COLLEGE CAMPUS, NEW MALLEPALLY, HYDERABAD-500 001.

Chapter outline

IN: HERBAL MEDICINE FOR HUMAN DISEASES: VOLUME-III, PAGES: 216-288

(EDITORS : IRFAN ALI KHAN AND ATIYA KHANUM), UKAAZ PUBLICATIONS - HYDERABAD (A.P)-INDIA

1. INTRODUCTION

Diabetes mellitus which was initially described as a single disease entity, is now regarded as a heterogeneous group of diseases that share the phenotype of hyperglycaemia, which in simple terms, is increased glucose levels in the body. It is emerging as one of the leading causes of end stage renal disease, heart attacks, non-traumatic amputations, and blindness, increasing the mortality and morbidity burden on the community.

The medical term 'diabetes mellitus' is derived from the Greek words 'syphon' and 'sugar', describing symptoms of uncontrolled diabetes, passing huge amounts of urine containing sugar-glucose. Diabetes is a condition where insulin is absent, deficient or defective, so that sugar-glucose cannot enter into the cells and remains in the blood in excessive amounts.

2. HISTORY

Diabetes is not a new disease but its spread in many affluent countries like an epidemic has made one aware of this deadly disease. It has been present since centuries, and the earliest recorded description of diabetes dates back to the year 1552 B.C., when Hesy-Ra, a Physician mentions polyuria(increased frequency of micturition) as a symptom of diabetes.

Arateus in the 1st Century A.D., related diabetes with the 'melting down of flesh and limbs into urine' which is reminiscent of diabetic nephropathy (diabetes induced damage to the kidney) wherein one loses proteins from the muscles which constitute the bulk of the limbs.

The word "mellitus" is a Latin word meaning 'honey' and was added to the term diabetes because the urine of diabetic people tasted sweet to the 'water tasters' who used to diagnose diabetes until the end of the 11th CenturyA.D.

It was not until the early part of the 19th CenturyA.D., when the first chemical tests were developed to indicate the presence and measure the glucose levels in urine. In the year 1908, a German scientist Georg Zuelzer, developed an injectable pancreatic extract to treat hyperglycaemia. This extract, however, was not used much because of its side effects, but it gave a new sense of direction to the many researchers and physicians, busy creating various diet charts and 'fad diets' for the diabetics.

The discovery of insulin in the year 1921, was a very big discovery of that time, and it shifted the whole focus of research towards the use of insulin for the treatment of diabetes. Then the development of insulin syringe in the year 1944, and the discovery of oral hypoglycaemic drugs in the year 1955, paved the way for further improvements in the treatment protocols which has made the control of hyperglycaemia possible.

3. EPIDEMIOLOGY

The chronic, world wide heterogeneous, life threatening disease, diabetes is growing at a faster rate. The prevalence of it will be 5.4% by the year 2025, with the global diabetic population reaching to 300 million. Among all the WHO regions, South East Asian regions are the highest affected with the maximum global burden of the disease. There will be nearly 80 million diabetic in the region by the year 2025.

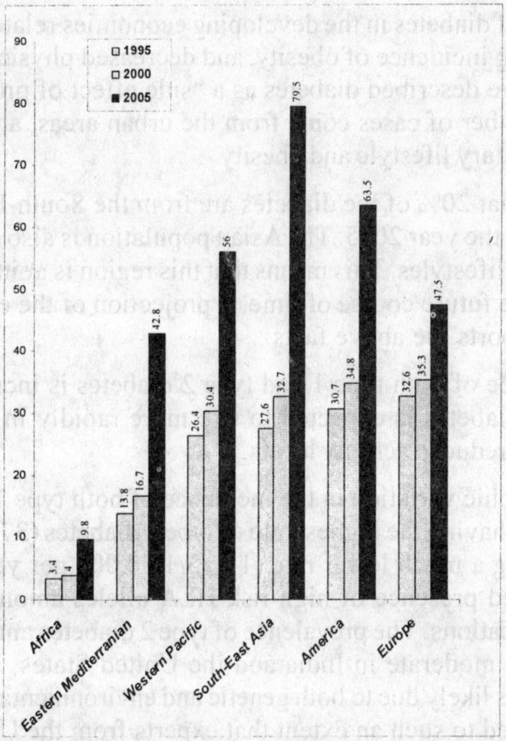

FIGURE 1: AN ESTIMATED PREVALENCE OF DIABETES MELLITUS BY WHO REGION, 1995-2005 [SOURCE: WHO (1999), HEALTH SITUATION IN THE SOUTH-EAST ASIAN REGION 1994-1997, REGIONAL OFFICE FOR SEAR, NEW DELHI]

The worldwide prevalence of diabetes has risen dramatically over the past three decades, and still it continues to rise. Recently compiled data shows that approximately 150 million people have diabetes mellitus worldwide, and that this number may well double by the year 2025. Of these 18.2 million people are in the United States, an estimated 13 million of them are 'diagnosed cases of diabetes'. Unfortunately, 5.2 million people (or nearly one-third) are unaware that they have the disease. In India, it is estimated that presently 19.4 million individuals are affected by this deadly disease, which is likely to go up to 57.2 million by the year 2025. The superior standard of healthcare facilities in the United States when compared to that in India makes the number of 'undiagnosed' cases in India rise to as high as 10 million, or nearly half of those affected by the disease. Thus, diabetes is an "iceberg" disease, with the small tip of iceberg denoting the "diagnosed cases", and a large submerged part of the iceberg representing the "undiagnosed cases".

Initially diabetes was known as the disease of the elderly. A dramatic rise in both the incidence and prevalence of type 2 diabetes in all age groups in the affluent, and newly industrialised countries has major implications on the countries economy as the young and the adolescent age forms the most productive period of life.

The rising prevalence of diabetes in the developing economies relates to the change in their lifestyle with increasing incidence of obesity, and decreased physical activity. Thus, many eminent physicians have described diabetes as a "side effect of prosperity". Studies have shown that a large number of cases come from the urban areas, and this could in part be attributed to their sedentary lifestyle and obesity.

It has been estimated that 20% of the diabetes are from the South-East Asia Region and it is estimated to triple by the year 2025. The Asian population is also said to be vulnerable to diabetes with changing lifestyles. This means that this region is going to bear the maximum burden of disease in the future course of time. A projection of the estimated prevalence of diabetes by WHO supports the above facts.

Although the prevalence of both type 1 and type 2 diabetes is increasing worldwide, the prevalence of type 2 diabetes is expected to rise more rapidly in the future, because of increasing obesity, and reduced activity levels.

A considerable geographic variation in the incidence of both type 1 and type 2 diabetes is seen, with Scandinavia having the highest rate of type 1 diabetes (37/1,00,000 per year) and Japan and China having a much lower rate (1 to 3/1,00,000 per year) of type 1 diabetes. This is due to increased presence of high-risk HLA alleles among the ethnic groups in different geographic locations. The prevalence of type 2 diabetes and pre-diabetes is high in certain Pacific islands, moderate in India and the United States, and low in Russia and China. This variability is likely due to both genetic and environmental factors. The incidence of diabetes has increased to such an extent that experts from the United States Centre for Disease Control (CDC) have said that one third of children born in the United States are at risk for developing diabetes. The lifetime risk of developing diabetes for persons born in the year 2000, is 33 percent for males and 39 percent for females. The main reason for such high rates of diabetes is the rapid increase in type 2 diabetes, which is being driven by the rising rates of inactivity and obesity. This rise in type 2 diabetes which was earlier restricted to 'above forty' age groups has now increased alarmingly in the pre-pubertal age group and the teenagers. There have also been instances of neonates being affected by diabetes in high risk areas.

4. PANCREATIC HARMONE

Diabetes is a life long disease marked by a high levels of sugar in the blood. It develops due to the body's inability to make appropriate use of food as a result of insufficient insulin, a hormone produced by the pancreas to regulate blood sugar level, resistance to insulin or both. To understand diabetes, it is important to understand the normal process of food metabolism. Normally the food eaten is converted within the body into a form of sugar called glucose, which cells use as a source of energy or fuel . Glucose cannot enter the cell alone and needs insulin to aid in its transport into the cells. Glucose causes an increase in blood glucose level which in turn signals the release of hormone insulin. The role of insulin is to move glucose from the blood stream into muscle, fat and liver cells where it can be used as a fuel. Without insulin, cell becomes starved of glucose energy despite the presence of abundant glucose in the blood.

People with diabetes have high blood glucose level, as their muscle, fat, and liver cells do not respond to insulin normally, or both. So the cell's inability to utilize glucose give rise to ironic situation of starvation in the midst of plenty. The abundant unutilized glucose is waste fully executed in the urine .Insulin is produced in the pancreas . Pancreas has islets of langerhans, which produce four different types of hormones.

4.1 SOMATOSTATIN

Somatostatin inhibits GH secretion, and regulates the secretion of insulin and glucagon from the islets.It is a cyclic peptide with a molecular weight of 1640. It is secreted by D cells of the islets. It is secreted as a prohormone and broken down into final size of 14 amino acids.

4.2 PANCREATIC POLYPEPTIDE

Pancreatic polypeptide regulates gastrointestinal secretion , by increasing calcium absorption by the small intestine and reabsorbtion of calcium by kidney.It has 36 amino acids and molecular weight of 4200. It is produced by F cells of the pancreas .

4.3 GLUCAGON

Glucagon is the hyperglycaemic, glycogenolytic factor of the pancreas. The hyperglycaemic effect of some pancreatic extracts due to presence of this hormone was first noted by Kimball and Murin, in the year 1923. Glucagon is a polypeptide with a molecular wieght of 3485. The polypeptide consists of 29 amino acid residues arranged in a straight chain. Glucagon and insulin are free from zinc.In addition to the alpha cells of pancreas, the gastric and mucosa cells also produce glucagon like substance .

4.3.1 PHYSIOLOGY OF GLUCAGON

Ingestion of carbohydrate in food stimulates the release of intestinal glucagon which in turn stimulates the pancreatic β cells to secrete insulin. Glucagon is transported in the blood in free state and is destroyed in the liver by the enzyme glucagonase. The stimulus to glucagon production is lowering of blood glucose levels. Glucagon stimulates hepatic adenyl cyclone enzyme, leading to increase of cyclic AMP level in the viscera, which in turn stimulates dephosphorylase kinase enzyme in reactivation of phosphorylase. The result is increased in breakdown of liver glycogan and rise in blood sugar level (hyperglycaemia).

4.4 INSULIN

Banting and Best (1922) succeeded in extracting insulin from pancreas. Insulin is a small protein comprising 51 amino acids residues synthesised in the beta cells of the islets of langerhans *via* its precursor, proinsulin . One molecule of proinsulin is cleaved by enzymes to give one molecule of insulin and one molecule of c-peptide. C- peptide can be measured in some diabetic patients to show that the insulin production has occurred.

4.4.1 PHYSIOLOGY OF INSULIN

We eat rice, bread, fruit, vegetables, sweets, meat, butter, eggs, *etc.* Of these, the group called carbohydrates, found usually in wheat, rice, fruits and potatoes is converted into glucose or sugar. Glucose is the energy supplier to all the cells of the body, which in turn powers and runs the whole human body. The extra glucose is stored in the liver and muscles.

Now, glucose cannot go straight into the cells on itself, as on the surface of the cell wall, there are protein receptors. Hormones in the body can act on cells through receptors. Glucose enters into the cells only if insulin, which is a hormone, attaches itself as magnet to the receptors, insulin helps cells to extract glucose from the blood.

When there is absolutely no insulin supply or if it is insufficient or the quality is poor or abnormal, the glucose cannot enter into the cells. Consequently, there is not enough energy to run into the body and everything begins to shut down and a person becomes diabetic.

In a diabetic person, the pancreas produces no insulin or not sufficient enough or the quality of insulin produced is not good. Indicating that there is something wrong with the system, it is not normal. The end result being glucose floats around in the bloodstream, at different levels, unable to enter the cells. So, all this excess sugar remains in the blood.

4.4.2 CHEMISTRY OF INSULIN

Insulin is a protein harmone, which can be purified and separated in a crystalline form. Traces of zinc are associated with insulin. Human insulin is made up of two polypeptide chains (A and B) linked together by two disulphide linkage and has a total of 51 amino acids. Chain A is made up of 21 amino acids and chain B is made up 30 amino acids. It has a minimum molecular weight of 5734. Insulin from different sources like pig , cattle, sheep and horse, show minor differences in the amino acid composition and immunological activity. Insulin is destroyed by the action of digestive enzymes and is, hence, inactive when administered by mouth. It is active when administered by injection.

4.4.3 BIOSYNTHESIS OF INSULIN

The primary translation product of the mRNA for insulin is a proinsulin (84 amino acid). This large molecule migrates to the endoplasmic reticulum,where peptidases remove the extra peptides to release "proinsulin"which is made up of A and B chains linked(51) together by another polypeptide containing 33 amino acid. It undergoes proteolytic cleavage and the insulin molecule separates out. The human pancreas is said to contain about 250 units of insulin at anytime. The daily requirement of the hormone is only about 50 units. Increase in the glucose concentration of the blood is a direct stimulus to insulin secretion. Glucose not only stimulates the release of the performed hormone, but can also stimulate further synthesis of the hormone by the beta cells.

4.4.4 MODE OF ACTION OF INSULIN

Muscle, adipose tissue and liver are the major sites of the action of insulin. It is also active on the lens and leukocytes. It has little action on the metabolism of the renal tissue, erythrocytes and the gastrointerstinal tract.

Insulin acts in several ways to reduce circulating blood glucose levels. It enhances cellular uptake of glucose from the blood in many tissues, particularly skeletal muscle and adipose tissue. It also stimulates glycogen production and inhibits glycogen breakdown in muscle and hepatocytes. Insulin is a potent anoblic agent, it enhances body mass by promoting muscle and fat deposition and inhibiting the break down of these tissues.

4.4.5 METABOLISM OF INSULIN

Insulin is degraded primarily in the liver and kidney by the enzyme glutathione insulin transhydrogenase which cleaves the –s-s- linkages, thus, separating the A and B chains. The A and B chain undergoes further hydrolysis by the enzyme " insulinase".

ACTION OF INSULIN ON DIFFERENT ORGANS

Action	Tissue/Organ
Effect on carbohydrate metabolism	
Enhances glucose uptake into cells	Adipose and muscle
Increases glycolysis	Adipose and muscle
Increases glycogen synthesis	Muscle and liver
Reduces glycogen break down	Muscle and liver
Effects on lipid metabolism	
Reduces fat breakdown	Adipose
Increases fatty acid synthesis	Adipose
Increases low density lioprotein synthesis	Liver
Increases cholesterol synthesis	Liver
Effects on protein metabolism	
Increases amino acid transport	Many tissue
Increases protein synthesis	Muscle and others
Reduces protein breakdown	Muscle and others

5. GENERAL SYMPTOMS OF DIABETES

- Increased thirst.
- Frequent urination, passing large quantities of urine, hence dehydration.
- Increased hunger.
- Feeling very tired without any particular reason.
- Blurred vision due to dehydration of eye lens.
- Continuous ache, pain in legs and feet including numbness, burning sensation, or no sensation.
- No healing of cuts, wounds, boils, and sores.
- Skin infections, especially around genital area, vaginal infections in women, urinary tract infections.
- Impotence.
- Weight loss.

6. TYPES OF DIABETES

Diabetes basically can be categorized into two types (WHO, 1985). Diabetes insipides and Diabetes mellitus.

6.1 DIABETES INSIPIDUS (DI)

It is due to the deficiency of hormone vasopressin, produced by the middle or intermediate lobe of the pitutary gland . Vasopressin is synthesized in the cells of specialized neurons and combines with a large polypeptide called neurophysin and a small glycoprotein to form granules. The granules are discharged into circulation from the blood plasma or decreased in blood volume. They reach the distal convoluted tubules and bind to receptors on the tubular cells and cause an activation of the adenylate cyclase and release of 3', 5' – cyclic AMP. This, in turn, causes the terminal membrane to become water permeable and leads to reabsorption of water by the distal convoluted tubules. Deficiency of vasopressin results in polyuria condition where large amount of urine of low specific gravity is passed.

6.2 DIABETES MELLITUS (DM)

Von Mering and Minkowski (1890), demonstated the relationship of pancreatic hypo-function and diabetes mellitus. Diabetes mellitus is a group of metabolic diseases characterized by high blood sugar (glucose) level, which results from defects in insulin secretion or action or both. Diabetes mellitus means sweet urine where elevated levels of blood glucose (hyper glycaemia) lead to spillage of glucose into urine, hence, the term sweet urine. Normally blood glucose levels are tightly controlled by insulin. Insulin lowers the blood glucose level when the blood glucose elevates, insulin is released from pancreas to normalise the glucose level. In patients with diabetes mellitus, the absence or insufficient production of insulin causes hyperglycaemia.

Diabetes mellitus in India is slowly becoming a killer disease next to coronary heart disease and has attacked 40 million persons. Nearly 10-13% of urban population and 4 to 6 % of the rural population of India have diabetes. The rising prevalence of diabetes is closely associated with the industrialization and socio -economic development. It is estimated that during the year 1997 about 102,800 persons died of diabetes mellitus in India.

6.2.1 TYPES OF DIABETES MILLITUS

There are several types of diabetes. The following classification system for diabetes was endoned by the board of directors of the American Diabetes Association at its 1979 annual meeting and also by the World Heath Organization (1994).

6.2.1.1 TYPE I: INSULIN DEPENDENT

Insulin dependent diabetes mellitus (IDDM) is characterized by beta cell destruction caused by an autoimmune process usually leading to absolute insulin deficiency. Type I diabetes occurs in 20% of all diabetic patients. Type I is insulin-dependent diabetes, and it can occur at any age, though it mostly occurs in youth. This type of diabetes used to be known as juvenile-onset diabetes. About one out of every 2,500 children has this disease, because the pancreas produces little or no insulin, such patients become dependent on outside sources of insulin. Before the discovery of insulin in the year 1921, children with insulin-dependent diabetes had a short life expectancy. Now the disease can be controlled with insulin, proper diet and exercise, and careful monitoring.

The onset of IDDM is usually acute, developing over a period of a few days to weeks. Over 95 percent of persons with type I diabetes mellitus develop the disease before the age of 25, with an equal incidence in both sexes and an increased prevalence in the white population. Most of the patients have the "immune mediated" form of type I diabetes mellitus with islet cell antibodies and often have other autoimmune disorders such as *Hashimoto's thyroiditis, Addison's disease*, Vitiligo or pernicious anemia. A few patients from Africa or Asia have no antibodies, but have similar clinical presentation and are included under "idiopathic form" of type I diabetes mellitus.

The pathological process of type I occur in genetically predisposed individual over many years, and appears to be triggered by environmental factors such as viral infection and nutritional factors, such as, ingestion of Cow's milk in early childhood.

SYMPTOMS OF TYPE I DIABETES MELLITUS

- Increased thirst
- Increased urination
- Weight loss inspite of increased appetite
- Fatigue
- Irritability
- Nausea
- Vomiting

Patient with type I of diabetes usually develops symptoms over a short period of time. In addition to high glucose level, type I diabetic patients have high levels of ketones. Ketones are produced by break down of fat and muscle, and are toxic at high level. Ketones in the blood cause a condition called 'acidiosis' which results in lowering of blood pH.

6.2.1.2 TYPE 2: NON-INSULIN DEPENDENT

Type 2 DM or NIDDM is characterized by insulin resistance in peripheral tissue and an insulin secretory defect of the β cell. Insulin resistance and hyper insulinimia eventually lead to impaired glucose tolerance. Defective β cells become exhausted, further fueling the cycle of glucose intolerance and hyperglycaemia. Resistance to the action of the insulin results in decrease in the ability of skeletal muscle to store glucose.

Type 2 occurs in 75% of all diabetic patients. The American Diabetes Association further divides this category into subtypes that include obese non-insulin dependent diabetes and non-obese, non-insulin-dependent diabetes (Estimates are that 60 – 90 % of those with non-insulin –dependent diabetes in western societies are obese). Non- insulin- dependent diabetes used to be called *maturity – onset diabetes.* Type 2 diabetes is much more common than Type I. If you have non-insulin diabetes you are one of the 5 million patients with the disease.This type is less severe than insulin- dependent diabetes and starts more slowly.

Patients with this type of diabetes produce some, or at times even excessive, insulin in their pancreas. Insulin produced in these patients is either is not enough for proper function or is not being produced quickly enough to influence glucose levels in the blood effectively. This type of disease usually occurs in middle or older age and frequently in overweight people. It is more common in women, especially woman with a history of gestational diabetes and in Blacks, Hispanics and native Americans. It can most often be controlled by diet alone, or by the combination of diet, exercise and oral medication.

SYMPTOMS OF TYPE 2 DIABETES MELLITUS

- Increased thirst
- Increased urination
- Increased appetite
- Fatigue
- Blurred vision
- Slow healing infection
- Impotence in men
- Itching
- Drowsiness
- Tingling and numbness in hands and feet
- Excess weight

7. CHARACTERISTIC OF INSULIN- DEPENDENT DIABETES AND NON-INSULIN DEPENDENT DIABETES

	Insulin-dependent (Type –I)	Non-Insulin-dependent (Type –II)
Age of onset	Usually during youth, but can occur at any age	Usually during adulthood;more common in older people
How noticed	Usually appears abruptly and progress rapidly	Gradual in onset; the disease may go unnoticed for years
Family background	Diabetes not always present in other family members	Often diabetes present in other members of the family
Treatment	Insulin injections are necessary. Diet, exercise and emotional control are necessary.	Insulin injections are not always necessary. Oral medications are sometimes recommended. Diet, exercise and emotional control are necessary.
Complications	Problems affecting blood vessels, eyes, kidneys, and nerves may occur at any age.	Problems affecting blood vessels, eyes, kidneys, and nerves may occur at any age.
Linked to obesity	Not necessarily.	80 percent of all patients are overweight at time of diagnosis.

8. TEST FOR URINE-SUGAR OR BLOOD-SUGAR

- Urine or blood sugar tests are common tests performed to know the state of diabetes.
- Blood contains some amount of sugar (80 to 140 mg%) round the clock, since certain tissues like brain can not survive without readily available glucose.

When the blood sugar exceeds 180 mg%, sugar appears in urine. Urine test is only a rough guide and if there is no sugar in urine it can only mean that blood sugar at that time is less than 180 mg%, (it can be between 60 to 180%). Urine sugar approximates with blood sugar in the ways mentioned below.

Urine sugar	Blood sugar mg%
+	200
++	250
+++	300
++++	350

- Since urine is secreted drop by drop by the kidney and stored in the bladder to be evacuated at longer intervals, if we wish to correlate urine sugar with blood sugar level we must test the second sample of urine *i.e.*, first evacuate the bladder and, dicard the urine and then after half an hour, pass the urine and collect the sample for the test. It will give better idea of blood sugar level at that time.

- Blood sugar is more accurate parameter for assessing diabetes.

GLUCOSE CONCENTRATION VALUE CHART (Mg per ml OF BLOOD)

	Fasting value	2 hrs.after meals
Normal	065-100	100-120
Impaired Glucose Tolerance*	105-120	120-150
Diabetes mellitus**	e"120	e"180

* These values are the boarderline cases of mild high blood sugar and can be recommended for further investigations/tests by the doctor so that the person with such condition should take necessary precaution to control it in time.

** e"Stands for equal to and greater than.

According to Harrison's 15th edition "Principles of Internal Medicine" Volume -2, pp 2111, the revised criteria reflect new epedemiologic and metabolic evidence and are based on the following premises :

- The spectrum of fasting plasma glucose (FPG) and the response to an oral glucose load varies in normal individuals,

- DM defined as the level of glycaemia at which diabetes-specific complications are noted and not on the level of glucose tolerance from a population based viewpoint. For example, the prevalence of retinopathy in Native Americans (Pima Indian population) begins to increase at a FPG>6.4 mmol/L (116mg/dL).

GLUCOSE TOLERANCE IS CLASSIFIED INTO THREE CATEGORIES BASED ON THE FPG

1. FPG < 6.1mmol/L (110 mg/dL) is considered normal;
2. FPG > 6.1 mmol/L (110 mg/dL) but < 7.0 mmol/L (126 mg/dL) is defined as IFG; and

3. FPG > 7.0 mmol/L (126 mg/dL) warrants the diagnosis of DM. IFG is a new diagnostic category defined by the Expert Committee on the Diagnosis and Classification of Diabetes mellitus. It is analogous to IGT, which is defined as plasma glucose levels between 7.8 and 11.1 mmol/L (140 and 200 mg/dL) 2h after a 75-g oral glucose load. Individuals with IFG or IGT are at substantial risk for developing type 2 DM and cardiovascular disease in the future, though they may not meet the criteria for DM.

9. CRITERIA FOR THE DIAGNOSIS OF DIABETES MELLITUS

- Symptoms of diabetes plus random blood glucose concentration >11.1 mmol/L (200mg/dL).
- Fasting plasma glucose >7.0 mmol/L (126 mg/dL)[b]
- Two-hour plasma glucose >11.1 mmol/L (200 mg/dL) during an oral glucose tolerance test[c]

In the absence of unequivocal hyperglycaemia and acute metabolic decompensation, these criteria should be confirmed by repeat testing on a different day.

- Random is defined as without regard to time since the last meal.
- Fasting is defined as no caloric intake for at least 8 hours.
- The test should be performed using a glucose load containing the equivalent of 75g. anhydrous glucose dissolved in water; not recommended for routine clinical use.

Source : Adapted from American Diabetes Association, 2000.

OPTIMUM WEIGHT* CHART RELATED TO HEIGHT FOR ADULTS

Women				Men			
Height			Weight/kgs	Height			Weight/kgs
Ft	Ins	cms	Range	Ft	Ins	cms	Range
4	10	147.3	43.5-48.5	--			--
4	11	149.3	44.5-49.9	--			--
5	0	152.4	45.8-51.3	5	0	152.4	50.0-55.0
5	1	154.9	47.2-52.6	5	1	154.9	52.2-57.7
5	2	157.5	48.5-54.0	5	2	157.5	53.5-58.5
5	3	160.0	49.9-55.3	5	3	160.0	54.9-60.3
5	4	162.6	57.3-57.2	5	4	162.6	56.2-61.7
5	5	165.1	52.6-59.0	5	5	165.1	57.6-63.0
5	6	167.6	54.4-61.2	5	6	167.6	59.0-64.9
5	7	170.2	56.2-63.0	5	7	170.2	60.8-66.7
5	8	172.7	58.1-64.9	5	8	172.7	62.6-68.9
				5	9	175.3	64.4-70.8
				5	10	177.8	66.2-72.6
				5	11	180.3	68.0-74.8
				6	0	182.9	69.9-77.1

* For without clothes and shoes, subtract, 2.7 kg for women and 4.5 kg for men.

SOURCE: *You Can Prevent Heart Attack* by Dr.O.P.Jaggi, published by Orient Paperbacks

10. SPECIFIC GROUPS OF DIABETES

Specific groups of diabetes accounts for 5% of all diabetic patients. These are categorized further as :

1. Malnutrition related diabetes mellitus (MRDM)
2. Diabetic associated with other condition and syndrome
   - Pancreatic disease
   - Disease of hormonal aetiology
   - Chemical induced diabetes
   - Abnormalities of insulin or its reception
   - Certain genetic syndrome
   - Miscellaneous

There are also many types of diabetes associated with certain conditions and syndromes, such as diabetes induced by drugs or chemicals, diabetes secondary to pancreatic disease such as pancreatic or cystic fibrosis, and diabetic secondary to endocrine disease acromegaly. This specific group includes persons with genetic defects of beta cell functions and this type was formerly called MODY or maturity onset diabetes in youth.

10.1 GESTATIONAL DIABETES

Refer to hyperglycaemia occurring for first time in pregnancy. During normal pregnancy insulin sensitivity is reduced through the action of placental hormone and this impairs glucose tolerance. The insulin secreting cells of pancreatic islets are unable to meet this demand in woman predisposed to develop diabetes. Repeat pregnancy may increase the likelihood of developing irreversible diabetes, particularly in obese woman.

CLINICAL CLASSIFICATION OF DIABETES MELLITUS

Clinically diabetes mellitus has been classified into two main groups

10.1.1 PRIMARY (IDIOPATHIC)

Constitute the major group, exact cause is not known but metabolic defect due to insufficient insulin is one of the reason. The idiopathic DM is of two clinical types:

(i) "Juvenile" onset diabetes : called as type I IDDM (insulin dependent)

(ii) Maturity- onset diabetes : Type 2 NIDDM (non- insulin dependent)

- **FACTORS RESPONSIBLE FOR IDIOPATHIC DIABETES MELLITUS**

HEREDITY

Diabetes mellitus has a heredity component and often runs in families. If both mother and father are diabetic, there are more than 80% chances that their children will also be diabetic.

AUTOIMMUNITY

Insulin dependent juvenile type may be an autoimmune disorder and has found to co-exist with other autoimmune disoder like lymphocytic and plasma cells infiltrations in pancreas.

INFECTIONS

Certain viral infection may precipitate juvenile type. Antibodies to coxsackie Bu virus have been found in young juvenile type.

OBESITY

Majority of middle ages maturity-onset diabetes are "obese", and "stress" during pregnancy may also precipitate.

DIET

Over eating and under activity are also predisposing factors in elderly middle aged maturity onset diabetes.

INSULIN ANTAGONISM

In maturity onset diabetes, the deficiency of insulin is relative and glucose induced insulin secretion may be greater and more prolonged than normal. The relative deficiency may be due to insulin antagonism. The various factors governing insulin antagonism may be either insulin antibodies, secretion of abnormal and less active insulin or altered insulin , receptor deficiency and lack of cellular response to insulin.

10.1.2 SECONDARY

This forms an inner group. Diabetes is secondary to some other disease. The different types of secondary diabetes are as follows:

PANCREATIC DIABETES

Pancreatic diabetes leads to pancreatites, haemochromatosis and malignancy of pancreas.

ABNORMAL CONCENTRATION OF ANTAGONISTIC HORMONES

The abnormal concentration of antagonistic hormones develop due to diabetes leads to hyperthyroidism, hypercorticism like Cushing's disease and syndrome, hyper pitutarism like acromegaly and increased glucagon activity.

IATROGENIC

Iatrogenic diabetes may be genetically susceptible and is precipitated by therapy like corticosteroids.

11. GENES FOR DIABETES MELLITUS

GENES OF DIABETES MELLITUS

Recently researchers have discovered two genes, called "MODY I" and "MODY III", that appear to contribute to the 2% to 5% of diabetes, that are clearly inheritable.

MODY 1 GENE

Mody I gene is located on chromosome 20, makes hepatocyte nuclear factor 4α(HN,4α), a cell receptor that plays a role in HNF-1α production.

MODY III GENE

Mody III gene is located on chromosome 12 produces hepatocyte nuclear factor-1α (HNF,1α), a protein found in the liver and β cells of the process.

12. HOMEOSTASIS

REGULATION OF BLOOD GLUCOSE (HOMEOSTASIS)

Blood glucose level is maintained within physiological limits 60 to 100 mg% (true glucose) fasting state and 100 to 140 mg% following ingestion of a carbohydrate containing meal by a balance between two sets of factors: Rate of glucose entrance into the blood stream and rate of removal from the blood stream.

RATE OF GLUCOSE ENTRANCE INTO THE BLOOD

The blood glucose is derived directly from the absorption of glucose from the intestine, breakdown of glycogan of liver, by gluconeogenesis in liver and from carbohydrate sources like fructose, galactose *etc.*

RATE OF REMOVAL FROM THE BLOOD STREAM

The removal of glucose from the blood is by the following sources:

- Oxidation of glucose by the tissues to supply energy
- Glycogen formation from glucose in liver and from glucose in muscles
- Conversion of glucose to fats specially in adipose tissues
- Formation of compounds containing blood glucose *i.e.,* formation of fructose in seminal fluid, formation of lactose in lactating mammary gland, synthesis of glycoprotein and glycolipid.
- Formation of ribose sugars from glucose required for nucleic acid synthesis
- Extraction of glucose in urine "glycosuria" when blood glucose level exceeds the normal range.

13. ABNORMALITIES IN BLOOD GLUCOSE LEVELS

Increase in blood glucose level above normal is called hyperglycaemia. Decrease in blood glucose level below normal is called hypoglycaemia.

13.1 HYPERGLYCAEMIA

Chronic hyperglycaemia causes damage to the eyes, kidneys, nerves, heart and blood vessels.

CAUSES OF HYPERGLYCAEMIA

The most common cause is that diabetes mellitus in which the highest values for fasting blood glucose is obtained, vary from normal to 500 mg% and over, depending on the severity of the disease.

- There may be increased incidence of diabetes mellitus in hyperthyrodism and hyperpituitarism. Emotional stress can increase the blood glucose level.
- In pancreatitis and carcinoma of pancreas, some increase in fasting blood glucose may occur. Increase in blood glucose in appreciable amount may be seen in sepsis and in a number of infectious diseases.
- A moderate hyperglycaemia may also be found in some intracramial disease such as meningitis, encephalitis, intracramial tumors and haemorrhage.

- Anaesthia can also increase blood glucose depending on the degree and duration of anaesthia. Asphyxia may also increase blood sugar level.

13.2 HYPOGLYCAEMIA

Hypoglycaemia may be considered to be present when the blood glucose is below 40 mg% (true glucose).

CAUSES OF HYPOGLYCAEMIA

- Most common cause is the overdosage of insulin in the treatment of diabetes mellitus.
- Low blood glucose are often found in severe liver disease, hypopitutarism (Simmond's disease) and hypoadrenalism (Addison's disease).
- Spontaneous hypoglycaemia in childhood may be due to deficiency of glucagon production.
- Severe exercise may produce hypoglycaemia due to depletion of liver glycogen. Hypoglycaemia is also found in some of the glycogen storage diseases (GSDs) as in VonGierke's disease.
- Hypoglycaemia has also been found to be associated with alcohol ingestion.

14. GLYCOSURIA

Glycosuria is defined as the excretion of glucose in the urine. In normal individuals, glycosuria occurs when the venous blood glucose exceeds 170 to 180 mg/100 ml. This level of the venous blood glucose is termed as the "Renal threshold", for glucose. Excretion of abnormal amounts of glucose in the urine may be due to two types of abnormalities.

- Increase in the amount of glucose entering in the tubule/ml.
- Decrease in the glucose reabsorption capacity of the renal tubular epithelium.

14.1 TYPES OF GLYCOSURIA

Glucosuria can be divided into two main groups.

14.1.1 HYPERGLYCAEMIC GLYCOSURIA

Different types of hyperglycaemic glycosuria exists:

ALIMENTARY GLYCOSURIA

When a large carbohydrate diet is taken, blood sugar rises and crosses as renal threshold in occasional cases may produce glycosuria.

NERVOUS OR EMOTIONAL GLYCOSURIA

Stimulation of the sympathetic nerves to the liver or of the splanchnic nerves, breakdown of liver glycogen occurs and produces hyperglycaemia and glycosuria. The excitement that stimulates sympathetic system such as emotion, stress *etc.,* may produce glycosuria. Nearly 1.6% of students going for examination show glycosuria.

GLYCOSURIA DUE TO ENDOCRINE DISORDER

Deranged function of a number of endocrine glands produces hyperglycaemia which may result in glycosuria.

14.1.2 RENAL GLYCOSURIAS

HEREDITARY

A milder glycosuria occurs spontaneously, as hereditary familiar traits, persisting throughout life, due to absence of "Carrier protein" or altered kinetics of the carrier system due to failure of development.

ACQUIRED

In some cases of kidney diseases, the renal tubules may be grossly damaged, thus, the tubule fail to reabsorb glucose producing glycosuria. The heavy metals like lead (pb), cadmium(cd), mercury (Hg) *etc.,* can damage the renal tubules, thus, interfering with the reabsorption of glucose, resulting to glycosuria.

LOWERING OF RENAL THRESHOLD

15 to 20% cases of pregnancy may be associated with the physiological glycosuria with advancement of pregnancy, due to lowering of renal threshold. But pregnancy may be associated with diabetes mellitus in which there will be hyperglycaemic glycosuria.

RENAL GLYCOSURIA

It may also occur in association with evidences of other renal tubular transport defects *e.g.,* amino acidurias, renal tubular acidosis, hyperphosphoturia as in Fanconi syndrome.

15. GLYCAEMIC INDEX (GI)

The glycaemic index is a ranking of carbohydrates based on their immediate effect on blood glucose levels. It compares food, gram for gram of carbohydrates. Carbohydrates that break down quickly during digestion have the highest glycaemic indexes. The blood glucose response is fast and high. Carbohydrates that break down slowly, releasing glucose gradually into the blood stream, have low glycaemic indexes.

Low glycaemic index means a smaller rise in blood glucose levels after meals. Low glycaemic diets can help people lose weight and improve body's sensitivity to insulin.It can improve diabetic control and can prolong physical endurance. High glycaemic index foods help to refuel carbohydrate stores after exercise.

16. GLYCAEMIC LOAD (GL)

Glycaemic load builds on the glycaemic index to provide a measure of total glycaemic response to a food or meal.

Glycaemic load =GI (%) × grams of carbohydrate per serving

One unit of GL is similar to glycaemic effect of one gram glucose.

17. METABOLIC CHANGES IN DIABETES MELLITUS

17.1 HYPERGLYCAEMIA

Occurs as a result of:

- Decreased and impaired transport and uptake of glucose into muscles and adipose tissues.
- Representation of key glycolytic enzymes like glucokinase, phosphofructokinase and pyruvate kinase.

- Depression of key gluconogenic enzymes like pyruvate carboxylase, phosphoenol pyruvate carboxykinase, fructose –bi-phosphatase and gluco-6-phosphatase, promoting gluconeogenesis in liver. This further contributes to hyperglycaemia.
- Elevated aminoacid level in the blood particularly alanine provides fuel for gluconeogenesis in liver.

17.2 AMINOACIDS LEVEL

- Transport and uptake of amino acids in peripheral tissues is also depressed causing an elevated circulating level of amino acids, particularly alanine. Glucocorticoid activity predominates having catabolic action peripheral tissue proteins, releasing more amino acids in blood.
- Amino acids breakdown in liver results in increased production of urea .

17.3 PROTEIN SYNTHESIS

Protein synthesis is decreased in all tissues due to:

- Decreased production of ATP.
- Absolute or relative deficiency of insulin.

17.4 FAT METABOLISM

- Decrease extramitochondrial '*de Novo*' synthesis of FA is due to decrease in acetyl CoA from carbohydrates, ATP, NADPH and α-glycero-(p) in all tissues.
- Stored lipids are hydrolyzed by increased lipolysis liberating free fatty acids (FFA). Increased FFA interferes at several steps of carbohydrate phosphorylation in muscles, further contributing to hyperglycaemia.

17.4.1 EFFECTS OF INCREASED FFA LEVEL

- FFA reaching the liver in high concentration inhibits further F.A. synthesis by a feedback inhibition at the acetyl CoA carboxylase step.
- Fats are mobilized for energy, increased fatty acid oxidation increases acetyl CoA level, which in turn activates *Pyruvate carboxylase*, stimulating the gluconeogenic pathway required for conversion of aminoacids to glucose.
- F.A. also stimulates gluconeogenesis by entering T.C.A. cycle and increasing production of citrates. Citrate in turn inhibits glycolysis at *Phosphofructokinase* level.
- Eventually F.A. inhibits T.C.A. cycle at the level of citrate synthase and possibly pyruvate dehydrogenase complex and Isocitrate dehydragenase level.
- AcetylCoA while no longer can be channelized to T.C.A cycle or be used for F.A synthesis are diverted to:
- Cholesterol synthesis, and
- Excessive production of ketone bodies,increases the concentration of ketone bodies in blood (ketonaemia) and excretion of ketone bodies in urine (ketonuria) and leads to acidosis.

17.5 EFFECTS ON GLYCOGEN SYNTHESIS

Glycogen synthesis is depressed as a result of:

- Decreased glycogen synthase activity due to deficiency of insulin.
- By activation of phosphorylase producing glycogenolysis through the action of epinephrine and/or glucagon (antagonistic) hormones.
- By increased ADP: ATP ratio.

18. COMPLICATIONS IN DIABETES MELLITUS

The complications occurred during diabetes mellitus are either immediate or late complications.

18.1 IMMEDIATE

Diabetic ketoacidiosis and coma is one of the most important and dreaded complication specially in type-1.

18.2 LATE COMPLICATIONS

Other complications during diabetes mellitus are late to appear and are due to changes in blood vessels. Two types of blood vessels are involved.

- **Large vessels involvement:** Involvement of coronary vessels can produce myocardial infarction and involvement of cerebral vessel can produce stroke.
- **Small vessels involvement :** Small vessels involvement results in thickening of basement membrane and microvascular changes.

The late complications of diabetes mellitus can further be of following types:

18.2.1 PANCREATIC COMPLICATIONS

The islets of langerhans are destroyed in Type I diabetes mellitus. This occurs probably as a consequence of a genetic susceptibility, followed by the onset of autoimmune destruction triggered by some environmental factor such as viral infection. Heavy lymphocytic infiltratesates appear in and around islets are eventually reduced, leading to decreased insulin production and glucose intolerance. The islets of langerhans are normal in number or somewhat reduced with Type 2 Diabetes mellitus. Fibrosis and deposition of amylin polypeptide with islets are most characteristic of the chronic states of Type 2 diabetes.

18.2.2 RENAL COMPLICATIONS

There are a variety of complications, involving the kidney, the nodular and diffuse glomerulosclerosis can lead to chronic renal failure. Diabetics are prone to infections, particularly pyelonephritis. Both bacterial and fungal infections can occur.

18.2.3 OCULAR COMPLICATIONS

Ocular complications during diabetes mellitus are :

18.2.3.1 DIABETIC CATARACT

Cataracts are more common in diabetes. The predilection for development of cataracts is felt to result from hyperglycaemia due to non- enzymatic glycosylation of lens, leading to accumulation of sorbitol that results in osmotic damage of the crystalline lens.

18.2.3.2 DIABETIC RETINOPATHY

70% of the diabetic patients are affected by diabetic retinopathy and diabetic retinopathy is one of the leading cause for irreversible blindness in the United States. This retinopathy can occur with either Type I or Type 2 diabetes mellitus, usually a decade or so after the onset of diabetes. Most persons with Type I diabetes and many of those with Type 2 diabetes develop some non-proliferative retinopathy. Proliferative retinopathy is more omnious and is more likely to occur when diabetes mellitus is poorly controlled. In severe retinopathy, vascularization may lead to adhesions between iris and cornea or iris and lens. Neo vascularization of the iris leads to secondary glaucoma with blindness. Tiny haemorrhages, punctate or flame shaped, exudates occur. Haemorrhage in vitreous humour can cause sudden blindness.

18.2.3.3 DIABETIC NEPHROPATHY

50% cases of diabetic nephropathy are recognised in diabetic mellitus patient, characterized by proteinuria, hypertension and oedema. Diabetic nephropathy causes Kimmelsteil Wilson syndrome. Microscopic lesions are called as Kimmelsteil- Wilson lesions disease. Lesions are often present when syndrome is not developed. Sometimes kidney lesions may be shown as papillary necrosin which is a dangerous complication and pyelonephritis, when secondary infections occur.

18.2.3.4 DIABETIC NEUROPATHY PERIPHERAL NEURITIS

Diabetic neuropathy is manifested by loss of sensation and twigling. Biochemically the cause is myoinositol deficiency associated by myopathes or weakness of muscles.

18.2.3.5 DIABETIC GANGRENE

Diabetic gangrene is due to diminished blood supply due to other osclerotic changes in blood vessels. Also associated tissue hypoxia due to formation of glycosylated Hb, which has less oxygen carrying capacity.

18.2.3.6 ATHEROSCLEROSIS

Persons with diabetic mellitus either Type I or Type 2 , have early and accelarated atherosclerosis. The most serious complication of this are atherosclerotic heart disease, cerabro vascular disease, and renal disease. The most common cause of death with diabetes mellitus is myocardial infarction.

18.2.3.7 MUCOR MYCOSIS

Mucor mycosis is feared complications of Diabetic mellitus. Diabetic ketoacidosis helps to potentiate the growth of mucor. The site of involvement is typically the nasopharyngeal region,but the infection can spread to involve soft tissue and bone of the face, orbit, skull and brain.

18.2.3.8 SKIN LESIONS

There may be boils/ulcers , carbuncle and necrosis of skin which causes necrobiosis.

18.2.3.9 DIABETIC PULMONARY TUBERCULOSIS

The patients will be susceptible to pulmonary tuberculosis.

18.2.3.10 GENETIC SYNDROMES

A number of genetic syndromes sometimes associated with diabetic are as follows:

- Down syndrome
- Cushing's syndrome

- Klinefelter's syndrome
- Turner's syndrome
- Wolfram syndrome
- Friedreich's ataxia
- Huntingtons chorea
- Lawrence –meon beidel syndrome
- Myotonic dystrophy
- Porphyria, and
- Prader – willi syndrome.

19. MANAGEMENT OF DIABETES

19.1 GOALS OF THERAPY

Although glycaemic control is central to diabetes therapy, comprehensive diabetes care should also detect and manage diabetes specific complications, and modify risk factors for diabetes-associated diseases.

The goals of therapy for diabetes are :

- To try to attain euglycaemic levels for as long a period of time as possible,
- To eliminate symptoms related to hyperglycaemia,
- To decrease the risk of the development of the long-term microvascular and macrovascular complications of diabetes, and
- To make the patient achieve as normal a life-style as possible.

For the patient to have a near normal life, the physician should try to attain a state of glycaemic control as near to the euglycaemic level as possible, provide the patient and his family with the education about the lifestyle changes, and pharmacologic resources necessary to reach this state, and to look out for the long term complications. Most of the hospitals now have a multidisciplinary team for diabetes care; the core group comprising a diabetologist / endocrinologist, a nutritionist and educator for diabetes. The specialists like ophthalmologists, nephrologists, neurologists, dermatologists, cardiologists, general surgeons, *etc.,* are a part of the group who regularly monitor the patients for the emergence of long term complications.

19.2 PATIENT AND FAMILY EDUCATION

Education about diabetes is essential not only to the patients but also to his/her family members as they have an important part to play in diabetes management. Education about nutrition, exercise, care of diabetes during illness, and medications to lower the plasma glucose improves patient compliance; and allows diabetics to assume greater responsibility in diabetes management. The incidence of long term as well as most of the short term complications of diabetes like hypoglycaemia, DKA and HHS has decreased in patients who/whose family had diabetes education.

A certified diabetes educator, educates the patient and his/her family about issues central to good diabetes care, which includes self-monitoring of blood glucose, urine ketone monitoring, foot and skin care, insulin administration, management of hypoglycemia, exercise management, and risk factor-modifying activities.

19.3 NUTRITION

A well balanced nutritious diet forms the basis of diabetes therapy. The dietary charts or schedules should be related to the type of diabetes. The nutrition therapy in individuals with type 1 diabetes should match the caloric intake with the appropriate amount of insulin. It must be flexible enough to allow for exercise, and for deviations in the caloric intake. Obese patients with type 2 diabetes should be advised a weight reduction programme that incorporates calorie restricted diet and regular exercise. The risk factors for cardiovascular disease such as hyperlipidemia and hypertension should be kept under control.

DIET FOR TYPE 1 DIABETIC AND NON-OBESE TYPE 2 DIABETICS

Weight maintenance diet

- Ideally high in carbohydrate and low in fat

Carbohydrates	**50-55%**
Fat	**30-35%**
Saturated fat	< 10%
Monounsaturated fat	10-15%
Polyunsaturated fat	< 10%
Protein	**10-15%**

ET FOR OBESE TYPE 2 DIABETICS

Low calorie, Weight reducing diet

- Ideally a daily deficit of 500 kcal inducing a weight loss of 0.5 kg/week
- Diets rich in fibre are preferred

Carbohydrates	**45-50%**
Fat	**25-30%**
Saturated fat	< 10%
Monounsaturated fat	10-15%
Polyunsaturated fat	< 10%
Protein	**15-20%**

A 'PLATE MODEL' OF DIABETIC DIET

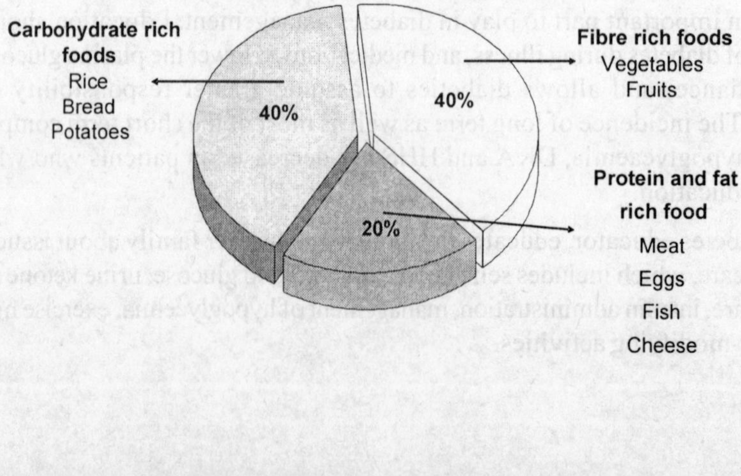

ADA recommends that the carbohydrate content for type 1 patients should be regulated, based on the presence of obesity, insulin regimens, and exercise pattern. In type 2 diabetics who are obese, the carbohydrate content should be reduced considerably. Current recommendations in both types of diabetes include limiting the cholesterol intake to 300 mg/day, and a daily protein intake of 10-20% of total calorie intake. The saturated fat should be < 10%. Poultry, veal, and fish are recommended as a substitute for red meats for keeping the saturated fat content low. Further data on meal planning can be obtained from www.eatright.org

19.4 FIBRE

Fibre is the term used to describe indigestible plant components such as cellulose, gum and pectin. Cellulose and hemicellulose form the insoluble fibre, and they increase the intestinal transit time. Gums and pectins are soluble fibres that tend to retard the nutrient absorption, thereby decreasing the amount of glucose absorbed. High fibre in diet prevents the absorbtion of cholesterol from the gut, decreasing the blood cholesterol levels.

19.5 ALCOHOL

Although the recommendations for alcohol use are the same as for the general population, individuals with diabetes are advised to restrain from alcohol because of its high calorigenicity, risk of development of lactic acidosis in patients taking metformin, potentiation of action of sulphonylureas causing hypoglycaemia, and confusion of inebriation with hypoglycaemic symptoms.

19.6 ARTIFICIAL SWEETENERS

Aspartame, a product of two amino acids aspartic acid and phenylalanine, is a widely used non-nutritive sweetener. It should not be used for baking and cooking as it is heat liable. Individuals having phenylketourea should avoid this as it contains phenylalanine.

Nutritive sweeteners like fructose and sorbitol are also available in the market. High doses of fructose cause a massive increase in the blood sugar levels, and so its use has been discouraged by the ADA. Ingestion of sorbitol too in a high quantity leads to osmotic diarrhea. The presence of side effects has decreased the popularity of these two agents to a certain extent, but nonetheless they still are being used in low doses.

Sucralose, marketed as *Splenda* in the U.S. is the latest non-nutritive sweetener that is quite popular because of its heat stable nature, making it suitable for cooking and baking purposes.

19.7 EXERCISE

Physical exercise is a modification of the sedentary lifestyle that is an integral component of comprehensive diabetes care. It is particularly recommended for type 2 obese patients with insulin resistance. It has multiple benefits which include reduced glucose levels, weight loss, reduction in body fat, reduced blood pressure, *etc.*

Individuals with type 1 diabetes are prone to hypoglycaemia during exercise, and so should be advised not to exercise on an empty stomach. They can sometimes develop hyperglycaemia due to the increased action of counter regulatory action of cathecholamines. In individuals with type 2 diabetes, exercise-related hypoglycaemia can occur rarely in individuals taking either insulin or sulfonylureas.

There is no cure for diabetes. The immediate goals is to stabilize blood sugar level and eliminate the symptoms of high blood sugar. The long term goals of treatment are to prolong life ,relieve symptoms , and prevent long term complications , such as heart disease and kidney failure . Basic diabetes management skills will help to prevent the need for emergency care. The skills include:

- How to recognize and treat low blood sugar (Hypoglycaemia) and high blood sugar (Hyperglycaemia)
- What to eat and when
- How to take oral medication or insulin
- How to test and record blood glucose
- How to test urine or ketones
- How to handle sick days, and
- Where to buy diabetes supplies and how to store them

The specific meal plans of the diabetic should be tailored to their food habits. People with type I diabetes should eat at about the same time each day, and try to be consistent with types of food they choose. This will help to prevent blood sugars from becoming extremely high or low. Type 2 diabetes should follow a well balanced and low fat diet.

Medications to treat diabetes include insulin and glucose lowering pills called oral hypoglycaemic agents. The people with type 1 diabetes can not make their own insulin, so daily insulin injections are required. The people with type 2 diabetes make insulin but can not use it effectively. Insulin is delivered by injections one to four times a day. Some times different types of insulin are mixed together in a single injection.

There are several other hypoglycaemic agents that lowers blood glucose in type 2 diabetes.

- Medications that increase insulin production by the pancreas, example: Amaryl, Glucotrol, Glucotrol XL, Micronase, Diabeta, Glynase, Prandin and Starlix.
- Medications that increase sensitivity to insulin, example: Glucophage, Avandia and Actos.
- Medications that delay absorption of glucose from gut, example: Precose and Glyset.

Most type 2 diabetic will require more than one medication for good blood sugar control within three years of starting their first medication. Some people with type 2 diabetes find they no longer need medication, if they lose weight and increase activity, because when their ideal weight is reached, their own insulin and a careful diet can control their blood glucose levels.

Oral hypoglycaemic agents are not safer during pregnancy. Modern therapies are far too costly to be practical for the majority of diabetic sufferers. This information has been presented in order to provide to the researchers, whose goal is to develop indigenous, renewable, medicinal plant resources as practical cost effective alternatives.

20. ALTERNATIVE MEDICINE FOR DIABETES

People all over the world are now switching to alternative or herbal medicine for the treatment of various ailments. Herbal medicine is gaining popularity not just because of its effectiveness but also by clever marketing of the herbal drugs, describing them as 'natural products' which can do no harm. On the other hand the so called herbal specialists describe insulin as addictive, the other drugs as 'pills of side effects' which can do more harm to the body than any benefit. Inspite of all these claims the fact remains that herbs contain active substances that can trigger side effects and that can interact with other herbs, supplements, or medications causing serious toxicities. Many of the available plant products used for 'the herbal therapy' have been found to contain hepatotoxic compounds or compounds that are biotransformed into toxic metabolites in the body. A recent ban on various herbal extracts and products in the U.K. is a 'breath of fresh air' for those opposing the random and indiscriminate use of various herbs and plant products. This ban brings forth many questions regarding the validity of the various herbal products available in the market, as many products banned in the U.K. were tested, and found to have hepatotoxic (toxic to liver) metabolites.

In spite of all these developments, one can still not deny the fact that the early developing phase of modern medicine relied on herbs as a major source of drugs. With years of extensive research and isolation of the active agents, herbs had given way to the 'pills of modern medicine'. With immense flora present on the earth, one can not keep a track of all the herbs, and so there can be many herbs and plants whose products may be beneficial in treating diseases. Such herbs or plant products should be analysed for their active ingredients which can be used for the manufacture of future drugs.

It is not the herbal products that physicians of modern medicine are wary of; it is the irrational and indiscriminate use of herbal products without proper knowledge of its action or its side effects. This indiscriminate use has lead to toxic reactions involving organs/organ systems whose function has been already compromised by the disease process itself. As practitioners of evidence based modern medicine, most physicians believe that herbal products could be effectively used for treating diseases only after these products are thoroughly tested for the benefits and validated for medical use, by the concerned agencies. For all these reasons herbs should be taken with care, under the supervision of a practitioner knowledgeable in the field of botanical medicine.

Plants based medicinal products have been popular all over the world for centuries. In the U.S, the popularity of herbal products began to decline in the year 1940, after the end of World war II, with the rise of synthetic drugs. The increased popularity of synthetic drugs in recent years has been attributed to their clinically proven efficacy and easy patentability. However, more recently, herbal approaches have regained their popularity, with their efficacy and safety aspects being supported by control clinical studies.

In diabetics, some herbal alternatives are proven to provide symptomatic relief and assists in the prevention of the secondary complications of the disease. Some herbs have also been proven to help in the regeneration of beta cells and in overcoming insulin resistance.

Besides helping to maintain normal blood sugar level, several of these herbs are also reported to posses antioxident and cholestrol lowering action. These herbs therefore, have multi-faceted roles to play in the management of diabetes. The herbal preparations are also free from side effects commonly encountered with conventional therapies. This is evidenced by their long history of safe use and the lack of undesirable side effects observed in clinical trials performed with therapeutically effective doses on diabetes.

The importance of antidiabetic plants in the development of economic and effective treatment for diabetes, currently estimated to affect over 30 million people worldwide, has been recognized by the World Health Organisation.

As more than 1300 plants representing 725 genera in 183 families extending from the marine algae and fungi, shows the antidiabetic activity. Over half of these plants have been used ethnopharmocologically in traditional medicine as antidiabetic. The plants which have been used represent a wide range of families , out of these 127 species are found in Fabaceae, 98 in the Asteraceae ,36 in the Lamiaceae ,35 in the Liliaceae ,30 in the Poaceae and 30 in the Euphorbiaceae. Screening these plants for the hypoglycaemic activity , has shown that 81% of the plants show positive results. This result reflects the great variety of possible active constituents and mechanism of action and illustrates the excellent potential for discovering new sources for antidiabetic drugs.

Basically the need is to develop cost effective, easily available and not life threatening antidiabetic drug, for this efforts have to be made on medicinal plants which aims at the development of medicine with modern standards of efficacy and safety, to combat diabetes which is relatively inexpensive and relevant to the present economic conditions. Therefore, the present chapter is aimed at discussing the plant based resources, available for treating the silent epidemic diabetes, increasing at a very fast rate. The antidiabetic plants contain the following compounds with antidiabetic activity. The compounds are inorganic ions , coumarins, lipids, flavonoids, steroids, peptides, amines, terpenoides, glycopeptides, alkaloids, complex carbohydrates and others.

21. ANTIDIABETIC PLANTS AND THEIR CURATIVE PROPERTIES

1. *Abelmoschus esculentus (L.) Moench*

Family : Malvaceae
Common name : Bhindi, Lady's finger.
Uses : 2 fresh seedless tender fruits are given twice daily till cure.

2. *Abroma augusta* L.f.

Family : Sterculiaceae
Common name : Devil's cotton
Uses : 10 ml juice of root bark or fresh stem bark and 10 ml flower juice is given once in a day for 7 days.

3. *Abrus precatorius* L.

Family : Papilionaceae
Common name : Wild liquorice, Indian liquorice, Rosary pea
Uses : Leaf juice is taken twice a day for 20 days.
: About 15 ml of fresh leaf juice is recommended once early in the morning.

4. *Abutilon indicum* (L.) Sweet.

Family : Malvaceae
Common name : Jhampi, Country mallow
Uses : 7 raw leaves are taken for seven days.
: Leaf juice is taken twice a day for 20 days.

5. *Acacia catechu* (L.f.) Willd.

Family : Mimosaceae
Common name : Katha/Khair, Cutch tree
Uses : 5 ml aqueous solution of the heartwood powder is prescribed early in the morning daily for 15 days to reduce the high sugar content in blood.

6. *Acacia farnesiana* (L.) Willd.

Family : Mimosaceae
Common name : Gund-Babul, Sweet acacia/Scented Babul
Uses : 5 g decoction of bark along with 2 black pepper (*Piper nigrum*) seeds is given once in a day for 5 days to lower blood sugar.

7. *Acacia leucophloea* (Roxb.) Willd.

Family : Mimosaceae
Common name : Tellatumma
Uses : Stem bark powder is taken twice a day for 30 days.

8. *Acacia nilotica* (L.) Willd. ex Del.

Family : Mimosaceae
Common name : Babul, Indian Gum Arabic
Uses : 100 g of the bark is taken in 500 ml of water and is boiled to get 100 ml of decoction and this is used in doses of 50 ml for about 21 days.
: Aqueous extract of bark 2 teaspoonfuls is given twice a day for 1 month.
: Gum obtained from the bark is used till cure.

9. *Acacia polyantha* Willd.

Family : Mimosaceae
Common name : Swetakhair, White cutch tree
Uses : 5 g of powdered heartwood is left overnight in a glass of water. Next day water is decanted and given on empty stomach in the morning for 10 days to check diabetes.

10. ***Acalypha indica*** **L.**

Family : Euphorbiaceae
Common name : Kuppi
Uses : Leaf juice 2 teaspoonfuls is given daily for one month.

11. ***Achyranthes aspera*** **L.**

Family : Amaranthaceae
Common name : Chirchir/Laljiri, Prickly chaff flower
Uses : 5 g of roots is recommended before breakfast for seven days against obesity caused due to diabetes.

12. ***Aconitum heterophyllum*** **Wall. ex Royle.**

Family : Ranunculaceae
Common name : Atis, Atis root
Uses : 5 g of roots is ground into paste with 2 seeds of 'Ela' (*Elettaria cardamomum*) and is given every morning for 3 days to reduce blood sugar content and high blood pressure.

13. ***Aconitum napellus*** **L.**

Family : Ranunculaceae
Common name : Mithavis/Mitha-zahar, Indian aconite/Monk's hood
Uses : 5 g of roots of this plant and that of 'Pippali' (*Piper longum*) is made into a paste and given for 7 days to reduce the sugar content in urine during the disease.

14. ***Acorus calamus*** **L.**

Family : Araceae
Common name : Ghorbach, Sweet flag
Uses : 5 g rhizome or root powder along with 2-3 g old jaggery is given against obesity caused due to diabetes.
: Roots contain tricyclic sesquiterpene-callaminone, aclamendiol and isoaclamendiol.
: Rhizome and roots contain volatile oil, where asarone and b-asarone are the important constituents.
: Rhizome also contains phenyl indane derivatives.

15. ***Actinopteris dichotoma*** **Bedd.**

Family : Polypodiaceae
Common name : Morpankhi, Peacock's tail
Uses : The paste of one entire plant with 5 black peppers (*Piper nigrum*) and 5 g dried ginger powder (Zingiber officinale) is prescribed to be eaten for 7 days to reduce excessive urination.

16. ***Aegle marmelos*** **(L.) Correa**

Family : Rutaceae
Common name : Bael, Holy fruit tree, Bael fruit tree
Uses : One teaspoonful of dried leaf powder is administered with a cup of water daily once till cure.

: About 10 ml of leaf juice is given with 5 black pepper seeds twice a day for about 2 months to control.

: 10 ml of leaf juice is taken internally 3 times a day for 20 days.

: Dry leaves, powdered and mixed with leaf powder of 'neem' and 'tulsi' is given 3 times a day for 15 days.

: Tender leaf juice of 10 ml mixed with 2-3 drops of honey is given twice daily (evening and morning) on empty stomach to reduce blood sugar within 3-4 weeks.

: Leaves of bel, Azadirachta indica and Ocimum sanctum are dried and powdered. 10 g powder is given thrice a day for 15 days for the treatment and control of diabetes.

: One tea spoon of leaf powder is given to the patient in empty stomach daily for seven days (Batra *et al.,* 2002).

: Leaves of Aegle (7), fruit of black pepper (7), seeds of almond (7), seeds of barley (2 table spoons) are soaked in water and kept for two hours. These are then grinded and prepared drink is given to the patient daily for 7-10 days (Batra *et al.,* 2002).

17. *Aerva lanata* (L.) Juss.

Family : Amaranthaceae

Common name : Kapuri jadi

Uses : Whole plant paste in 2 spoonfuls is taken twice a day for 30 days.

: Leaves are taken daily till cure.

: 5 g root paste or 10-15 ml decoction of the whole plant is given 2 times a day for 10 days to correct cardiac problem caused due to diabetes.

18. *Ailanthus excelsa* Roxb.

Family : Simarubaceae

Common name : Maharukh, The tree of heaven

Uses : 20 g bark decoction with 10 g rhizome of ginger is given for 7 days.

19. *Alangium salvifolium* (L.f.) Wang.

Family : Alangiaceae

Common name : Akola, Sage leaved alangium

Uses : 10-15 ml of leaf leachate is given twice daily to reduce sugar in urine.

20. *Allium cepa* L.

Family : Liliaceae

Common name : Piyaz, Onion

Uses : 2 spoons of whole plant paste is taken twice a day for 30 days.

: The leaf juice is given 2 teaspoonfuls twice a day for a long time.

21. ***Allium sativum L.***

Family : Liliaceae

Common name : Garlic, Lahsan

Uses : Regular use of garlic is effective in the treatment of diabetes

22. ***Aloe vera* (L.) Burm. f.**

Family : Liliaceae

Common name : Gheekunwar, Indian Aloe

Uses : 1 spoonful of leaf powder with hot water is taken twice a day after food for 30 days.

: About 5 ml of leaf juice mixed with 8-10 drops of 'Tulsi' juice (*Ocimum sanctum*) is given twice a day for 15 days in acute cases.

23. ***Aloe barbadensis Mill.***

Family : Liliaceae

Common name : Ghikanvar, Indian Aloe

Uses : 1 spoonful of leaf powder with hot water is taken twice a day after food for 30 days.

: About 5 ml of leaf juice mixed with 8-10 drops of 'Tulsi' juice (Ocimum sanctum) is given twice a day for 15 days in acute cases.

24. ***Alpinia galanga* (L.) Willd.**

Family : Zingiberaceae

Common name : Barakulanjan, Greater galanga

Uses : 15 g of soft portion of the rhizome is ground with 10 g of rhizome of 'Vacha' (*Acorus calamus*) and given every morning to the patient to lessen the sugar content of the blood.

25. ***Andrographis elongata* T. And.**

Family : Acanthaceae

Common name : Nelavemu

Uses : Entire plant decoction is taken 3 times per day.

26. ***Andrographis paniculata* (Burm. f.) Wall. ex. Nees**

Family : Acanthaceae

Common name : Kiryat, King of bitters.

Uses : Decoction of whole plant is taken 2 times a day till cure.

: Leaves crushed with the roots of *Calotropis procera* and the paste is made into pills. 2 pills are given twice a day for 21 days.

: Leaves crushed to powder along with the leaves of *Syzygium jambos*, *Ziziphus rugosa*, *Aegle marmelos*, Gymnema sylvestre and tubers of Corallocarpus epigaeus (leaf, tuber powder in 2:1 ratio). 1 spoonful of powder along with hot water is taken twice a day for 7 days.

: About 10 ml of leaf/root decoction is given once a day for 6 months against hyperglycaemia.

27. *Aphanamixis polystachya* (Wall.) Parker

Family : Meliaceae
Common name : Harinhara, Rohituka tree
Uses : A decoction of the bark is given twice a day for 1 month.

28. *Aquilaria agallocha* Roxb.

Family : Thymeleaceae
Common name : Agar, Aloe wood/Eagle wood
Uses : 15 g decoction of the fragrant resinous wood is given twice daily for 10 days.

29. *Areca catechu* L.

Family : Arecaceae
Common name : Supari/Kasali, Betel nut/Areca nut
Uses : 15 g decoction of nuts mixed with 5 g of old jaggery is given once daily for 10-20 days to correct nervous system disorder and urinary disorder caused by diabetes.

30. *Argyreia cuneata* (Willd.) Ker- Gawl.

Family : Convolvulaceae
Common name : Samudra pala
Uses : Leaves are powdered in water with black pepper and 2 spoonfuls of it is drunk twice a day for 15 days.

31. *Argyreia nervosa* (Burm.f.) Boj.

Family : Convolvulaceae
Common name : Samundarka-pat, Elephant creeper
Uses : Pills made from the leaf paste are given for a long time.
: 10-15 g roots or seeds (2-5 g) made into a paste and is given once daily for 10 days in the early stage of the disease.

32. *Aristolochia bracteolata* Retz.

Family : Aristolochiaceae
Common name : Gadidagadapaku
Uses : 2 spoonfuls of whole plant paste is eaten twice a day for 30 days.

33. *Aristolochia indica* L.

Family : Aristolochiaceae
Common name : Isarmul, Serpent root plant
Uses : Roots are ground with 9 black pepper seeds and made into pills and administered 1 pill thrice a day for 15 days. Avoid non-vegetarian during this period.

34. *Asparagus gonocladus* Baker

Family : Liliaceae
Common name : Shakakul

Uses : Tuberous root powder is mixed with leaf powder of *Gymnema slyvestre* in water and taken twice a day till cure.
: Tuberous root powder is mixed with leaf powder of *Gymnema sylvestre* in hot milk and is drunk twice a day for 40 days.

35. *Asparagus racemosus* Willd.

Family : Liliaceae
Common name : Pilli tegalu
Uses : 2 spoonfuls of leaf tuber is taken once a day for 30 days.
: Boiled tuberous roots are eaten once a day for a long time.
: 5 g tuberous root powder mixed with 5 drops of honey is given to the patient once in a day for 1 month to restore potency.

36. *Azadirachta indica* A. Juss.

Family : Meliaceae
Common name : Nim, Neem tree, Margosa tree
Uses : Leaf paste with black pepper is given once a day for 1 month.
: Pinch of dried tender shoot powder is administered daily once for a month.
: 1 g of seed powder is administered twice a day for 1-2 months.
: Roasted flowers/bark powder is taken with buttermilk for 40 days.
: 7 tender leaves of the plant are prescribed daily to the person suffering from diabetes.
: 6 seeds of the plant made into a paste with 50 ml rice wash and 1 ml ghee should be given after meal in case of long standing diabetes.

37. *Bacopa monnieri* (L.) Penn.

Family : Scrophulariaceae
Common name : S: Brahmi, Sarasvati, T: Sambrani Chettu
Uses : Aqueous leaf juice is given twice a day for 1 month.
: Leaf juice of 15 ml along with equal amount of leaf juice of 'Bilva' (*Aegle marmelos*) is prescribed for 1 month to reduce blood sugar.

38. *Balanites aegyptiaca* (L.) Del.

Family : Balanitaceae
Common name : Hingan, Zachun-oil tree
Uses : 5 ml of unripe fruit juice along with 2 g of jaggery is given to control excessive thirst during this disease. This preparation should be used atleast for 15 days before breakfast.

39. *Baliospermum montanum* (Willd.) Muell-Arg.

Family : Euphorbiaceae
Common name : Danti
Uses : 10 g root paste is given after mixing with a cup of cow milk. This preparation is usually given 1 hour before breakfast for 1 month.

40. *Bambusa arundinacea* (Retz.) Willd.

Family : Poaceae

Common name : Kantabams, Thorny bamboo

Uses : Young leafy shoots contain cyanogenetic glucoside.

: 20 g decoction of the roots or 15 g leaves is given once daily for 10 days.

41. *Barleria cristata* L.

Family : Acanthaceae

Common name : Thinte, Tandrelu

Uses : 5 mg of root powder along with equal amount of the leaf powder of 'Nimbah' (*Azadirachta indica*) is given early in the morning on empty stomach for 7 days.

42. *Bauhinia variegata* L.

Family : Caesalpiniaceae

Common name : Kanchar/Mohata, Camel's foot

Uses : 2-4 g root powder is mixed with 5 g of powdered 'Haritaki' (*Terminalia chebula*) and is given to check loss of weight during diabetes.

43. *Bauhinia purpurea* L.

Family : Caesalpiniaceae

Common name : Lal kachnar, Pink Bauhinia

Uses : 10 g stem powder is soaked in 20 ml water overnight and the filtrate is given with 100 ml goat's milk against obesity.

44. *Benincasa hispida* (Thunb.) Cong.

Family : Cucurbitaceae

Common name : Petha, White gourd melon

Uses : 20 ml fruit juice along with 1 g seed powder of 'Jambuh' (*Syzygium cuminii*) is given 2 times a day for 1 month in acute case.

45. *Berberis aristata* DC.

Family : Berberidaceae

Common name : Dar-hald/Rasant/Kilmora, Indian berberry

Uses : About 5 g of roots along with 3 black peppers (*Piper nigrum*) is made into a paste with water and given once in the morning for 7 days.

: 15 ml decoction of the stem is given to the patient 2 times a day for 3 days to stop excessive appetite (Polyphasia).

46. *Berberis lycium* Royle

Family : Berberidaceae

Uses : Decoction of roots is taken internally 3 times a day for 13 days.

47. *Biophytum nervifolium* Thw.

Family : Oxalidaceae
Common name : Lakchana
Uses : Decoction of leaves is given in diabetes.

48. *Boerhaavia diffusa* L.

Family : Nyctaginaceae
Common name : Thikri, Pig weed
Uses : 10 ml leaf or root juice is used to reduce sugar in urine. The patient is also recommended to eat the leaves and tender branch tips as vegetables.
: Leaf contains crystalline acids.

49. *Bombax ceiba* L.

Family : Bombacaceae
Common name : Semul, Red silk cotton tree
Uses : 10 g roots of a young plant is made into a paste with 3 black peppers (*Piper nigrum*) and 100 ml curd and is given once in a day for 10-20 days to restore potency.

50. *Bombax pentandrum* L.

Family : Bombacaceae
Common name : Tella buruga
Uses : Stem bark powder is administered twice a day after meals for 1 month.

51. *Boswellia serrata* Roxb. ex Colebr.

Family : Burseraceae
Common name : Anduga
Uses : Stem bark paste is taken twice a day for 30 days.
: Decoction of resin (1 g) is given once daily for 7 days against cardiac problems due to diabetes.

52. *Bougainvillea spectabilis* Willd.

Family : Nyctaginaceae
Common name : Kagitamu puvvulu
Uses : Leaf paste is made into pills of Bengal gram seed size and 3 pills are administered orally twice a day for 20 days.

53. *Brassica juncea* Czern. and Cross.

Family : Brassicaceae
Common name : Rai, Indian Mustard
Uses : About half teaspoon of powdered seeds, mixed with half teaspoon of lime juice is given daily for 5 days to lessen the sugar content in blood.

54. *Butea monosperma* (Lamk.) Taub.

Family : Papilionaceae
Common name : Dhak, Flame of the forest, Bengal king
Uses : Aqueous extract of leaves and fruits is given 2 teaspoonfuls once a day for a long time.
: 10 ml of leaf juice is administered once a day for 5-10 days on empty stomach. This reduces blood sugar and is also useful in glycosuria.

55. *Buchanania lanzan Spreng.*

Family : Anacardiaceae
Common name : Piyar, Almondette tree, Cheronjee
Useful parts : Seeds and leaves
Uses : Powder of leaf or seed helps in controlling glucose levels at early stage of diabetes.

56. *Caesalpinia bonduc* (L.) Roxb.

Family : Caesalpiniaceae
Common name : Karanju, Fever-nut
Uses : 15 g of seeds are pounded and given early in the morning with 100 ml goat's milk for 15 days.

57. *Caesalpinia sappan* L.

Family : Caesalpiniaceae
Common name : Patanga, Sappan wood/ brazil wood
Uses : 50-60 ml decoction of heartwood powder is given once in the morning for 15-20 days. This helps in checking the excessive thirst caused by diabetes.

58. *Cajanus cajan (L.) Millsp.*

Family : *Papilionaceae*
Common name Arhar, Tuar, Red gram, Pigeon pea,
Uses : 10-15 g decoction of leaves is given twice daily for one month to restore potency during the disease.

59. *Calamus rotang* L.

Family : Arecaceae
Common name : Bet/ Chachibet, Common rattan
Uses : 50 g juice of fresh bark is prescribed twice a day for 7 days for dysuria.
: 25-30 ml of the decoction of 10 g flowers is given once daily for 10 days.

60. *Callicarpa macrophylla* Vahl.

Family : Verbenaceae
Common name : Priyangu

Uses : 10 g infusion of flowers with 5-10 ml of curd is prescribed twice a day for 7 days to check excessive appetite caused due to diabetes.

61. *Calotropis gigantea* (L.) R. Br. ex Ait.

Family : Asclepiadaceae

Common name : Ak/Mudhar, Giant milk weed/Madar/Swallow wort

Uses : 10 ml decoction of flowers along with the rhizome juice of 3 ml of 'Haridra' (*Curcuma longa*) is given twice daily for 15 days.

62. *Calotropis procera* (Ait.) R. Br.

Family : Asclepiadaceae

Common name : Tellajilledu

Uses : Roots pound with the leaves of *Andrographis paniculata* and paste is made into pills. 2 pills are taken twice a day for 21 days.

63. *Cardiospermum halicacabum* L.

Family : Sapindaceae

Common name : Kanphuti/Kapalphoti, Heart's pea/Balloon vine

Uses : 2-3 g root powder is recommended to check obesity.

64. *Carica papaya* L.

Family : Caricaceae

Common name : Papeeta, Papaya

Uses : Juice of green fruits is drunk twice a day for 3 weeks.

: Green fruits are boiled and made into a paste and given with a pinch of common salt and jeera (*Cuminum cyminum*) powder for 6 months.

65. *Carissa carandas* L.

Family : Apocynaceae

Common name : Kauranda, Bengal current/Jasmine flowered carissa

Uses : 5 g fruit paste is given for 1 month to alleviate nervous disorder caused due to diabetes.

66. *Cassia auriculata* L.

Family : Caesalpiniaceae

Common name : Taroda, Tarval, Tarvar, Tarwar, Tanner's Cassia

Uses : Leaves and flower juice with triphala churnum (mixture of *E.officinalis, T.chebula, T.pallida*) is taken for 15 days.

: 2 spoons of dried flower buds powder along with honey once a day is taken for 1 month.

: 30 ml decoction of buds and flowers is taken orally 3 times a day for 40 days.

: Leaves and flower juice with fruit powder of *Terminalia pallida* is drunk daily 2 teaspoonfuls for 40 days.

: 1 teaspoonful of tender shoot paste is administered daily once till cure.

: 10 ml of leaf juice is mixed with 5 g old jaggery and given once daily for 1 month at early stage of the disease.

67. ***Cassia fistula*** **L.**

Family : Caesalpiniaceae

Common name : Amaltas, Bandarlauri, Grimalah, Indian laburnum, Golden shower

Uses : Fruit is eaten once a day for 30 days.

: 5 ml juice of fresh root sheath along with that of 3 ml rhizome of ginger (*Zingiber officinale*) and 2 black pepper seeds powder is prescribed for 15 days.

68. ***Cassia occidentalis*** **L.**

Family : Caesalpiniaceae

Common name : Kasondi

Uses : Leaf powder with milk is taken twice a day for 40 days.

: 15 ml leaf decoction is given twice a day to reduce the sugar content of blood within 7 days.

69. ***Cassia sophera*** **L.**

Family : Caesalpiniaceae

Common name : Kasamanda, Senna sophera, Kasamarda

Uses : Bark and powdered seeds mixed with honey is given once a day for 10 days.

70. ***Cassia tora*** **L.**

Family : Caesalpiniaceae

Common name : Chakunda, Foetid cassia

Uses : 5 g of seeds are powdered with 2 pepper seeds and powder administered daily once for a month.

71. ***Catharanthus roseus*** **(L.) Don.**

Family : Apocynaceae

Common name : Sadabahar, Madagascar periwinkle

Uses : 5 spoonfuls of leaf decoction on empty stomach once a day for 45 days.

: Leaf powder is used till cure.

: Fresh twig with 2 leaf buds is given daily for 7 days on empty stomach. During this administration, using sugar is strictly prohibited.

72. ***Cedrus deodara*** **(Roxb. Ex D.Don) G.Don**

Family : Pinaceae

Common name : Debdar/Deyodar, Deodar/Himalayan cedar

Uses : The heartwood is rubbed on a piece of stone with water and 10 g of paste is given early in the morning for 10 days.

73. ***Centella asiatica*** **(L.)**

Family : UrbanApiaceae
Common name : Brahmi, Indian Penny wort
Uses : 2 spoonfuls of leaf juice is taken twice a day for 30 days.

74. ***Centrantherum anthelminticum*** **(L.) Kuntze**

Family : Asteraceae
Common name : T: Kampurodda
Uses : Leaves are crushed into paste and is made into pills of Bengal gram seed size. These pills are administered in doses of 3 pills twice a day for 40 days.

75. ***Ceratophyllum demersum*** **L.**

Family : Ceratophyllaceae
Common name : Sevara, Hornwort
Uses : 20 g juice of the flowers mixed with a teaspoon of limejuice and a pinch of common salt is given every morning for a month for the treatment of glycosuria.

76. ***Chloroxylon swietenia*** **DC.**

Family : Flindersiaceae
Uses : About 100 ml gum powder mixed with water is given for about 1 month.

77. ***Cicer arietinum*** **L.**

Family : Papilionaceae
Common name : But/Chana, Horse pea/ Gram, Chick pea
Uses : Germinated seeds are given as a prophylactic against general weakness due to diabetes in particular.
: Experiments have shown that the intake of water extract of Bengal gram, enhances the utilization of glucose in both diabetic and normal persons. Tests were conducted at the Central Food Technological Research Institute in Mysore. When patients were kept on a diet which included liberal supplements of Bengal gram extract, the condition of the patient improved considerably and his insulin requirement was reduced to about twenty units per day. (T. Pullaiah and K. Chandrasekhar Naidu)

78. ***Cinnamomum tamala*** **(Buch-Ham.) Nees**

Family : Lauraceae
Common name : Tejpatta, Cassia cinnamon
Uses : 10 g decoction of leaves mixed with 5 g old jaggery is given to check excessive thirst caused by diabetes.

79. ***Cinnamomum verum*** **Presl.**

Family : Lauraceae
Common name : Dalchini, Cinnamon/Ceylon cinnamon
Uses : 5 g inner bark and 10 g roots are made into a paste and given once a day for 5 days at early stage of the disease.

80. ***Cissampelos pareira*** **L.**

Family : Menispermaceae
Common name : Patha, Velvet-leaf pariera, False pariera brava or root.
Uses : About 60 g of the root is boiled in half a litre of water for 20-30 min in a closed vessel. About 30-60 ml of this preparation is given 2 or 3 times daily to correct the kidney disorder caused by diabetes.
: Root powder with water is taken once a day for 40 days.

81. ***Citrullus colocynthis*** **(L.) Schrad.**

Family : Cucurbitaceae
Common name : Indrayan, Colocynth, Bitter apple
Uses : Fruit paste is eaten once a day for 45 days.

82. ***Cichorium intybus L.***

Family : Asteraceae
Common name : Kasni, Chicory
Uses : Infusion of Root powder twice a day normalizes blood sugar level.

83. ***Clerodendrum multiflorum*** **(Burm.f.) Ktze**

Family : Verbenaceae
Uses : Aqueous extract of the plant is taken.

84. ***Clerodendrum serratum*** **(L.) Mo.**

Family : Verbenaceae
Common name : Barangi
Uses : 15 g root paste and 7 black peppers (*Piper nigrum*) is given in 3 doses at half an hour intervals to cure chest pain and heart palpitation due to acute diabetes.

85. ***Clitoria ternatea*** **L.**

Family : Papilionaceae
Common name : Senkupuvvu
Uses : 1 spoonful of flower juice is given once a day for about 30 days.

86. ***Coccinia grandis*** **(L.) Voigt**

Family : Cucurbitaceae
Common name : Adavidonda
Uses : The extract of roots, leaves and young fruits are taken in doses of 2 spoonfuls once a day for 30 days.

87. ***Coccinia indica* Wight & Arn**

Family : Cucurbitaceae
Common name : Kunduri, Ivy Gourd
Uses : The fruits and leaves of the bitter variety are useful in the treatment of diabetes.
: Powder of leaves and roots is used 3 times a day for the treatment of diabetes.

88. ***Cocculus hirsutus* (L.) Diels**

Family : Menispermaceae
Common name : Jamtikibel
Uses : 5 ml leaf juice mixed with equal amount of stem juice of 'Guduchi' (*Tinospora cordifolia*) is prescribed to be consumed daily for 15 days.

89. ***Cocos nucifera* L.**

Family : Arecaceae
Common name : Nariyal, Coconut
Uses : 2 spoonfuls of flower juice is taken twice a day for 30 days.
: Fresh coconut milk of a very young fruit is prescribed every alternate day for 1 month to restore potency.

90. ***Commiphora wightii* (Arn.) Bhandari**

Family : Burseraceae
Common name : Guggul, Indian bdellium tree/Guggul
Uses : 2 g of the resinous gum in hot water is given to the patient for 1 month to reduce the blood sugar content (verified clinically).

91. ***Corallocarpus epigaeus* (Rottl and Willd.) Clarke**

Family : Cucurbitaceae
Common name : Akash gaddah, Bryons
Uses : The tuber crushed to powder and mixed with the leaf powder of *Syzygium jambos, Ziziphus rugosa, Aegle marmelos, Andrographis paniculata* and *Gymnema sylvestre* in 1:2 ratio. 1 spoonful powder is taken with hot water twice a day for 1 week.

92. ***Coscinium fenestratum* (Gaertn.) Colebr.**

Family : Menispermaceae
Common name : Thar-I-haldi, Tree turmeric/ False calumba
Uses : 5 g stem powder is soaked in 10 ml water overnight and the filtrate is given with 50 ml goat's milk against obesity.

93. ***Crataeva magna* (Lour.) DC.**

Family : Capparaceae
Common name : Barun, Three-leaved caper

Uses : 5 g decoction of the bark and 10 g juice of the leaves of 'Madhunasini' (*Gymnema sylvestre*) is given to reduce the sugar content in urine and blood.

94. *Cressa cretica* L.

Family : Convolvulaceae
Common name : Rudravanti
Uses : The infusion of the whole plant, sweetened with jaggery is prescribed thrice daily after meals for impotency and loss of weight caused by diabetes.

95. *Cucumis sativus* L.

Family : Cucurbitaceae
Common name : Khira, Common cucumber
Uses : 2 g seeds made into paste with liquorices (*Glycyrrhiza glabra*) is given daily for 15 days to reduce sugar level in blood. Liberal intake of cucumber is recommended to reduce body weight.

96. *Cucumis trigonus* Roxb.

Family : Cucurbitaceae
Common name : Indrayan, Colocynth/Bitter cucumber/Bitter apple
Uses : About 2-3 g of root powder mixed with 10 ml of curd is prescribed daily for 15 days to reduce the sugar content in urine and also to check excessive urination.

97. *Curculigo orchioides* Gaertn.

Family : Hypoxidaceae
Common name : Kali musli, Black Musli
Uses : 10 g roots or rhizome paste with fermented rice water is recommended daily for 7 days on empty stomach to reduce blood sugar.

98. *Curcuma longa* L.

Family : Zingiberaceae
Common name : Haldi, Turmeric
Uses : 15-20 ml fresh juice of the rhizome with equal amount of fruit juice of 'Amalaki' (*Phyllanthus emblica*) is given 3 times a day for 15 days against glycosuria.

99. *Curcuma pseudomontana* Graham

Family : Zingiberaceae
Common name : Adavi pasupu
Uses : Tuber extract with juice of *Phyllanthus emblica* is administered 2 spoonfuls twice a day for 7 days.

100. *Curcuma zedoaria* (Berg.) Rosc.

Family : Zingiberaceae
Common name : Kachura, Zedoary/Indian arrow root
Uses : 20 g paste of rhizome and 5 black peppers (*Piper nigrum*) is given daily atleast for 7 days.

101. ***Cyamopsis tetragonoloba*** **(L.) Taub.**

Family : Papilionaceae
Common name : Gowar, Guar gum, Cluster bean
Uses : Fruit decoction is drunk or fried as a curry or chutney and taken for 40 days.

102. ***Cymbopogon martinii*** **(Roxb.) Wats**

Family : Poaceae
Common name : Gandhbel, Palmarosa grass
Uses : Decoction of the young terminal vegetative parts of the plant (20 g) mixed with 5 g of butter is given once a day for 7 days to check excessive appetite caused by diabetes.

103. ***Cynodon dactylon*** **(L.) Pers.**

Family : Poaceae
Common name : Dub/Hariali/Durba, Conch grass/Dhub grass
Uses : Juice of the whole plant along with 15 ml rhizome is given 2 times a day for 15 days.

104. ***Cyperus platystylis*** **R. Br.**

Family : Cyperaceae
Uses : 15 g paste of tuber and 3 black peppers (*Piper nigrum*) is given along with rice wash water twice daily for 7 days to restore potency in diabetic patients.

105. ***Cyperus rotundus*** **L.**

Family : Cyperaceae
Common name : Mutha, Nut grass
Uses : The tuber is sliced and dried in sun and powdered. 5 g of this powder is mixed with 2 black pepper (*Piper nigrum*) seeds and prescribed in diabetes especially during excessive thirst.

106. ***Cyperus squarrosus*** **L.**

Family : Cyperaceae
Common name : Tunga gaddi
Uses : 2 spoonfuls of powder of tuberous roots are taken internally once a day for 45 days.

107. ***Cyperus triceps*** **(Rottb.) Endl.**

Family : Cyperaceae
Common name : Nirbishi
Uses : 10 ml root decoction is given during excessive thirst caused due to diabetes.

108. ***Datura innoxia*** **Mill.**

Family : Solanaceae
Common name : Nalla ummetta
Uses : Seed paste of 2 spoonfuls is taken once a day for 30 days.

109. ***Daucus carota*** **L. var. sativa DC.**

Family : Apiaceae
Common name : Gajar
Uses : 1 teaspoonful of root powder is given twice a day with hot water for 20 days.

110. ***Decalepis hamiltonii*** **Wight and Arn.**

Family : Asclepiadaceae
Common name : Sariba
Uses : Tuberous root powder 1 teaspoonful twice a day with hot water for 40 days.

111. ***Desmodium dalbergioides*** **Benth.**

Family : Papilionaceae
Common name : Sandan
Uses : 2-5 ml aqueous extract of the bark mixed with the 10 g stem juice of 'Guduchi' (*Tinospora cordifolia*) is prescribed for excessive urination caused by diabetes.

112. ***Dioscorea alata*** **L.**

Family : Dioscoreaceae
Common name : Khamalu, Chupri-alu, Asiatic yam
Uses : The tuber is boiled and pounded with a pinch of black salt and mustard oil. 1 teaspoon of paste is given twice a day regularly for 2 weeks.

113. ***Diospyros peregrina*** **(Gaertn.) Guercke**

Family : Ebenaceae
Common name : Gabh, Indian persimmon
Uses : Decoction of the bark 10 g mixed with that of 'Jambuh' (*Syzygium cuminii*) and 'Pitasara' (*Pterocarpus marsupium*) is given once daily for 4-5 days against high blood sugar and drying of mouth caused by diabetes.

114. ***Eclipta alba*** **(Linn)**

Family : Asteraceae
Common name : Bhamgra, Trailing Eclipta
Uses : The leaves powder should be taken in empty stomach for a period of 30-45 days for reducing the blood sugar level.

115. ***Eleusine coracana Gaertn.*** **F**

Family : Poaceae
Common name : Ragi, Mandva, Ragulu.
Uses : The grains are sweet and are very useful if taken in cooked form for treating diabetic.

116. *Embelia ribes* Burm.f.

Family : Myrsinaceae
Common name : Baberang, Embelia
Uses : 5-10 g fruit powder mixed with 3 black pepper (*Piper nigrum*) seeds in hot water is recommended.

117. *Enicostemma axillare* (Lam.) Royal.

Family : Gentianaceae
Common name : Nagaguha, Indian Gentian
Uses : Whole plant is used till cure.

118. *Ephedra gerardiana* (Wall.) Stapf.

Family : Gnetaceae
Common name : Asmania, Ephedra
Uses : About 15 g of crushed Ephedra plant put in a litre of water and evaporated to 500 ml. This decoction is then strained and preserved in a tightly corked bottle for use. 30-50 ml decoction is given as a drink once daily for 10 days to check loss of body weight and excessive urination caused by diabetes.

119. *Euphorbia bombiensis* Sant.

Family : Euphorbiaceae
Uses : A paste made out of about 24 g of the whole plant and 3 g black pepper seeds is taken with 250 ml of cow's milk for 8 days.

120. *Euphorbia ligularia* Roxb.

Family : Euphorbiaceae
Common name : Sehund, Common milk hedge
Uses : 10 g root juice mixed with 5 ml stem juice of 'Guduchi' (*Tinospora cordifolia*) is given every morning for 15 days. This preparation enhances glucose utilization and checks release of glucose from liver.

121. *Feronia limonia (Linn). Swingle*

Family : Rutaceae.
Common name : Wood apple.
Uses : Leaves powder is useful if it is taken on empty stomach every day for 30 days.

122. *Ferula narthex* Boiss.

Family : Apiaceae
Common name : Hing, Asafoetida
Uses : About 2 g of oleo-gum-resin of the rhizome of this plant (Hengu of commerce) is used daily for 5 days to check excessive urination during diabetes.

123. ***Ficus arnottiana* (Miq.) Miq.**

Family : Moraceae

Common name : Paras papal

Uses : 5 ml leaf juice along with equal amount of fruit juice of 'Amalaki' (*Phyllanthus emblica*) is given 2 times a day for 15 days to reduce the sugar content in blood.

124. ***Ficus bengalensis* L.**

Family : Moraceae

Common name : Bargad, Banyan tree

Uses : An infusion of the bark (10 g) mixed with 5 g of old jaggery is an effective and specific medicine for diabetes. This should be given once daily for 10-15 days to reduce blood sugar. The laticiferous sap of this tree is also effective in controlling the diabetes and increasing the pancreatic cells.

: Stem bark contains leuco-anthocyanins.

: The bark of this tree is found to be effective in controlling diabetes. During preliminary trials in uncomplicated cases, normal blood sugar level was achieved within six weeks.

: Either finely ground powder(1-3 gm taken three times daily) or the water extract (100 gm soaked in three cups of cold water for 24 hours, the bark squeezed and taken 1 cup twice daily) is effective in controlling diabetes. Interestingly, it has also proved to be effective in controlling the cholesterol levels.

: Aqueous extract of bark and aerial roots is given for treatment.

: Root bark soaked in a cup of water overnight and infusion administered daily in the morning for a month.

: An infusion of the bark (10 g) mixed with 5 g of old jaggery is an effective and specific medicine for diabetes. This should be given once daily for 10-15 days to reduce sugar.

: The laticiferous tissue of this tree is also effective in controlling the diabetes and increasing the pancreatic cells.

: Aqueous extract of aerial root along with salt 5ml once a day in the morning is given for 2 months for the treatment of diabetes.

125. ***Ficus carica* L.**

Family : Moraceae

Common name : Anjir, Common figure

Uses : Decoction of leaves as supplement to breakfast in IDDM could be help to control postprandial glycemia.

126. *Ficus hispida* L. f.

Family : Moraceae
Common name : Dagarin, Wild fig, Devil fig
Uses : One new fruit is eaten one per day for 20 days.
: 2 spoonfuls of root decoction in cold water is taken twice a day for 30 days.

127. *Ficus microcarpa* L. f.

Family : Moraceae
Common name : Kamrup
Uses : 15 g decoction of bark or 10 g leaves is given thrice a day for promoting health and vigour and restoring absolute fitness of the body. This preparation is administered during acute loss of weight caused by diabetes.

128. *Ficus racemosa* L.

Family : Moraceae
Common name : Gular, Gular fig, Cluster fig
Uses : Latex of root mixed with ragi powder is made into small pills of Bengal gram seed size and 2 pills are administered once a day for 15 days.
: 50 g paste made out of the boiled unripe fruit and equal quantity of fine rice, given with normal meal for 2-3 months, reduces sugar level in urine.

129. *Ficus religiosa* L.

Family : Moraceae
Common name : Pipal, Peepal tree
Uses : Bark extract is taken till cure.
: Unripe fruits are boiled and made into a paste (10 g) with a pinch of rock salt and 'jeera' (*Cuminum cyminum*) powder. This is given once daily for atleast 15 days.

130. *Garuga pinnata* Roxb.

Family : Burseraceae
Common name : Garngudi
Uses : 8 g of bark and black peppers pounded and given twice daily for over 15 days.

131. *Glycosmis pentaphylla* (Retz.) DC.

Family : Rutaceae
Common name : Gulimi
Uses : 2 new epimeric pentacyclic triterpenes-arborinol, isoarborinol from leaves.
: 3 new acridone alkaloids from root bark.
: Leaf paste in doses of 3 spoonfuls twice a day for about a month.
: Leaf oil is taken till cure.

132. ***Glycyrrhiza glabra*** **L.**

Family : Papilionaceae
Common name : Jathimadh, Liquorice
Uses : 3-5 g stem powder mixed with one long pepper powder (*Piper longum*) is prescribed once daily for 10-15 days.

133. ***Gmelina arborea*** **Roxb.**

Family : Verbenaceae
Common name : Gamhar/Khambhari, Gumbar tree/Coomb tree
Uses : Juice of the young leaves with 2-3 drops of honey is given 3 times a day after food, for 10 days to rectify the eye sight problems due to diabetes.

134. ***Gossypium herbaceum*** **L.**

Family : Malvaceae
Common name : Kapas
Uses : 5 ml decoction of the seeds is taken orally 2 times a day for 40 days.

135. ***Grewia tiliifolia*** **Vahl.**

Family : Tiliaceae
Common name : Dhamni/Dhaman
Uses : 10 ml decoction of the bark with 5-6 drops of rhizome juice of ginger (*Zingiber officinale*) is given to check obesity.

136. ***Gymnema sylvestre*** **(Retz.) R.Br. ex Schultes**

Family : Asclepiadaceae
Common name : Meshasingi, Periploca of woods, sugar killer
Uses : 10 g each of the leaves of this plant and *Syzygium cuminii* are boiled in half litre of water till it reduces to about 60 ml. The filtered extract is then mixed with 1 teaspoonful of honey and is given twice daily for 2 months.
: Shade dried leaves are ground, a teaspoonful of infusion given orally on empty stomach for 1 month. Ragi malt diet is preferred.
: Leaves are chewed.
: Aqueous extract of leaves and fruits in combination with leaves of *Tinospora cordifolia* is taken for a long time.
: Root/leaf decoction is taken orally till cure.
: Dried leaves ground with coriander (3:1 ratio) and extract administered orally.
: Leaves crushed to powder along with the leaves of *Andrographis paniculata, Syzygium jambos, Ziziphus rugosa, Aegle marmelos* and also with the leaves of *Corallocarpus epigaeus* (leaf, tuber powder in 2:1 ratio). This powder of 1 spoonful is taken along with hot water twice a day for 7 days.

: Fresh leaves/dried leaf powder is taken twice a day till cure.
: 2-3 g dried leaf powder is given with water.
: 7 fresh leaves are recommended daily in the morning for 15 days.

137. *Helicteres isora* L.

Family : Sterculiaceae
Common name : Maraphali, East Indian Screw tree
Uses : Root contains cucurbitacin-B and isocucurbitacin-B.
: 2 spoonfuls of root bark decoction is mixed with fruit powder of 'somp' (*Foeniculum vulgare*) and is administered for about a month.
: 1 teaspoonful root/bark powder is recommended once daily for 15 days early in the morning before breakfast.
: 20 g of root bark paste is given daily once for a month.

138. *Helleborus niger* L.

Family : Ranunculaceae
Common name : Khorasani
Uses : An unani drug 'QS' containing *Helleborus niger* and *Anacyclus pyrethrum* (3:1) reduced the cholesterol levels in patients of diabetes mellitus. Use of the drug in patients with insulin dependent diabetes reduced the dose of insulin.

139. *Hemidesmus indicus* (L.) R. Br.

Family : Asclepiadaceae
Common name : Sugandhipala, Gudipala
Uses : Aqueous extract of the root 1 teaspoonful is given for 9 days.
: 5 g of powdered roots is given 2-3 times a day in a cup of hot milk for 1 month to reduce sugar content in the blood and urine.

140. *Hibiscus rosa-sinensis* L.

Family : Malvaceae
Common name : Jasat/Jasum, China rose/Chinese hibiscus/Shoe-flower
Uses : 5-10 ml infusion of petals is given in diabetes to lessen the quantity of sugar.

141. *Holarrhena pubescens* Wall. ex G. Don.

Family : Apocynaceae
Common name : Kurchi/Indrajaba, Easter tree
Uses : 10 g decoction of the bark and of 10 g leaves of 'Madhunasini' (*Gymnema sylvestre*) is given 2 times a day for 1 month to reduce blood sugar content.

142. *Holoptelea integrifolia* (Roxb.) Planch

Family : Ulmaceae

Common name : Papri/Kanju, Indian elm

Uses : 20 g juice of the boiled bark mixed with the leaf juice of 'Nimbah' (*Azadirachta indica*) is given once daily for 5-10 days. Alternatively, either bark or leaves may be soaked in a cup of luke-warm water at night and the water is given in the morning.

143. *Homalomena aromatica* L.

Family : Araceae

Common name : Gan-kachu.

Uses : Rhizomes of plant advised to consume regularly in chronic pain and diabetes.

144. *Hordeum vulgare* L.

Family : Poaceae

Common name : Jav, Barley

Uses : 1 or 2 chapati's are taken daily till cure.

145. *Hybanthus enneaspermus* (L.) F.V.Muell

Family : Violaceae

Common name : Ratanpurus

Uses : 20 g of whole plant (including roots) is ground with 3 black peppers (*Piper nigrum*) and the paste is given in the morning on empty stomach for 1 month.

146. *Hydnocarpus laurifolia* (Dennst.) Sleumer

Family : Flacourtiaceae

Common name : Chalmogra, Marothi tree

Uses : 20 g roots of this plant and fruit juice of 'Jambuh' (*Syzygium cuminii*) combinedly is effective in reducing the sugar content in blood. About 15-20 ml of this if taken daily, cures acute diabetic condition within 2-6 months. However rice, sugar products and meat have to be eliminated from the diet.

: Seed paste prepared with the leaf juice of 'Nimbah' (*Azadirachta indica*) is applied externally on the ulcers of a diabetic patient for speedy recovery.

147. *Hygrophila auriculata* (Schum.) Heine

Family : Acanthaceae

Common name : Gokula-kanta, Long-leaved barleria

Uses : 5 ml leaf juice along with 5 drops of honey is given at evenings for 15 days.

148. *Ichnocarpus fruetescens* (L.) R.Br.

Family : Apocynaceae
Common name : Nallateege
Uses : 2 spoonfuls of leaf powder twice a day after meals is administered for 20 days.
: 10 ml fresh juice of leaf and fruit along with 2 black pepper (*Piper nigrum*) seeds is given early in the morning on empty stomach.

149. *Indigofera arrecta* Hochst

Family : Papilionaceae
Common name : Bengal Indigo
Uses : Root powder is taken 3 times a day till cure.

150. *Indigofera trifoliate (Linn).*

Family : Fabaceae
Common name : Jangli-methi, Baragadamu.
Uses : Seeds powder is useful in reducing the blood sugar level.

151. *Inula racemosa* Hook.f.

Family : Asteraceae
Common name : Pohakarmul
Uses : 10-15 ml decoction or infusion of roots is given twice a day for 5 days against nervous exhaustion and debility caused by diabetes.

152. *Ipomaea maxima* Roxb.

Family : Convolvulaceae
Uses : 10 g of roots is made into a paste and given with sugar candy twice daily for 2-3 days.

153. *Ipomaea nil* (L.) Roth.

Family : Convolvulaceae
Common name : Jharmarich, Morning glory
Uses : Seed oil contains palmitic, stearic, archidic, oleic, linoleic and linolenic acids.
: 5 g fresh seed powder is given daily with slightly hot milk.

154. *Justicia adhatoda* L.

Family : Acanthaceae
Common name : Aduladsa/Arusha
Uses : 10 ml leaf juice along with the equal amount of the leaf juice of 'Nimbah' (*Azadirachta indica*) is given once in a day on empty stomach for 15 days to reduce blood sugar.

155. *Lablab purpureus* (L.) Sweet

Family : Papilionaceae
Common name : Sem, Indian Butter bean/Carpet legume
Uses : Tender pods are cooked and recommended for inclusion in the regular diets of the patient.

156. *Lagenaria siceraria* (Molina) Standley

Family : Cucurbitaceae
Common name : Kadutumbi, Bottle gourd
Uses : 10-20 g fruit pulp boiled with cow's milk is given daily for 6 months to reduce sugar content in blood.

157. *Lagerstroemia reginae* Roxb.

Family : Lythraceae
Common name : Jarul, Pyinma
Uses : Decoction of the leaves and fruits contain an amorphous, slightly bitter insulin-like substance with a hypoglycaemic activity.

158. *Lawsonia inermis* L.

Family : Lythraceae
Common name : Mehndi, Cypress shrub, Henna
Uses : Decoction of equal quantity of flowers and seeds (2-5 g each) is given once in a day for 10-15 days to reduce sugar level in urine.

159. *Limonia acidissima* L.

Family : Rutaceae
Common name : Bilin, Wood apple
Uses : 10 g pulp of ripe fruit along with 5 g of jaggery is given once a day for 1 month.

160. *Linum usitatissimum* L.

Family : Linaceae
Common name : Alsi/Tisi, Linseed/Lint/Common flax
Uses : 10 ml decoction of flowers or 5 g roasted seeds is prescribed to the patient during excess urination (polyuria).

161. *Luffa acutangula* (L.) Roxb.

Family : Cucurbitaceae
Common name : Torai/Jinga, Ribbed gourd
Uses : 10 g juice of the fruit skin and 5 g roots is given once daily on empty stomach to reduce blood sugar.

162. *Lycopersicon esculentum* Mill.

Family : Solanaceae
Common name : Tamatar, Tomato
Uses : Raw fruits are prescribed in daily diet of a patient suffering from general weakness caused due to diabetes.

163. *Macrotyloma uniflorum* (Lam.) Verdc.

Family : Papilionaceae
Common name : Kulthi, Horse gram
Uses : 50 g of seeds are boiled with water for about half an hour. The water is drunk on empty stomach everyday to control blood sugar level.

164. ***Madhuca indica*** **Gmel.**

Family : Sapotaceae
Common name : Mohua, Butter tree
Uses : 15 g decoction of bark is prescribed.

165. ***Madhuca longifolia*** **(Koen.) Macbride**

Family : Sapotaceae
Common name : Mohwa, Butter tree
Uses : 50 g decoction of bark is boiled in a glass of water and the decoction is administered twice a day till cure.

166. ***Mallotus philippinensis*** **(Lam.) Muell-Arg.**

Family : Euphorbiaceae
Common name : Kambila/Kamala, Monkey face tree/Spoon weed
Uses : 5 ml fruit juice mixed with 10 ml of goat's milk is given once daily for 3 days to lessen the sugar content in urine.

167. ***Mangifera indica*** **L.**

Family : Anacardiaceae
Common name : Aam, Mango tree
Uses : A small piece of kernel is taken in the morning with water for a period of 1 month.
: Basal part of 7 leaf petioles is made into a paste and given with a glass of water for 21 days to check increased urination and sugar in urine.
: An infusion is prepared by soaking 15 g of fresh leaves into 50 ml of water, overnight and squeezing them well in the water in the morning. This filtrate is taken every morning to control early diabetes.
: 1/2 teaspoonful of shade dried leaves is taken twice a day till cure.

168. ***Marsdenia tenacissima*** **(Roxb.) Moon**

Family : Asclepiadaceae
Common name : Tongus
Uses : 5 ml root leachate is mixed with a pinch of date palm jaggery and given twice a day after food for 10 days to correct the kidney disorder due to diabetes.

169. ***Maytenus emarginatus*** **(Willd.) D. Hou.**

Family : Celastraceae
Common name : Vingar
Uses : 5-10 ml root juice is prescribed in the early morning for 10-15 days.

170. ***Melia azedarach*** **L.**

Family : Meliaceae
Common name : Mahanimb, Persia lilac/Bread tree
Uses : 5 g root powder mixed with 10 ml fresh juice of 'Amalaki' (*Phyllanthus emblica*) is an effective medicine for diabetes. This is given twice a day for 10-15 days.

171. *Mesua ferrea* L.

Family : Clusiaceae

Common name : Nag kesar, Mesua tree

Uses : Flower buds made into a paste with butter and 10 g is administered 2 times a day for 5 days to rectify the eyesight defect due to diabetes.

172. *Mimosa pudica* L.

Family : Mimosaceae

Common name : Lajwanti, Sensitive plant

Uses : 1 teaspoonful of leaf juice is given 2 times a day till cure.

: Leaf powder mixed with that of *Gymnema sylvestre* is used till cure.

173. *Mimusops elengi* L.

Family : Sapotaceae

Common name : Tedu

Uses : Leaf powder mixed in milk is drunk twice a day for 40 days.

: 2 teaspoonfuls of fruit juice is given once a day early in the morning regularly.

174. *Mitragyna parviflora* (Roxb.) Korth

Family : Rubiaceae

Common name : Kaddam/Kayim, Kaim

Uses : 10 ml root decocton is given 2 times a day for atleast 15 days.

175. *Momordica charantia* L.

Family : Cucurbitaceae

Common name : Kareli, Bitter gourd

Uses : Fruit juice in doses of 5 spoonfuls is given once a day early in the morning regularly for about 30-45 days.

: Green fruit juice is taken daily in the morning.

: Decoction of the fruits is given to the patient in the morning on empty stomach atleast for 1 month. The patient is also advised to include the fruit as vegetable in his daily diet.

: Green fruit juice is taken daily in the morning. Decoction of the fruits is given to the patient in the morning in empty stomach atleast for 1 month. A mixture of leaf powder of 'Karavellam', 'Jambuh', (*Syzygium cuinii*), 'Madhunasini' (*Gymnema sylvestre*) and 'Nimbah' (*Azadirachta indica*) in the ratio 2:1:1:1 is an effective remedy for diabetes.

176. *Morinda pubescens* Sm.

Family : Rubiaceae

Common name : Ach, Togari wood of Madras

Uses : Fried fruit is taken for 20 days.

: Fruit juice (15-20 ml) along with a pinch of old jaggery is given once daily for 15 days. Patients are advised to eat fruits and leaves as vegetables in daily diet.

177. ***Moringa pterigosperma*** **Gaertn.**

Family : Moringaceae

Common name : Mungna, Drum stick tree

Uses : Fried fruit is taken for 20 days.

: Fruit juice (15-20 ml) along with a pinch of old jaggery is given once daily for 15 days. Patients are advised to eat fruits and leaves as vegetables in daily diet atleast 15 days per year.

178. ***Mukia maderaspatana*** **(L.) Roem.**

Family : Cucurbitaceae

Common name : Agumaki

Uses : Leaf juice and seed powder are mixed and given for treatment.

179. ***Murraya koenigii*** **(L.) Spreng**

Family : Rutaceae

Common name : Katnim, Curry leaf tree

Uses : Eating 7 fresh fully grown curry leaves every morning for 3 months is said to prevent diabetes due to hereditary factors and also due to obesity as the leaves have weight reducing properties.

180. ***Musa paradisiaca*** **L.**

Family : Musaceae

Common name : Kela, Banana

Uses : Flowers are made into curry and is taken twice a week for about 5 weeks.

181. ***Naringi crenulata*** **(Roxb.) Nicolson**

Family : Rutaceae

Common name : Mullaluka, Vaickandlaaku

Uses : Leaf along with fruits of *Syzygium cuminii* is made into decoction and is taken internally 2 times a day for 40 days.

182. ***Neolamarkia cadamba*** **(Roxb.) Bosser**

Family : Rubiaceae

Common name : Kadamb, Kadam

Uses : 5-6 g of powdered bark or extracted juice of the fresh bark or 50-100 ml of unripe fruit is prescribed 2 times a day after meals for atleast 7 days to control diabetes.

183. ***Nelumbo nucifera*** **Gaertn.**

Family : Nymphaeaceae

Common name : Kanwal, Sacred lotus

Uses : About 10 g of seeds fried in ghee and mixed with 2 g of jaggery eaten once daily for 30 days before sunrise to check impotency during this disease.

184. ***Nepenthes khasiana Hook.f.***

Family : Nepenthaceae
Common name : Pitcher plant.
Uses : The local herbal doctors in Khasi and Jantia Hills of Meghalaya prescribe the fluid of the pitcher to diabetic patients and to the patients suffering from difficulty in urination.

185. ***Nepeta cataria L.***

Family : Lamiaceae
Common name : Catnip, Catmint.
Uses : Leaves and flowering tops are considered carminative, tonic, diaphoretic, refrigerant and saporific. Leaves are chewed to relieve tooth ache.

186. ***Nyctanthes arbor-tristis* L.**

Family : Oleaceae
Common name : Harsinghar, Coral jasmine/Sad tree
Uses : The juice obtained by rubbing a few leaves with a little water and strained through a clean piece of cloth is useful for control of excessive thirst and loss of weight caused by diabetes. About 5 ml of the leaf juice is given twice a day for 15-20 days.

187. ***Ocimum tenuiflorum* L.**

Family : Lamiaceae
Common name : Kala-tulsi, Sacred basil
Uses : Decoction of roots or leaves or both is given daily at evening for 1 month during excessive urination caused due to diabetes.

188. ***Operculina turpethum* (L.) Silva Manso**

Family : Convolvulaceae
Common name : Pitwori, Indian Jalap
Uses : 10 g powdered roots mixed with juice of 20 g unripe fruits of 'Amalaki' (*Phyllanthus emblica*) is given twice a day for 10 days to check weight loss caused by diabetes.

189. ***Orchis latifolia* L.**

Family : Orchidaceae
Common name : Salam-panja, March orchid
Uses : 10 ml rhizome juice is mixed with equal amount of 'Jambuh' (*Syzygium cuminii*) fruit juice and given twice a day for 5 days to reduce the blood sugar.

190. ***Oxalis corniculata* L.**

Family : Oxalidaceae
Common name : Amrul, Indian Sorrel
Uses : 1 tablespoon of fresh juice mixed with butter of cow's milk is given once daily for 15 days to curb excessive thirst caused by diabetes or severe heat.

191. ***Orthosiphon aristatus (Blume) Miq***

Family : Lamiaceae
Common name : Java tea, Kidney tea plant
Uses : Leaf extract lowers the blood sugar in diabetic patients. It stimulates glycogen formation.

192. ***Panax ginseng*** **C. X. Meyer**

Family : Araliaceae
Common name : Ginseng
Uses : The dried root powder is taken orally twice a day till cure.
: B-sitosterol, oleanolic acid and 2 unknown triterpenes.

193. ***Panax pseudo-ginseng*** **Wall.**

Family : Araliaceae

194. ***Pandanus fascicularis*** **Lam.**

Family : Pandanaceae
Common name : Keora, Screw pine
Uses : 10 ml decoction of roots or rhizome is given at the time of excessive urination.

195. ***Passiflora foetida L.***

Family : Passifloraceae
Common name : Stinking passion flower, tagua passion flower, hispid granadilla.
Uses : The whole plant is considered to have sedative properties and is used in the treatment of diabetes. It should be used in the form of powder.

196. ***Pennisetum typhoideum (Burm. F) Stapf and C.E. Hubbard***

Family : Gramineae/ Poaceae.
Common name : Bajra, Pearl millet, Bulrush Millet, Spiked Millet Herb.
Uses : Plant tonic useful in diseases of heart and appetizer. The powder leaf base is very useful in reducing the blood sugar level of a diabetic patient as reported by Dr. Shaik Imam, CRIUM, Hyderabad.

197. ***Phaseolus vulgaris L.***

Family : Fabaceae
Common name : Bakla, Lobia, French bean, Kidney bean
Uses : Beans are found to be more effective in reducing plasma glucose levels. It is advised to take overnight soaked fresh or cooked beans.

198. ***Paspalum scrobiculatum*** **L.**

Family : Poaceae
Common name : Kodaka/Kodra, Kodo-millet
Uses : 10 g mature grains of this plant are made into paste with 1ml latex of banyan prop roots (Ficus bengalensis) and is recommended for ingestion once daily for 7 days to lessen the excessive appetite during diabetes.

199. ***Pergularia daemia* (Forsk.) Chiov.**

Family : Asclepiadaceae

Common name : Juttipala teega

Uses : 2 spoonfuls of root paste is taken once a day for 30 days.

200. ***Phoenix sylvestris* (L.) Roxb.**

Family : Arecaceae

Common name : Khejur, Wild date palm/Date sugar palm

Uses : About 20 ml of fresh juice of stem extracted early in the morning is given to the patient (immediately after extraction) to restore potency during the disease.

201. ***Phyllanthus amarus* Schum. and Thonn.**

Family : Euphorbiaceae

Common name : Jaramal, kirinelli

Uses : 1 spoon of shade dried whole plant powder is administered once in a week for 5 weeks.

: Whole plant is ground with 4 black pepper seeds and taken twice a day till cure.

202. ***Phyllanthus emblica* L.**

Family : Euphorbiaceae

Common name : Amla, Indian Gooseberry

Uses : 2 spoonfuls of fruit paste is taken twice a day for 30 days.

: Dry fruit powder 1 teaspoonful with milk is taken twice per day.

: Paste of fresh leaves (5 g) is given daily for 1 month on an empty stomach.

: Paste prepared from equal quantity of boiled fruits of this plant and the fruit of 'Bibhitaki' (*Terminalia bellerica*) is given with 50 ml cow's milk twice daily 1 hour before food.

203. ***Phyllanthus fraternus* Webster.**

Family : Euphorbiaceae

Common name : Jarmla

Uses : Juice of the whole young plant is prescribed during every stage of the disease.

204. ***Phyllanthus virgatus* Forst f.**

Family : Euphorbiaceae

Common name : Nelausiri

Uses : 2 spoonfuls of whole plant extract in cold water is taken twice a day for 45 days.

205. ***Picrorhiza scrophulariiflora*** **Pennel**

Family : Scrophulariaceae
Common name : Kuru/Kutti, Picrorhiza
Uses : 5 ml of root juice along with 2 seeds of black pepper (*Piper nigrum*) is given 2 times a day for 7 days against loss of weight.

206. ***Pinus roxburghii*** **Sarg**

Family : Pinaceae
Common name : Chir/Chil, Three-leaved pine, Himalayan-long leaved pine
Uses : Decoction of the wood dust along with 3 black pepper (*Piper nigrum*) seeds is given for the treatment of diabetes, especially during the symptom of excessive thirst.

207. ***Piper chaba*** **Hunt.**

Family : Piperaceae
Common name : Chab, Wild pepper
Uses : 5 g root decoction and 10 g fruits decociton is given for 7 days.
: A paste prepared out of 10 g roots of this plant and 5 g roots of 'Gaja pippali' (*Scindapsus officinalis*) is given 2 times in a day for atleast 7 days during dry mouth caused by diabetes.

208. ***Piper longum*** **L.**

Family : Piperaceae
Common name : Pipli, Indian long pepper
Uses : 5 ml immature fruit juice mixed with fresh turmeric juice (*Curcuma longa*) is given once in a day for 10-15 days to check excessive urination caused by diabetes.

209. ***Piper nigrum*** **L.**

Family : Piperaceae
Common name : Golki, Black pepper
Uses : 5 g fruits are pounded with 10 g roots of 'Bimbi' (*Coccinia indica*) and the paste is administered for 1 month to improve the general health condition of the patient.

210. ***Pistia stratiotes*** **L. var. cuneata Engl.**

Family : Araceae
Common name : Jalakumbhi, Tropical duck-weed
Uses : 10 ml juice of young plants mixed with equal amount of green coconut milk is given to reduce sugar content in blood.

211. ***Plumbago indica*** **L.**

Family : Plumbaginaceae
Common name : Chitra/Rakta chitra, Fire plant/Rosy-flowered lead-wort

Uses : 5 ml root leachate with 5 g of old jaggery is given 2 times (morning and evening) a day for 5 days during excessive appetite related to diabetes.

212. *Polyalthia longifolia* (Sonn.) Thw.

Family : Annonaceae
Common name : Asoka, Cemetry tree/Mast tree
Uses : 50 g decoction of the bark mixed with the leaf powder (2-3 g) of 'Madhunasini' (*Gymnema sylvestre*) gives good results in impotency caused by diabetes. This preparation should be given once in a day for 10 days on empty stomach.

213. *Pongamia pinnata* (L.) Pierre

Family : Papilionaceae
Common name : Karanj, Indian Beech
Uses : The flowers are used in decoction to quench thirst in diabetes.
: 3 teaspoonfuls of flower decoction administered daily once till cure.
: 10 ml juice of the roots is given along with equal quantity of coconut milk once a day for 3 days to check excessive urination during diabetes.

214. *Portulaca oleracea* L.

Family : Portulaceae
Common name : Khursa/Kulfa, Common parslone
Uses : A teaspoon of seed is given everyday with hot water for 2-3 months to increase the body's own insulin, which help in curing diabetes.

215. *Premna corymbosa* Rottl.

Family : Verbenaceae
Common name : Arni, Agetha
Uses : 10 g root paste and 2 black peppers (*Piper nigrum*) along with rice washed water twice daily for 15 days is used to reduce blood sugar.

216. *Prunus cerasoides* D. Don

Family : Rosaceae
Common name : Patmakh, Himalayan wild cherry
Uses : 10 g decoction of the bark and 5 g roots of 'Vrischikali' (*Tragia involucrata*) is given against excessive urination in diabetes.

217. *Psidium guajava* L.

Family : Myrtaceae
Common name : Amrud, Common Guava
Uses : Fresh flowers contain ellagic acid, guaijaverin, quercetin and oleanolic acid.
: Juice of leaves is taken thrice a day for 35 days.
: Fruit powder with buttermilk is taken twice a day for 13 days.
: About 10 ml juice of vegetative as well as reproductive buds is given daily once in the evening for atleast 1 month.

218. *Pterocarpus marsupium* Roxb.

Family : Papilionaceae

Common name : Bijasal, Indian kino tree

Uses : The decoction of stem bark is taken orally for 20 days.

: Aqueous extract of the heartwood is taken for a long time.

: Tumblers made of its wood are being marketed under trade name of "Rishi Glass" which are used for drinking water.

: 20 g of heartwood is taken and made into fine powder. This powder is kept in a clay pot to which 50 ml of water is added and kept overnight. In the morning this solution is filtered and the filtrate is taken. Same dosage is administered for about 30 days.

: Heartwood soaked overnight with water and the filtrate (10 ml) is given daily for 1 month. Seeds of this plant are also used but found less efficient than the wood.

: A pinch of stem bark powder is administered with a cup of hot water daily once till cure.

: It was found to reduce blood sugar levels in maturity onset diabetes. Water stored overnight in a tumbler made of heartwood showed encouraging hypoglycaemic activity from the second week of treatment and maintain the blood sugar levels till the drug was withdrawn during clinical trials on patients who consumed 20ml twice a day for two months. The solid extract of wood in the form of capsules (250 mg each) also proved efficacious.

: The decoction of heart wood taken for 10 days or heart wood powder in a dose of 5 gm, twice daily or extract obtained from overnight soaking of heart wood taken for a month will reduce blood sugar level.

219. *Pterocarpus santalinus* L.

Family : Papilionaceae

Common name : Lalchandan, Red sanders.

Uses : Water incubated in wooden cups is drunk twice a day or decoction is drunk.

: Aqueous extract with pieces of wood is taken twice per day.

: Heartwood is rubbed on a piece of stone and the paste of about 5 g is given with a glass of water.

220. *Pueraria tuberosa* DC.

Family : Papilionaceae

Common name : Vidarikanda, Indian kudzu

Uses : 2 g each of root powder of this plant and 'Satavari' (*Asparagus racemosus*) mixed with a banana and 100 ml of milk is given once daily for 1 month.

221. ***Punica granatum*** **L.**

Family : Punicaceae
Common name : Anar/Dhalim, Pomegranate
Uses : Root bark and fruit rind ground in equal proportions and 10 g paste is given twice a day to check excessive urination (polyuria).
: Fruit rind contains tannin-punicalagin and punicalin.

222. ***Quercus infectoria Olivier***

Family : Fagaceae
Common name : Gall oak, Dayer's oak, Maju-phal
Uses : The leaf galls are astringent because they contain tannins. The dry extract exhibits hypoglycaemic activity.

223. ***Raphanus sativus. Linn.***

Family : Brassicaceae
Common name : Radish, Muli, Mullangi.
Uses : The roots have been reported very useful in the raw form.

224. ***Rauvolfia serpentina*** **(L.) Benth. ex Kurtz**

Family : Apocynaceae
Common name : Chhotachand, Serpentine root
Uses : Roots of this plant, barks of *Syzygium cuminii, Acacia chundra, Aegle marmelos, Strychnos potatorum* and leaves of *Gymnema sylvestre* in equal parts are ground and a pinch of powder is administered once a day for 40 days.

225. ***Rhinacanthus nasutus*** **(L.) Kurz.**

Family : Acanthaceae
Common name : Palakjuhi
Uses : 5-10 ml juice of leaves along with 10 ml fruit juice of 'Amalaki' (*Phyllanthus emblica*) is given. Stem powder is also given with hot water for 10 days.

226. ***Rotula aquatica*** **Lour.**

Family : Boraginaceae
Uses : Half a teaspoon of the powder of the root mixed with a little of ghee can be given twice daily with milk on an empty stomach in case of impotency caused by diabetes.

227. ***Rubia cordifolia*** **L.**

Family : Rubiaceae
Common name : Manjeet, Indian Madder
Uses : 10 g roots made into paste with water collected after washing raw rice and given once in a day for 10 days to reduce sugar content in blood.

228. ***Salacia chinensis*** **L.**

Family : Hippocrateaceae
Common name : Nerani
Uses : Stem bark decoction is taken till cure.
: Root powder is taken till cure.

229. ***Salix tetrasperma*** **Roxb.**

Family : Salicaceae
Common name : Jalmala/Baisi, Indian willow
Uses : 50-75 ml decoction of bark once in the morning for 10-15 days is useful in controlling diabetes.

230. ***Santalum album*** **L.**

Family : Santalaceae
Common name : Chandan, Sandal wood
Uses : 5 g paste prepared from heartwood with water or heartwood oil mixed with seed powder of 'Menthi' (*Trigonella foenum-graecum*) is given for 7 days.

231. ***Saraca asoca*** **(Roxb.) de Wilde.**

Family : Ceasalpiniaceae
Common name : Asok , Asoka
Uses : Leachates of flowers along with 5 g of old jaggery is given with 50 ml cow's milk in the morning for 1 month against polyuria caused due to diabetes.

232. ***Saussurea lappa*** **Clarke**

Family : Asteraceae
Common name : Pachak/Kuth, Saussurea
Uses : 5 g root powder is mixed with 2 g of 'Nimbah' leaf (*Azadirachta indica*) is given once daily for 7 days to check loss of weight during the disease and also to lessen excessive urination.

233. ***Schrebera swietenioides*** **Roxb.**

Family : Oleaceae
H: Ban-palas E : Weaver's beam tree
Chemical constituents : Betulinic and oleanolic acids.
Uses : 10 g unripe fruits with 2-3 g jaggery is given once a day for 7 days to enhance potency during the disease.

234. ***Scindapsus officinalis*** **(Roxb.) Schott.**

Family : Araceae
Common name : Gajapipal/Bari-pippli
Uses : 5 g mature inflorescence powder with 2-3 g jaggery is given twice a day before meal for 15 days.

235. ***Scirpus grossus*** **L. f.**

Family : Cyperaceae
Common name : Kasuru
Uses : 5 g tuber powder along with 2 groundnut seeds is given daily for 1 month to check loss of weight during the disease.

236. ***Scoparia dulcis*** **L.**

Family : Scrophulariaceae
Common name : Ghoda-tulsi, Sweet broom-weed
Uses : Infusion of leaves or young green parts of the plant is given to rectify the eyesight affected due to diabetes. Amellin an antidiabetic compound found in leaves is said to be useful in anaemia, albuminaria, ketonuria, retinitis and other diabetic complications.

237. ***Semecarpus anacardium*** **L.f.**

Family : Anacardiaceae
Common name : Bhilawa, Marking nut tree/Oriental cashew
Uses : Fruit kernel is boiled and then crushed into a dilute paste for external application on skin ulcers due to long standing diabetes.
: 1-2 g processed fruit kernel is ingested on empty stomach once daily with milk, reduces blood sugar.

238. ***Sesamum orientale*** **L.**

Family : Pedaliaceae
Common name : Til, Sesame/Gingely, Nuvvulu
Uses : Seeds yield oil containing sesamin and sesamolin. Seeds especially the black ones along with equal quantity of dried fruits of 'Draksha' (*Vitis vinifera*), 'Amalaki' (*Phyllanthus emblica*) and 'Haritaki' (*Terminalia chebula*) are ground to prepare a mixture. About 5 g of this mixture is given after thoroughly mixing with the fruit juice of 'Avighnah' (*Carissa carandas*) for a period of 15 days.
: Handful of seeds taken daily for a week.

239. ***Sesbania sesban*** **(L.) Merr.**

Family : Papilionaceae
Uses : Fruit bark with seed juice is given till cure.

240. ***Sida cordifolia*** **L.**

Family : Malvaceae
Common name : Bariar/Khareti, Country mallow/Sida
Uses : 2-3 g root powder with 1 glass of milk is given daily for effective reduction in blood sugar level within a short period.

241. ***Sida spinosa*** **L.**

Family : Malvaceae
Common name : Culsakari, Prickly sida

Uses : 50 ml decoction of roots is given twice daily for 15 days to reduce sugar in blood.

242. *Solanum americanum* Mill.

Family : Solanaceae
Common name : Kaamanchi
Uses : The decoction of the whole plant is taken till cure.

243. *Solanum virginianum* L.

Family : Solanaceae
Common name : Kateli/Bhat-Kaliya, Yellow berried night shade
Uses : 1 g of powdered root is given twice a day with 250 ml goat's milk. This treatment should be continued till the weakness due to disease, is completely over.

244. *Sphaeranthus indicus* L.

Family : Asteraceae
Common name : Gorakh mundi, Tr: Indian Globe Thistle
Uses : The extraction of whole plant is taken once in a day for 30 days.
: 15 g paste of this plant is given with a little old jaggery twice a day for 3 days to check excessive urination.

245. *Spinacia oleracea* L.

Family : Chenopodiaceae
Common name : Palak, Spinach
Uses : Leaves and fruits are fried with cow's ghee and given daily in diet to reduce sugar content in urine.

246. *Spondias pinnata* (L.f.) Kurz.

Family : Anacardiaceae
Common name : Amra/Jungli-am, Wild mango/Hog-plum
Uses : 15 g bark of young branches and 3 black peppers (*Piper nigrum*) are ground in goat's milk and the paste is given on empty stomach once daily for 7 days to reduce the blood sugar.

247. *Striga densiflora* (Benth.) Benth.

Family : Scrophulariaceae
Common name : Laghu-kurandika
Uses : 5 g fruit powder is taken with warm water for 15 days.

248. *Strychnos nux-vomica* L.

Family : Loganiaceae
Common name : Bailewa, Snake wood, Poison nut
Uses : Seeds immersed in cow's urine for 40 days, shade dried, roasted with cow's ghee, ground, infusion mixed with honey and made into pills. 2 pills are given a day after dinner for week days.

: Seeds immersed in cow's urine for 40 days, ground, infusion given on empty stomach on alternate days.

: 50-100 mg seed powder mixed with 5 seeds of 'Ela' (*Elettaria cardamomum*) is given once daily for 5-10 days.

249. *Strychnos potatorum* L.f.

Family : Loganiaceae

Common name : Nirmali, Clearing nut tree

Uses : The mixture of seed paste and buttermilk are taken twice a day for 10 days.

: Seeds are rubbed with honey and a pinch of camphor and the mixture is recommended once a day to lessen the blood sugar.

250. *Swertia chirayita* (Roxb. ex Flem.) Karst.

Family : Gentianaceae

Common name : Chirayata/Nepalinim, Chirata

Uses : 20 g of decoction of whole plant is given along with 2 g black cumin (*Nigella sativa*) powder once in a day during excessive urination (polyuria).

: Chiratin and ophelic acid, a phenolic compound, oleic, palmitic, stearic acids and a phytosterol.

251. *Symplocos racemosa* Roxb.

Family : Symplocaceae

Common name : Lodh, Lodh tree

Uses : 10 g decoction of the bark with stem juice of 'Guduchi' (*Tinospora cordifolia*) is given with 50 ml cow's milk in acute condition of the disease.

252. *Syzygium alternifolium* (Wight) Walp.

Family : Myrtaceae

Common name : Mogi, Adavineredu

Uses : 1 teaspoonful of seed powder in water is taken 3 times a day after food along with root juice of *Asparagus racemosus.*

253. *Syzygium cuminii* (L.) Skeels

Family : Myrtaceae

Common name : Jamun, Black plum, Jaman

Uses : Seed kernel powder in doses of 1 teaspoonful once a day for about 2 months.

: 10 g each of the leaves of this plant and *Gymnema sylvestre* are boiled in half litre of water till it reduces to about 60 ml. The filtered extract is then mixed with 1 teaspoonful of honey and is given twice a day for about 2 months.

: 50 ml of decoction of fruits is taken internally thrice a day for 45 days.

: 1 teaspoonful of dried fruit powder with honey is taken daily once for 15 days.

: The stony endocarp of fruit and dried ginger (*Zingiber officinale*) is taken in equal proportions and made into fine powder. This powder is mixed with juice of Aloe vera and made into pills of Bengal gram seed size. 1 pill with honey is taken thrice a day for 21 days.

: 10 g each of the leaves of this plant and 'Madhunasini' (*Gymnema sylvestre*) are boiled in 500 ml of water till it reduces to about 50 ml. The filtered extract is then given along with 5 g of jaggery daily for 2 months.

: The fruit pulp (5 g) or dried powder (1-2 g) is given twice a day for 15 days. However the seed powder (1-2 g) given twice daily is more effective than the fruit.

: Bark juice along with milk is given till cure.

: Fruit of this plant and leaves of *Mangifera indica* are ground separately and the extracts mixed and taken orally for 41 days.

: The seeds are hypoglycaemic. Jambul fruit is regarded in traditional medicine, as a specific against diabetes, because of its effect on the pancreas. The fruit, the seeds and fruit juice are all useful in the treatment of this disease. The seeds contain a glucoside 'jamboline' which is believed to have the power to check the pathological conversion of starch into sugar in cases of increased production of glucose. The seeds should be dried and powdered. One teaspoon of this powder should be mixed, in one cup of milk or water or half a cup of curd, and taken twice daily.

: The inner bark is also used in the treatment of diabetes. The bark is dried and burnt. It will produce an ash of white colour. This ash should be pestled in mortar, strained and bottled. The diabetic patient should be given ten grams of this ash on an empty stomach with water in the morning and twenty grams in the afternoon, and in the evening an hour after taking meals.

: An equal quantity of Indian goosberry powder, Jamun powder and bitter gourd powder are useful for diabetes. A teaspoon of this mixture once or thrice a day is effective in checking the progress of this disease (Bakhru, 1998).

254. ***Syzygium jambos*** **(L.) Alston**

Family : Myrtaceae

Common name : Gulab jaman, Rose apple

Uses : Powder is prepared by pounding the leaves along with the leaves of *Aegle marmelos, Andrographis paniculata, Gymnema sylvestre, Ziziphus rugosa* and tuber of *Corallocarpus epigaeus* (leaves and tuber in 2:1 ratio). 1 spoonful of powder is taken along with hot water twice a day for 1 week. All tubers, pumpkin, brinjal and green gram should be abstained during the treatment.

255. *Talinum portulacifolium* (Forsk.) Asch. and Schweinf.

Family : Portulacaceae
Common name : Paalaku
Uses : Leaf powder mixed with boiled milk is taken twice a day for 60 days.
: Leaf powder mixed with leaf powder of *Gymnema sylvestre* is taken 1 spoonful in milk twice a day for 30 days.

256. *Tamarindus indica* L.

Family : Caesalpiniaceae
Common name : Imli/Ampli, Tamarind tree
Uses : Crushed seeds are over soaked overnight and 10 ml aqueous extract along with 20 ml curd is given once in a day for 7 days.

257. *Tecoma stans* L.

Family : Bignoniaceae
Common name : Pachagotla
Uses : Leaf decoction is drunk till cure.

258. *Tectona grandis* L. f.

Family : Verbenaceae
Common name : Sagwan, Teak
Uses : Bark and flowers are ground in equal proportions and 10 g paste is given twice a day for 7 days to check excessive urination caused due to diabetes.

259. *Tephrosia purpurea* (L.) Pers.

Family : Papilionaceae
Common name : Sarpanka, Wild Indigo
Uses : Roots crushed with those of *Chloroxylon swietenia, Gloriosa superba* and *Tamilnadia uliginosa* (equal proportions) and the paste made into pills (jowar seed size) and administered daily twice till cure.
: The dicoction of the whole plant is very useful, if it is taken on empty stomach for a period of 30-45 days.

260. *Terminalia arjuna* (Roxb.) ex DC) Wt. and Arn.

Family : Combretaceae
Common name : Tella maddhi

Uses : Decoction of stem bark is administered 1 spoonful along with a pinch of sugar twice a day for 21 days.
: Barks of *Terminalia arjuna, Pterocarpus marsupium, Azadirachta indica* and *Syzygium cuminii in* equal parts are boiled in 1/4 litre of water and the decoction is administered for 40 days.
: Bark powder (1 g) mixed with 10 ml decoction of the fresh bark and 5 drops of honey is given on empty stomach twice daily.

261. *Terminalia bellerica* (Gaertn.) Roxb.

Family : Combretaceae
Common name : Badami, Beleric myrobalan
Uses : 1 fruit per day is eaten for 30 days.
: 1-2 g fruit powder is given with hot water twice a day for atleast 6 months.

262. *Terminalia chebula* Retz.

Family : Combretaceae
Common name : Harara, Chebulic myrobalan
Uses : 2 spoonfuls of dried fruit powder with water is administered once a day for 20 days.
: 1 fruit per day is eaten for 30 days.
: 1 or 2 spoonfuls of dry fruit powder is taken with water for 20 days.
: 1 teaspoonful of leaf juice is administered daily once for 2 months.
: 10 ml of fruit juice with one black pepper (*Piper nigrum*) is given daily for 1 month.

263. *Terminalia paniculata* Roth.

Family : Combretaceae
Common name : Flowering murdah
Uses : A pinch of bark powder is used in soft drinks for reducing sugar content in urine.

264. *Thespesia lampas* (Cav.) Dalz. x Gibson

Family : Malvaceae
Common name : Adavipatti
Uses : The paste of seeds is taken twice a day for 15 days.

265. *Thespesia populnea* (L.) Sol. ex Corr.

Family : Malvaceae
Common name : Gajadanda/Paras papal, Portia tree
Uses : 5 g roots of this plant and 2 g seeds of 'Ela' (*Elettaria cardamomum*) are made into a paste and given to restore potency.
: One leaf with 3 seeds of black pepper (*Piper nigrum*) is given once daily atleast for 7 days.

266. *Tinospora cordifolia* (Willd.) Miers ex Hook.f.

Family : Menispermaceae
Common name : Gulancha, Gulonga
Uses : 2 spoonfuls of stem decoction with honey is taken on empty stomach for about a month.
: Dried powder of leaf is taken 3 times a day for 20 days.
: One teaspoonful of leaf powder mixed in milk is taken twice a day for 60 days.
: 15-20 ml stem juice with 2 drops of honey is given twice a day for 15 days.
: Stem powder (5 g) of this plant and 2-3 g of long pepper powder (*Piper longum*) are prescribed for 7 days to cure oral ulcers of diabetic patients.

267. *Trachyspermum ammi* (L.) Sprague

Family : Apiaceae
Common name : Ajowan, Caraway/Lovage
Uses : 5 g aqueous extract of dried fruits along with 5 g seeds of 'Methi' (*Trigonella foenum-graecum*) is given for 7 days to keep diabetes in control.

268. *Tragia involucrata* L.

Family : Euphorbiaceae
Common name : Barhanta, Indian Stinging-nettle
Uses : 1-2 g root powder mixed with 50 ml of curd is given twice a day for 3-5 days.

269. *Trapa natans* L.

Family : Trapaceae
Common name : Singhara, Water chest nut
Uses : 10 g fruit pulp along with 2 black pepper (*Piper nigrum*) seeds is given daily on empty stomach for 15 days for rectifying eyesight defect caused due to diabetes.

270. *Tribulus terrestris* L.

Family : Zygophyllaceae
Common name : Gokshri, Puncture Vine
Uses : Seeds of *T.terrestris* and seeds of Guar in equal quantities are crushed and ground and kept inside a vegetable. After 3 days it is taken out and eaten, 1 teaspoonful in the morning for 5 days.
: 15 ml of infusion of matured fruits is prescribed early in the morning on empty stomach to rectify the urinary troubles (diabetic neuropathy) and impotency.

271. ***Trichosanthes dioica*** **Roxb.**

Family : Curcurbitaceae
Common name : Parvar/Parval, Pointed gourd
Uses : 5 ml juice of leaves and roots is given daily on empty stomach for 10 days. This helps the diabetics indirectly by lowering down the total cholestrol.

272. ***Trigonella foenum-graecum*** **L.**

Family : Papilionaceae
Common name : Methi, Fenugreek
Uses : Seed powder with water is taken daily in the morning for 30 days.
: 5 g seeds are soaked in water overnight and made into paste. This paste is mixed with half cup of curd and taken daily in the early morning with empty stomach for 30 days.
: About 25 g seed powder is given with warm water daily in the morning on empty stomach. This is also prescribed as preventive measure for the disease. Alternatively, 2 teaspoons of the seeds may be soaked in a cup of water at night and this water is given in the morning.
: A report brought out of the Indian Council of Medical Research states that fenugreek seeds, when given in varying doses of 25-100 g daily, diminish reactive hyperglycaemia.

273. ***Valeriana wallichii*** **DC.**

Family : Valerianaceae
Common name : Mushkbala, Indian valerian
Uses : 10 g powdered rhizome or 5-10 g of powdered roots is given in hot water daily for 10-15 days to lessen the sugar content in blood. However, the juice of the fresh rhizomes or roots is more effective.

274. ***Vateria indica*** **L.**

Family : Dipterocarpaceae
Common name : Saphed dammar/Kahruba, Indian Copal Tree/Piney Varnish Tree
Uses : 2-3 g bark powder along with 5 g old jaggery is given once daily for 21 days.

275. ***Ventilago maderaspatana*** **Gaertn.**

Family : Rhamnaceae
Common name : Tellapoliki
Uses : 50 ml of decoction of bark of stem is taken internally 2 times a day for 45 days.

276. ***Vetiveria zizanioides*** **(L.) Nash**

Family : Poaceae
Common name : Khas, Vetiver/Khas-Khas

Uses : 10 g decoction of roots is given early in the morning atleast half an hour before breakfast for 15 days to check excessive thirst caused due to diabetes.

277. ***Vigna mungo*** **(L.) Hepper**

Family : Papilionaceae
Common name : Urd, Black gram
Uses : 2 teaspoonfuls of germinated black gram is taken with a half cup of fresh bitter gourd juice and a tablespoon of honey once in a day for 4 months.
: 10 g of black gram is soaked in 1/4 litre of milk overnight and taken in the morning for about a week.

278. ***Vigna pilosa*** **Baker**

Family : Papilionaceae
Common name : Ban-Mung
Uses : About 100 g of seeds with 1 'Karavella' fruit (*Momordica charantia*) is boiled and is given once in a day for 5 days to reduce sugar content in urine and check excessive urination.

279. ***Vitis vinifera*** **L.**

Family : Vitaceae
Common name : Angur, Grape vine/European grape/Wine-grape
Uses : 5 g roots are made into paste with 3-5 g jeera (*Cuminum cyminum*) and prescribed everyday morning on empty stomach for 1 month.

280. ***Withania somnifera Dunal***

Family : Solanaceae
Common name : Asgand, Asvagandha
Uses : Antiinflammatory, Antibacterial, Hypotensine, Cataract etc.

281. ***Woodfordia fruiticosa*** **(L.) Kurz.**

Family : Lythraceae
Common name : Dhawi/Dhai, Fire-flame bush/Woodfordia
Uses : 2-3 g dried flowers are given once in a day for 1 month.

282. ***Wrightia tinctoria*** **(Roxb.) R. Br.**

Family : Apocynaceae
Common name : Mitha indarjou, Pala indigo plant
Uses : 3-6 g bark powder or 20-30 g decoction of the seeds is given once a day for 15 days especially in acute case.

283. ***Xanthium indicum*** **Koen.**

Family : Asteraceae
Common name : Chhota-gokhru, Cocklebur/Burweed

Uses : 15-20 ml decoction of young twig or unripe fruits is given 2 times a day for 1 month against general weakness caused due to diabetes.

284. *Ximenia americana* L.

Family : Olacaceae
Common name : Nakkara
Uses : The fruit is taken directly once a day for 30 days.

285. *Zanthoxylum armatum* DC.

Family : Rutaceae
Common name : Tejphal, Toothache tree
Uses : 10 g infusion of bark mixed with 15 g juice of roots of 'Charati' (*Hybanthus enneaspermus*) is given once daily for 1 month to promote health and vigour and restore potency during diabetes.

286. *Zingiber officinale* Rosc.

Family : Zingiberaceae
Common name : Soth, Dry ginger
Uses : Half teaspoon of the rhizome powder with a half-boiled egg is prescribed at night for a month.

287. *Ziziphus rugosa* Lam.

Family : Rhamnaceae
Common name : Konda regu, Pedda regu
Uses : Leaves pounded along with the leaves of *Aegle marmelos, Syzygium jambos, Andrographis paniculata, Gymnema sylvestre* and tuber of *Corallocarpus epigaeus* (leaves and tuber in 2:1 ratio) is powdered. 1 spoonful of powder along with hot water is taken twice a day for 1 weeek.

HERBAL THERAPY FOR MENOPAUSE

FARHATH KHANUM
DEPARTMENT OF BIOCHEMISTRY AND NUTRITION DEFENCE FOOD RESEARCH LABORATORY,
SIDDHARTHA NAGAR, MYOSRE 570 011 INDIA

Chapter outline

1. INTRODUCTION

Menopause is the cessation of menstrual periods that occur in women sometime between the ages of 45 and 53. It happens when the ovaries stop releasing eggs, signifying the end of the female reproductive period of life which commences at adolescence in the early teens. It is usually a gradual process, and sometimes it happens all at once.

Perimenopause is the period of gradual changes that lead into menopause. It affects a woman's hormones, body, and feelings. It can be a stop-start process that may take months or years.

"Climacteric"is another word for the time when a woman passes from the reproductive to the non-reproductive years of her life.

IN: HERBAL MEDICINE FOR HUMAN DISEASES: VOLUME-III, PAGES: 289-296
(EDITORS : IRFAN ALI KHAN AND ATIYA KHANUM), UKAAZ PUBLICATIONS - HYDERABAD (A.P)-INDIA

2. CAUSES AND SYMPTOMS

At the time of menopause, the entire chain of endocrine glands is affected, particularly, the gonads, thyroid and pituitary glands. In some women, the menopausal change takes place without any unpleasant symptoms, the only change really being the cessation of menstrual flow. There are however, many women who develop disturbing symptoms such as hot flushes/flashes, night sweats, insomnia, tensions, diminished interest in sex, irritability and depression. Other symptoms are fatigue, palpitations, dizziness, headaches and numbness. In addition, weight gain and osteoporosis (a loss of bone density) are often encountered at the menopause. One may have only a few menopausal symptoms, or may have every symptom associated with it. Two hormones made in the ovaries, estrogen (the main female hormone) and progesterone (the female hormone that plays a major part in menstruation), help to keep a woman's monthly period going in a regular cycle. The levels of estrogen and progesterone produced by the ovaries are reduced in the body during menopause.

Induced menopause occurs if the ovaries are removed or damaged as in hysterectomy or chemotherapy. In this case, menopause begins immediately, with no perimenopause. The time after menopause is called postmenopause.

There are different kinds of menopause. If one has breast cancer, it is important to understand which kind of menopause one may be experiencing:

- Natural menopause, a normal part of the ageing process
- Medical or surgical menopause that is the result of chemotherapy or ovary removal
- "Cold turkey" menopause that is the result of being taken off menopausal hormone therapy after being diagnosed with breast cancer.

3. INDICATIONS OF MENOPAUSE

Aching joints, hot flushes, temporary and minor decrease in the ability to concentrate or recall, changes in sexual desire, extreme sweating, headaches, frequent urination, early wakening, vaginal dryness, mood changes, insomnia, night sweats, weight gain, loss of energy, and skin and hair changes –are the conditions commonly associated with perimenopause / menopause.. Long-range issues include osteoporosis, heart and vascular disease.

Hot flashes, are the sudden, intense, hot feeling on the face and upper body, perhaps preceded or accompanied by a rapid heartbeat and sweating, nausea, dizziness, anxiety, headache, weakness, or a feeling of suffocation. Hot flashes are mostly caused by the hormonal changes of menopause, but can also be affected by lifestyle and medications. A diminished level of estrogen has a direct effect on the hypothalamus, the part of the brain responsible for controlling the appetite, sleep cycles, sex hormones, and body temperature. Somehow, the drop in estrogen confuses the hypothalamus-which is sometimes referred to as the body's "thermostat"-and makes it read "too hot". The brain responds to this report by broadcasting an all-out alert to the heart, blood vessels, and nervous system: "Get rid of the heat!" The message is transmitted by the nervous system's chemical messenger, epinephrine, and related compounds:

norepinephrine, prostaglandin and serotonin. The message is delivered instantly. The heart pumps faster, the blood vessels in the skin dilate to circulate more blood to radiate off the heat, and the sweat glands release sweat to cool you off even more.

This heat-releasing mechanism is how our body keeps us from overheating in the summer, but when the process is triggered instead by a drop in estrogen, the brain's confused response can make you very uncomfortable. Some women's skin temperature can rise by six degrees centigrade during a hot flash. Body cools down when it should not, and you are miserable.

4. OTHER EFFECTS OF MENOPAUSE

4.1 BLOOD VESSELS

Quick body temperature changes (hot flashes) and waking during the night;

4.2 BRAIN/NERVES

Moods that change frequently or a tendency toward sadness or anger. Some women become more confused or notice they are not able to concentrate as well as usual;

4.3 GENITALS

Problems with dryness, itching, pain during sexual intercourse, or irritation of the tissues in and around the vagina;

4.4 URINARY SYSTEM

Problems with sudden or frequent urinating;

4.5 BONE

A higher risk of weaker bones, osteoporosis, and bone breaks;

4.6 HEART

Acceleration of risk factors associated with heart attacks and other heart problems, perhaps at least in part because levels of lipids (fat) in the blood may rise;

4.7 SKIN

Problems with thinner skin, wrinkling, and blemishes as estrogen levels drop.

How mild or severe your menopausal symptoms are, depends on how fast your transition to menopause occurs, how much time your body has to adapt to its changing hormones, and how much estrogen your body has from other sources. After menopause, most of your estrogen comes from androgens manufactured by the adrenal glands situated above the kidneys. The fat and muscle cells convert the androgens to estrogens. The more the fat and muscle that you have, the higher the level of non-ovary-produced estrogen.

5. TREATMENT, DIET AND LIFESTYLE

Dealing with menopause is best accomplished via, a combination of diet, healthy life styles and alternative or natural treatments. As with every big change in the body's chemistry, good nutrition is essential for a smooth transition. What you eat can help you deal with some of the unpleasant side effects of the menopause. The treatment, recommendations, that follow include a range of suggestions covering lifestyle choices, complementary therapy, and conventional medicine.

One should start with the simplest, mildest remedy with the broadest benefit and the least number of side effects, then gradually move on to stronger forms or amounts of treatment. Careful exercise is an ideal example of therapeutic measures with minimal drawbacks: It strengthens your bones and heart, controls weight, lessens hot flashes, improves your sleep, boosts your energy, revs up your sex drive, and makes your skin glow - without side effects.

Women have many choices, in the ways they can treat symptoms of menopause. All women, however, should aim for a healthy lifestyle: Eat a healthy diet, including 1500 mg of calcium along with vitamin D daily to prevent bone loss, lower the amount of fat in their diet, and the right balance of calories to maintain an active lifestyle; if overweight, weight reduction is advisable. A general advice would be

- Quit or try to cut down smoking;
- Use alcohol moderately;
- Exercise for 30 minutes at least three times a week;
- Avoid stressful situations; and
- Have a yearly mammogram and breast examination by a health professional.

Preventing disease will be a major concern after you go through menopause. Your risk of bone loss, bone fractures, heart disease, and other conditions increases as you age. Bone loss can be prevented by maintaing a healthy diet and exercise.

6. OTHER BONE TREATMENTS REQUIRE A PRESCRIPTION

- The hormone calcitonin is used to block bone breakdown.
- The bisphosphonate family of drugs blocks the breakdown of bone and results in an increased amount of bone.
- Hormone therapy is effective at preventing bone loss and fractures, but you should weigh the risks against the potential benefits.
- The "designer estrogens" (SERMs) tamoxifen and raloxifene also help to prevent bone loss; tamoxifen is also used to prevent breast cancer and its recurrence.
- Parathyroid hormone is used to add bone in severe cases of bone loss.

A healthy diet and regular exercise can also help to keep your heart healthy as you age. If your cholesterol is high, however, you may need cholesterol-lowering drugs. These drugs are called the "statin" drugs, such as lovostatin, simvastatin, and pravastatin.

Tamoxifen and raloxifene help to lower levels of bad cholesterol (LDL), which can block blood vessels and cause heart disease.

Treatment for the symptoms of menopause can be approached in two phases:

- Early in menopause, the problem/symptoms should be discussed with the doctor and treat the symptoms as they occur. One should be evaluated for one's risk of getting breast cancer, osteoporosis , and heart disease. If one is not at high risk for breast cancer, one may want to consider taking estrogen for a limited time, and using the lowest effective dose, which can help manage several symptoms at once. If one is at risk, other treatments are available.

- Later in menopause one should focus on effectively preventing the disease. The earlier symptoms will probably disappear.

7. TREATMENT FOR SYMPTOMS OF EARLY MENOPAUSE

Here are some ways to treat your symptoms without choosing hormone therapy:

- Blood-pressure-lowering drug that is also used to reduce the frequency and severity of hot flashes.
- Medroxyprogesterone acetate and megestrol acetate, progesterone-type drugs, may be used to treat hot flashes.
- The SSRI (Selective-Serotonin Reuptake Inhibitor) drugs are useful in two ways - treating depression and treating hot flashes.
- Counseling or support groups can also help you to handle sad, depressed, or confusing feelings you may be having as your body changes.
- Vaginal lubricants, can help women with thinning vaginal tissue or dryness.
- Low-dose vaginal estrogen is generally a safe way to take estrogen to solve vaginal thinning and dryness problems without substantially increasing the levels of estrogen in the blood.

8. HORMONE THERAPY

Estrogen therapy is recommended almost automatically by many physicians for most significant menopausal symptoms in women without breast cancer. Many women want to replace the estrogen their body is losing, because estrogen does relieve many symptoms of menopause. Women who still have a uterus usually take a combination of estrogen with a form of progesterone, called progestin. This is called hormone therapy (HT). Estrogen can help to reduce hot flashes, vaginal dryness, and skin changes. Estrogen is a good way to protect your bones from rapid weakening as you age. However, estrogen increases the risk of uterine cancer if taken alone. If a woman has had her uterus removed, she can take estrogen by itself. This is called estrogen therapy or ET. If you have a family history of breast cancer or have survived breast cancer, you probably should not take estrogen or HT, although not all studies support this conclusion. You also should not take estrogen if you have had cancer of the uterus, liver disease, history of blood clots, heart disease or unusual bleeding from the vagina. The role of estrogen in preventing heart disease is being debated by scientists. Recently, the American Heart Association announced that no woman should take estrogen only to prevent heart disease. Right now more studies are being conducted to learn whether estrogen prevents heart disease and stroke. Recent reports indicate that combined estrogen plus progestin do not reduce the risk of heart disease in women with or without previous heart disease, and may actually increase the risk of heart disease and stroke.

Some studies have shown other preventive roles for estrogen. More studies are needed to learn how effective estrogen might be in preventing these diseases. For example:

- Estrogen loss may be linked with Alzheimer's disease. Taking estrogen may help to prevent this disease after menopause. However, data from the WHI (Women's Health Initiative) suggest that women who initiate estrogen treatment at the age 65 or older, may not have improvement and may even have some mild cognitive decline and dementia. Whether this is the optimal age to initiate estrogen treatment, or whether the results would have been different if estrogen had been started at the time of the menopause remains to be determined.

- Taking estrogen may lower the risk of developing colon cancer.

Taking estrogen may lower the risk of developing age-related macular degeneration, a degeneration of the retina of the eye.

8.1 DESIGNER ESTROGENS

Tamoxifen (used to prevent breast cancer) and raloxifene (used to prevent osteoporosis) are drugs known as "designer estrogens." These drugs have been developed to act beneficially as estrogen on some tissue and to act as estrogen-blockers (anti-estrogens) on other tissue. These drugs also are known by the more technical name Selective Estrogen Receptor Modulators or SERMs.

8.1.1 THE SERMS

- help to protect your bones
- lower the levels of bad cholesterol; and
- may lower the risk of breast cancer.

Tamoxifen, however, acts like an estrogen on the uterus, increasing the risk of uterine cancer. Raloxifene blocks the harmful effects of estrogen on the breast, and does not stimulate the lining uterus, so women who still have a uterus may want to try raloxifene.

Estrogen dominance is also a factor in some of the more troublesome symptoms of menopause as well as perimenopause. Estrogen dominance is thought to occur when there is a drop in progesterone production during menopause.

The acceptance of Hormone Replacement Therapy (HRT) as a perimenopausal treatment has not been without controversy. Many women choose not to undertake HRT as a treatment of first choice, preferring instead to try what appear to them to be softer options offered by natural and complementary medicine. However, as with most drugs, hormonal therapy is not without risk. There is, in fact, an increased incidence of breast cancer, ovarian cancer, stroke, heart attack, and uterine fibroids. One might also experience irregular bleeding, perimenopause-like symptoms, increased incidence of migraine headaches, and effects such as facial hair, oily skin, and voice deepening. According to scientific research and observation, many women get as much relief from vitamins and herbs as they do from hormonal drugs. While such alternatives may not be for everyone, such as those with surgical menopause caused by removal of the ovaries (who need hormone therapy).

Medical science has an answer for those problems, but as often the case, the conventional remedy can cause more serious problems than those it is meant to relieve. For the last so many years, whatever modern medicine prescribed to deal with menopause, has produced complications like breast cancer, gall bladder disease, and high blood pressure; however, these side effects can be avoided by taking herbal medicines.

8.1.2 NUTRITION

DIET IS OF UTMOST IMPORTANCE IN MENOPAUSAL DISORDERS

During menopause lack of ovarian hormones can result in severe calcium deficiency. For this reason, a larger than usual intake of calcium may help greatly. Vitamin D is also essential for assimilation of calcium. Any woman experiencing disturbing symptoms at this time should supplement her daily diet with1000 units of vitamin D, 500 mg of magnesium, 2g of calcium daily which can be supplied by one litre of milk. Diet should comprise of seeds, nuts, grains, vegetables, with emphasis on vitamin E- rich foods and sprouted grains. Plenty of fresh fruit juices and seasonal vegetables should be included.

BEET JUICES

Beet juice has been found very useful in menopausal disorders. It should be taken in small quantities of 60 ml to 90 ml at a time, thrice a day. It has proved much more permanently helpful than the degenerative effects of drugs or synthetic hormones.

CARROT SEEDS

Carrot seeds have also been found valuable in menopausal tension. A teaspoon of the seeds should be boiled in a glass of cow's milk for about ten minutes and taken daily as a medicine in the treatment of this disorder.

LIQUORICE

Liquorice contains the natural female hormone, estrogen and can to some degree, compensate for the diminished hormone. One teaspoon of the powder should be taken daily.

INDIAN SPIKENARD

This should be taken in smaller doses of 2 g daily. It will smoothen the nervous system and induce tranquility of the mind.

BLACK COHOSH

Black cohosh (*Cimicifuga racemosa*) is one of the more thoroughly researched herbs which contains phytoestrogens. Because Black Cohosh has mild estrogen-like effects it will bind to estrogen receptors, without raising estrogen levels in the body - thereby lowering the estrogenic activity of the body. Phytoestrogens can compete with excess systemic estrogen and xeno-estrogens, and therefore help to balance systemic estrogen production. In addition, research suggests that Black Cohosh also suppresses Luteinizing Hormone (LH), high levels of which are responsible for hot flashes, among other things. Black Cohosh is a relaxing nerve tonic and has been used over the ages as a remedy for female gynecological problems. Recent clinical studies done in Germany have confirmed that Cimicifuga is strongly estrogenic and that it is effective in relieving menopausal symptoms. It has, as its main constituents, triterpene glycosides, cinnamic acid derivatives, chromone, isoflavones, tannins and salicylic acid.

PASQUE FLOWER

Pasque flower (*Pulsatilla vulgaris*) which is a well known tonic for the female reproductive system. Pasque Flower is an important nerve relaxant and mild sedative, which is also a soothing analgesic for the female reproductive organs.

DON QUAI

Don quai is also well researched and apart from its phyto-estrogenic properties, it has also been shown to be effective in the induction of progesterone receptor activity, thereby further balancing the estrogen/progesterone ratios.

ST JOHN'S WORT

This herb has been used traditionally for anxiety and mood disturbance particularly in the menopausal years. A number of controlled clinical trials have supported this claim, showing it to be effective in cases of mild to moderate depression. No significant side effects have been observed.

REMIFEMIN

A preparation of dried aqueous ethanolic extract, Remifemin=AE, was shown to significantly lower LH without affecting FSH, implying an oestrogenic effect. While no serious side effects have been observed, the British Herbal Compendium suggests that treatment should not exceed six months and that it be avoided during pregnancy and lactation.

WILD YAM

The use of wild yam (*Dioscorea villosa*) is not so clear cut. Traditionally viewed as of minor importance in menopausal problems, it is an effective antispasmodic to the gut and a gentle liver stimulant, with a reputed mild oestrogenic action. It is currently promoted as a useful source of progesterone when used externally as a cream. There is no history of traditional use in this form, nor has scientific research been undertaken to back up these claims. Herbalists who have investigated the constituent profile of wild yam have found no relationship between its known constituents and the claimed progestogenic action, either via ingestion or external application. Anecdotes suggest that women are benefitting from its use, and the creams are very popular, particularly it seems, in the Northern Rivers region.

Another estrogenic herb that also helps improve dry skin is flaxseed, which can be used as an oil, found in foods or taken as a supplement.

EVENING PRIMROSE OIL

Evening primrose oil (EPO) has also been shown to be very helpful.

9. CONCLUSION

Herbal medicine has much to offer women in the treatment of symptoms associated with menopause. For many it is the therapy of choice. In this area of herbal treatment, a blending of tradition and science has begun, which has the potential to allow practitioners and patients to be confident in a wider range of effective therapeutic interventions. The treatment of the symptoms of menopause by herbal medicine has a long history of usage, and is often clinically the only intervention required. Naturopaths and herbalists do not prescribe 'natural' HRT, but rather use remedies and supplements that ease the transition to and through menopause. Herbs and supplements are used to effectively facilitate the transition from the reproductive to the post-reproductive phase of life.